Pediatric Anesthesia Procedures

ANESTHESIA ILLUSTRATED
Keith J. Ruskin, MD and Barbara Burian, PhD
Series Editors

Published and Forthcoming Titles:

Pediatric Anesthesia Procedures, edited by Anna Clebone and Barbara Burian

Ultrasound Guided Procedures and Radiologic Imaging for Pediatric Anesthesiologists, edited by Anna Clebone, Joshua Finkle, and Barbara Burian

Emergency Anesthesia Procedures, edited by Lauren Berkow

Cancer Pain Procedures, edited by Amit Gulati

Radiologic Imaging for the Anesthesiologist, edited by Keith Ruskin and Abraham Dachman

Pediatric Anesthesia Procedures

EDITED BY

Anna Clebone, MD
Department of Anesthesia and Critical Care
The University of Chicago
Chicago, IL

Barbara K. Burian, PhD
Senior Research Psychologist
Human Systems Integration Division
NASA Ames Research Center
Moffett Field, CA

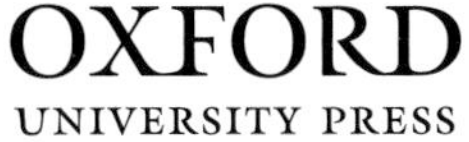

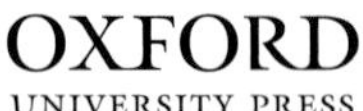

Oxford University Press is a department of the University of Oxford. It furthers the University's objective of excellence in research, scholarship, and education by publishing worldwide. Oxford is a registered trade mark of Oxford University Press in the UK and certain other countries.

Published in the United States of America by Oxford University Press
198 Madison Avenue, New York, NY 10016, United States of America.

Library of Congress Control Number: 2020950796
ISBN 978–0–19–068518–8

9 8 7 6 5 4 3 2 1
Printed by Sheridan Books, Inc., United States of America

Contents

PART III: REGIONAL ANESTHESIA 129

PART IV: PEDIATRIC EMERGENCIES 175

Preface

Procedures in pediatric anesthesiology were historically taught using actual patients, with little or no student preparation. In recent years, this has rightfully become unacceptable. The side effect, however, is that the performance of such procedures is pushed to later in training, with clinicians having fewer opportunities to perform them prior to independent practice. Simulation, including part-task trainers, have been used with some success, however, these sessions are often limited and, by nature, may not include the repetition or variation in presentation needed for learning and deep understanding.

In traditional textbooks, procedures are typically described at length, with much attention given to research findings that may have little direct or clear relevance to how a procedure ought to actually be carried out. Additionally, the lengthy paragraphs in which they are written do not readily translate into actual guidance for procedure execution. Furthermore, they are naturally restricted in the number of illustrations provided and may be narrow in the procedural skills described.

In this text, we address these shortcomings by providing well-illustrated and clearly defined and actionable guidance. This guide is intended as a ready resource for both experts and novices. It will be useful to both those with extensive training and experience as well as beginners and those with remote experience and training. A wealth of knowledge in the human factors of procedure design and use has been applied throughout to ensure that desired information can be easily located, that steps are clearly identified and comprehensible, and that additional information of high relevance to procedure completion is co-located and salient.

This book begins with the basics, but quickly progresses to advanced skill sets. It is divided into four parts. Part I focuses on the airway and breathing, and advances from the basics of airway management through specialty skills such as lung isolation. Part II covers vascular access, from the fundamentals of fluid management and programming several types of common pumps, to intraosseous line placement. Part III examines neuraxial regional anesthesia techniques as well as sympathetic blocks performed by those with an additional fellowship in pain management. This volume concludes with Part IV on emergencies and critical conditions including cardiopulmonary resuscitation for neonates and older children and treatment of local anesthetic systemic toxicity. It also includes four chapters which detail the anesthetic management for classic neonatal surgical pathologies, such as tracheoesophageal fistula, myelomeningocele, gastroschisis/omphalocele, and congenital diaphragmatic hernia.

A second book of serves as a companion volume to this one, and is titled 'Ultrasound Guided Procedures and Radiologic Imaging for Pediatric Anesthesiologists'. This second book includes a primer on ultrasound machine functionality as well as procedural chapters on lung ultrasound to detect a mainstem intubation or pneumothorax, gastric ultrasound, ultrasound guided peripheral intravenous line placement, ultrasound guided arterial line placement, ultrasound guided central line placement and several regional anesthesia techniques. That volume also includes an extensive guide to the basics of pediatric radiology for the pediatric anesthesiologist. Topics covered include radiology of the pediatric airway and mediastinum, lungs, gastrointestinal, genitourinary, musculoskeletal, and neurologic systems.

We hope that these volumes will serve as a guide for both beginners and experts to pediatric anesthesiology procedures, and will benefit children everywhere.

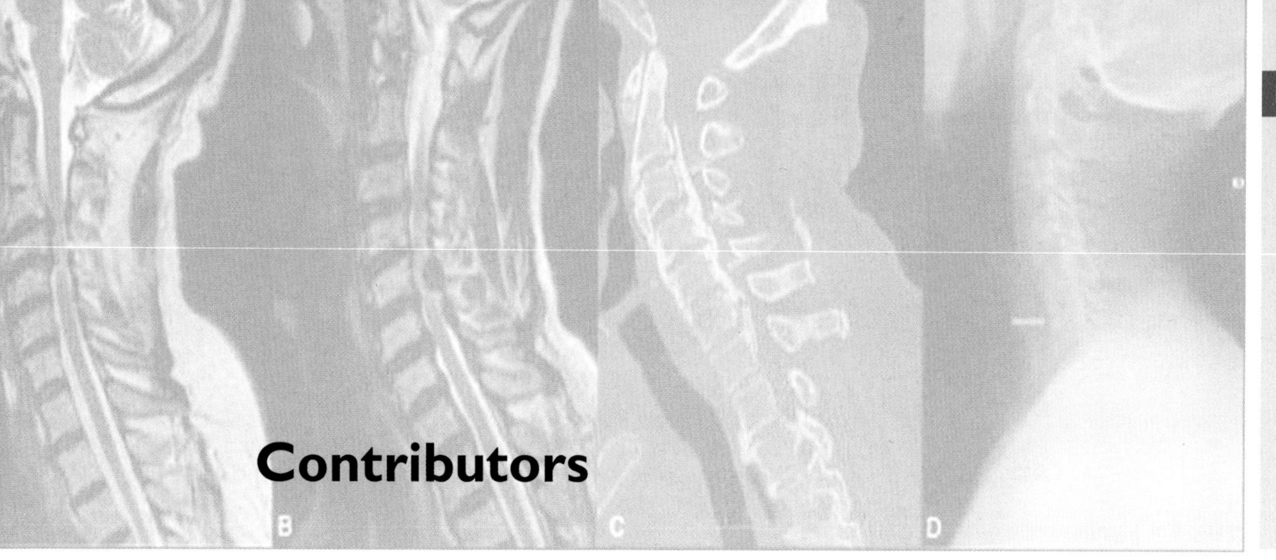

Contributors

Jennifer Anderson, MD
Visiting Associate Professor
Department of Anesthesiology
The University of Illinois Chicago
Chicago, IL, USA

Katiun Attarpour, BSN, MS, CRNA
Department of Anesthesia and Critical Care
University of Chicago
Chicago, IL, USA

Caitlin Aveyard, MD
Clinical Associate
Department of Anesthesia and Critical Care
University of Chicago
Chicago, IL, USA

Heather Ballard, MD
Assistant Professor of Anesthesiology
Pediatric Anesthesiology, Ann & Robert H. Lurie Children's Hospital of Chicago
Northwestern University Feinberg School of Medicine
Chicago, IL, USA

Sarah Choxi, MD
Pain Management
Garden State Medical Center
Whiting, NJ, USA

Anna Clebone, MD
Department of Anesthesia and Critical Care
The University of Chicago
Chicago, IL, USA

Ajay D'Mello, MD
Clinical Assistant Professor
Department of Anesthesiology and Pain Medicine
Nationwide Children's Hospital
The Ohio State University College of Medicine
Columbus, OH, USA

Elizabeth Dixon, MS, CRNA
Department of Anesthesia and Critical Care
University of Chicago
Chicago, IL, USA

John Faria, MD
Assistant Professor
Pediatric Otolaryngology
University of Rochester
Rochester, NY, USA

Amanda Foley, MD
Clinical Educator
NorthShore Medical Group
Chicago, IL, USA

Jared R. E. Hylton, MD, MS
Assistant Professor
American Family Children's Hospital
Department of Anesthesiology
University of Wisconsin School of Medicine and Public Health
Madison, WI, USA

Narasimhan Jagannathan, MD
Professor of Anesthesiology
Pediatric Anesthesiology, Ann & Robert H. Lurie Children's Hospital of Chicago
Northwestern University Feinberg School of Medicine
Chicago, IL, USA

Alina Lazar, MD
Assistant Professor
Department of Anesthesia and Critical Care
The University of Chicago
Chicago, IL, USA

Tristan Levey, MD
Resident
Department of Anesthesia and Critical Care
The University of Chicago
Chicago, IL, USA

Renata Miketic, MD
Clinical Assistant Professor
Director of Student and Resident Education
Department of Anesthesiology and Pain Medicine
Nationwide Children's Hospital, The Ohio State University Wexner Medical Center
Columbus, OH, USA

Sarah Nizamuddin, MD
Assistant Professor
Department of Anesthesia and Critical Care
The University of Chicago
Chicago, IL, USA

Jorge A. Pineda, MD
Assistant Professor
Anesthesiology & Perioperative Medicine
Oregon Health and Science University School of Medicine
Portland, OR, USA

Vidya T. Raman, MD, FAAP, FASA
Director, Preoperative Admission Testing (PAT)
Department of Anesthesiology and Pain Medicine
Nationwide Children's Hospital
Clinical Associate Professor
The Ohio State University Wexner Medical Center
Columbus, OH, USA

Samuel C. Seiden, MD, FAAP
Pediatric Anesthesiologist
Granite Bay, CA, USA

Chirag Shah, MD
Regional Anesthesia Fellow
University of Illinois at Chicago
Chicago, IL, USA

Aisha Sozzer, MD
Pediatric Anesthesiology Fellow
Department of Anesthesia and Critical Care
The University of Chicago
Chicago, IL, USA

Michelle Tsao, MD
Instructor in Anesthesiology
Pediatric Anesthesiology, Ann & Robert H. Lurie Children's Hospital of Chicago
Northwestern University Feinberg School of Medicine
Chicago, IL, USA

Audra Webber, MD
Assistant Professor
Department of Anesthesiology and Perioperative Medicine
University of Rochester School of Medicine and Dentistry
Rochester, NY, USA

Andrew Wuenstel, MD
Pediatric Anesthesiologist
Midwest Anesthesia Partners
Chicago, IL, USA

Pediatric Anesthesia Procedures

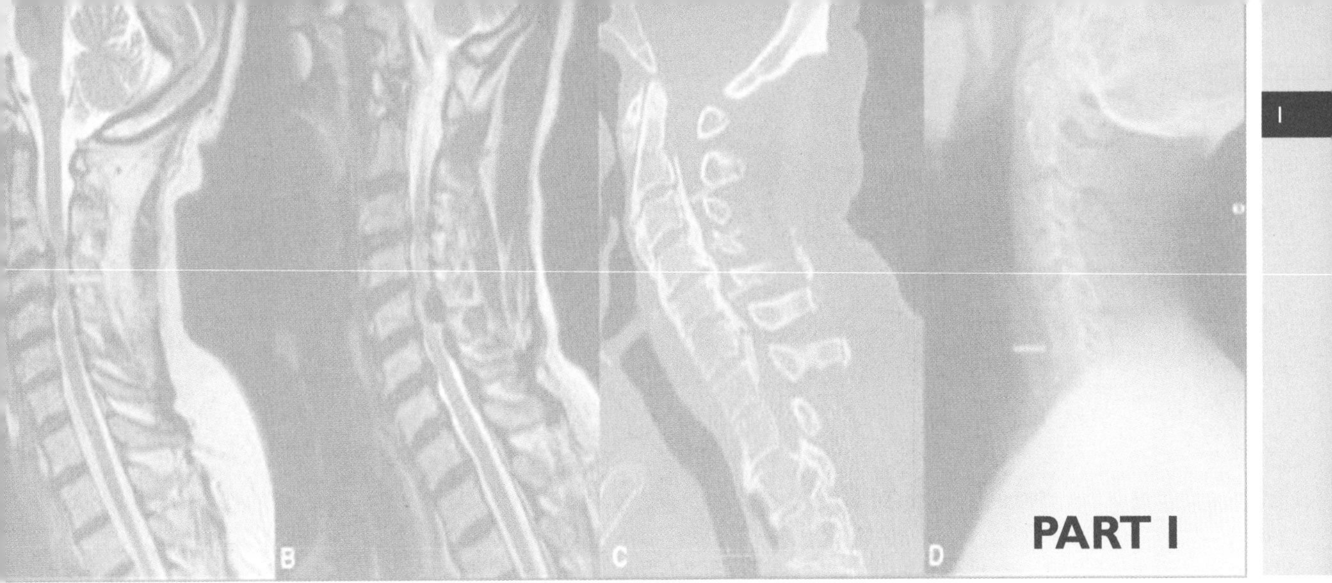

PART I

AIRWAY/BREATHING

Chapter 1

Pediatric Airway Fundamentals

Aisha Sozzer and Jennifer Anderson

Anatomy and Respiratory Physiology

Anatomic Differences—Comparing the Infant, Child, and Adult Airways

Compared with adults, infants and children have proportionately larger heads with a more prominent occiput (Figure 1.1). This causes significant neck flexion in the infant while lying supine.

>> **Tip on Technique:** A rolled towel underneath an infant's shoulders extends the neck, bringing the child into the sniffing position (Figure 1.2); see Chapter 2, Mask Ventilation, Direct Laryngoscopy, and Supraglottic Airway Placement Procedures.

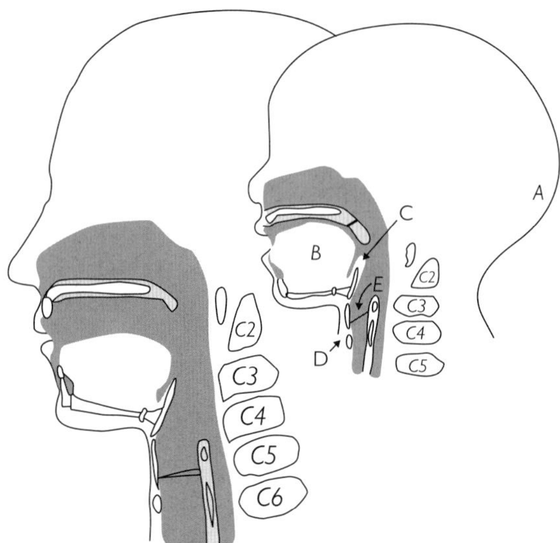

Figure 1.1 Adult versus pediatric airway anatomy. *Left*—adult anatomy. *Right*—infant anatomy. A: Large rounded occiput. B: Relatively large tongue. C: Floppy, omega-shaped epiglottis. D: Cephalad location of larynx. E: Acutely angled vocal cords. (Original illustration by Kira Okshewsky.)

Pediatric patients have relatively larger tongues and less upper airway muscle tone. As a result of these anatomic features, upper airway obstruction can occur quickly in infants during induction of anesthesia. Compared with adults, the larynx is located more cephalad in children.

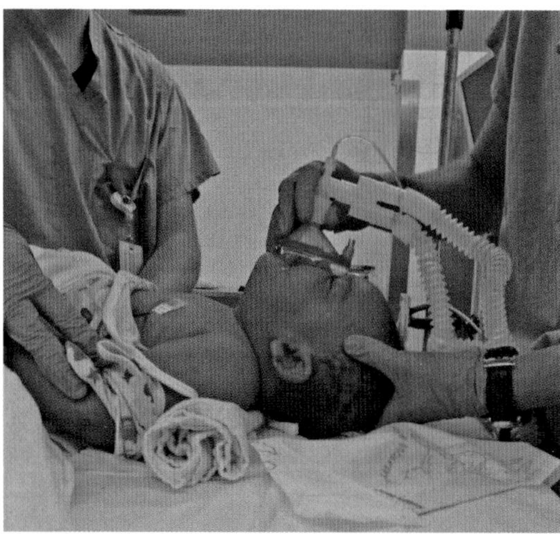

Figure 1.2 A shoulder roll reduces neck flexion and associated airway obstruction in the supine infant.

(a)

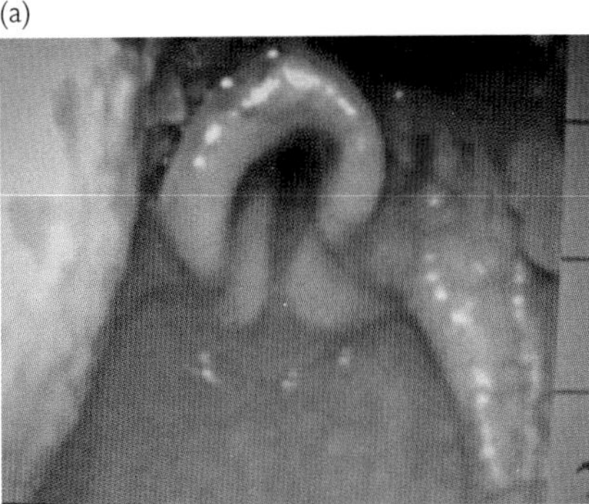

Figure 1.3a Infant larynx with an omega-shaped epiglottis.

It is at C3 in premature infants, C4 in infants born at a normal gestational age, C5 by the age of 6 years, and as caudal as C6 in the adult.[1] The relatively cephalad position of the larynx in infants can result in difficulty in visualizing the glottis during laryngoscopy because of an inability to align the oral and laryngeal axes. The omega-shaped epiglottis of the infant is narrower and more horizontally positioned than that of an adult (Figure 1.3a). Vocal cords (VCs) of infants are attached to the anterior larynx at an acute angle. The anterior downward slope of the VCs can make advancing an endotracheal tube (ETT) through the glottic opening challenging. By the age of 8 years, the anatomy of the child mimics that of the adult (Figure 1.3b).[2]

Note: Historically, the infant larynx was thought to be funnel shaped, narrowing down to a circular cricoid ring. New imaging and bronchoscopic evidence indicates that the narrowest portion of the infant larynx is just below the glottis. Additionally, in infants, the subglottic area is elliptical, not circular, with the transverse diameter as the narrowest portion.[3,4] This indicates that a circular uncuffed ETT may not be able to form a good seal without putting increased pressure on portions of the mucosa. Traditional ETTs do not solve this problem because they have a cuff that, to inflate, requires a lower volume but inflates to a higher pressure. Recently, the Microcuff ETT (Halyard, Alpharetta, GA), which has a cuff that inflates with a higher volume but to a lower pressure, has become commonplace.

(b)

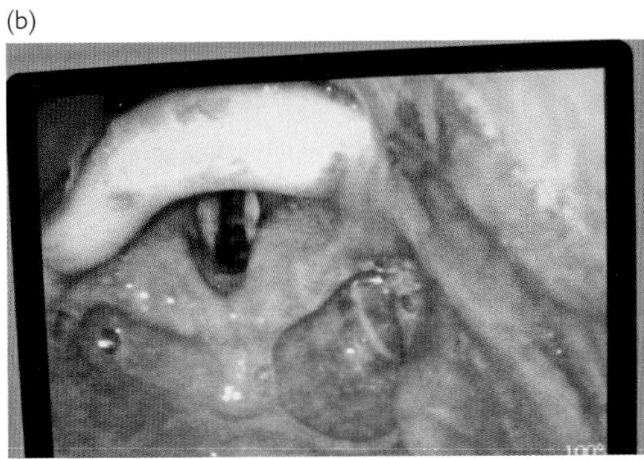

Figure 1.3b Adult larynx with a flat epiglottis.

Pediatric Respiratory Physiology

There are several differences in the respiratory system between children and adults. At birth, there are approximately 100 to 150 million immature alveoli. These alveoli continue to grow and increase in number until the adult number of 300 million alveoli is reached at about 3 years of age.[5,6] Because of a deficiency of type 1 muscle fibers, which assist in repetitive, continuous movement, the diaphragm is less efficient and fatigues easily in pediatric patients. Also, owing to the smaller diameter of the airway, resistance to airflow is higher in infants. Because resistance is proportional to the inverse of the fourth power of the radius, secretions and airway edema in an infant can severely impede airflow.

The major differences in pediatric ventilation stem from oxygen consumption, which is approximately 7 mL/kg/min at birth, two to three times higher than in adults. As a result, children require a higher minute ventilation (MV). MV is the product of respiratory rate (RR) and tidal volume (TV). Infants cannot significantly increase their TV. Therefore, a high RR is needed to meet metabolic demands. Adults breathe 12 to 18 times per minute, while infants breathe up to 35 times per minute.

Other smaller differences include the following: The compliant nature of the thoracic cage results in a lower outward recoil in infants; however, inward lung recoil is similar to that of adults. Lung volumes in pediatric patients per kilogram are slightly smaller than in adults. Although the functional residual capacity (FRC) is a larger percentage of lung volume in children, it is somewhat smaller in size proportional to the patient's body weight (Figure 1.4). The FRC in infants is 25 mL/kg and in adults is about 40 mL/kg. The closing volume is greater than the FRC until about 8 years of life (see Figure 1.4).[7] As a result, some alveoli are collapsed and unable to participate in gas exchange even during TV breathing.[8] Physiologic dead space is 30% of TV in children and adults, but owing to smaller lung volumes any increase in dead space has a larger effect on gas exchange in children.

WARNING!! Because of mostly to higher oxygen consumption, but also because of a lower FRC in children, hypoxia during apnea occurs much more rapidly in infants and children compared with adults.

Clinical Applications

- Children generally have compliant lungs, and 10 mmHg of positive pressure ventilation is often sufficient to produce adequate TVs.
- Some controversy exists as to TVs. Many experts recommend that TVs for healthy children be the same as those for adults, 5 to 6 mL/kg. Other experts recommend a TV of 10 mL/kg in pediatric patients to avoid atelectasis. Adequate chest rise and appropriate end-tidal carbon dioxide ($EtCO_2$) values should be verified because some older anesthesia machine ventilators may not account for compliance of the circuit tubing and may therefore deliver TVs lower than intended.
- Avoid allowing intubated infants to breathe spontaneously without ventilator support for long periods of time. Infants can fatigue quickly when breathing against the resistance of a small ETTs, given that infants have underdeveloped respiratory muscles.
- Use of positive end-expiratory pressure (PEEP) is advantageous in children to help keep alveoli open during TV breathing.
- Because of their much higher oxygen consumption, rapid desaturation occurs in infants during periods of apnea or suboptimal ventilation. **It is important to be prepared by gathering all primary and backup airway equipment ahead of time.** Multiple ETTs

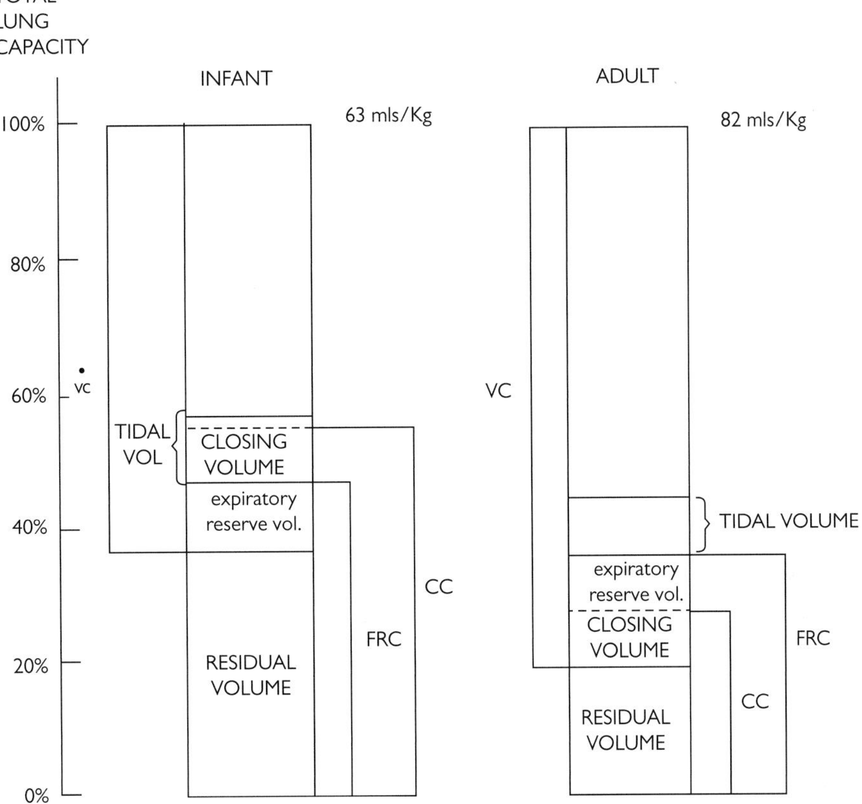

Figure 1.4 Adult and infant lung volumes. (Reproduced with permission from Moss DR. Pediatric anesthesia. In: Matthes K, Urman R, Ehrenfeld J, eds. *Anesthesiology: A Comprehensive Board Review for Primary and Maintenance of Certification*. New York: Oxford University Press; 2013:143.)

of various sizes, laryngoscope blades of different types and sizes, and supraglottic airways (SGAs) should be immediately available. If you are anesthetizing a child in an adult location, the pediatric anesthesia cart, as well as advanced airway equipment (e.g., video laryngoscope), should be brought to your anesthetizing location. Atropine or glycopyrrolate should also be drawn up into a syringe and the appropriate dose calculated ahead of time because hypoxia in infants and children rapidly leads to bradycardia.

Airway Management Equipment

Types of Laryngoscopes and Best Uses

The size and structure of the pediatric airway change as the child develops. For most children, direct laryngoscopy is the most straightforward and expedient method of viewing the larynx for intubation. The two most common laryngoscope blades are the Miller (straight) blade and the Macintosh (curved) blade. Miller blades are available in sizes 00 to 4. Macintosh blades are available in sizes 0 to 4. Both blade styles have a flange that keeps the tongue from obstructing the clinician's line of sight.

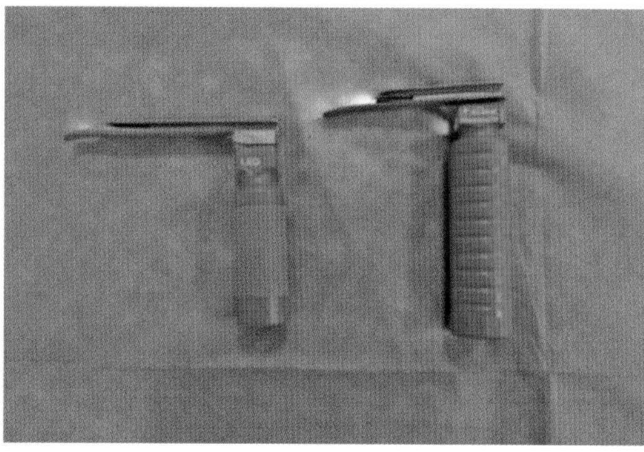

Figure 1.5 Size 1 (*left*) and size 0 (*right*) Miller blades.

Clinical Applications

Choice of Blade Type

The Miller blade (Figure 1.5) is often preferred for infants and small children because the clinician can use the tip to lift the floppy epiglottis to obtain a view of the VCs. The Macintosh blade (Figure 1.6) has some advantages, including the fact that it has a larger flange, which may be useful for sweeping the tongue out of the visual field in patients who have large tongues, such as patients with Down syndrome. To use the Macintosh blade, insert into the vallecula and lift upward at a 45-degree angle, taking care to avoid hitting the upper teeth or gum. When the Macintosh blade is used correctly, the epiglottis will be indirectly lifted upward as the hyoepiglottic ligament is pressed inward by the tip of the blade. This technique avoids trauma to the surface of the epiglottis and causes less sympathetic stimulation.

Choice of Blade Size

The choice of an appropriate blade size is generally based on patient age (Table 1.1). Alternatively, a blade approximately the length of the distance between the lips and angle of the jaw can be selected.

If the distance between the lips and angle of the jaw does not correlate with an available blade, a longer blade is generally preferred. The blade should then be gently inserted only as far as necessary while being cautious not to damage the patient's teeth, gums, or lips. Children with Down syndrome and those with certain congenital disorders are often small for age, necessitating a

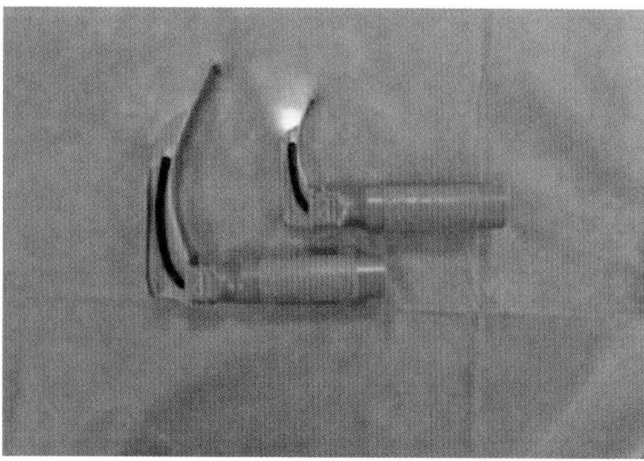

Figure 1.6 Size 2 (*left*) and size 1 (*right*) Macintosh blades.

Table 1.1 Suggested Laryngoscope Blade Types and Sizes Based on Patient Age

Age	Miller	Wis-Hippel	Macintosh
Small premature infant	00		0
Premature infant	0		0
Term neonate	0–1		1
1–12 months	1		1–2
1–2 years	1	1.5	2
2–6 years	2		2

smaller blade and ETT. The Wisconsin, Phillips, and Wis-Hipple laryngoscope blades are additional straight blades commonly used for intubating infants and small children. The Wisconsin blade has a slightly wider tip than the Miller blade, which is designed to help lift the epiglottis. The flange has a relatively large semicircular cross section. This feature aims to create more space for placing an ETT (Figure 1.7). Wis-Hipple laryngoscope blades are a modified version of the Wisconsin blade with a wider, straighter spatula and straighter flange.

Endotracheal Tubes and Best Uses

The smallest standard uncuffed ETT has an internal diameter of 2.5 mm, and the smallest cuffed ETT has an internal diameter of 3.0 mm (Figure 1.8). Size 2.0-mm ETTs are also manufactured but are not commonly available. Specialized ETTs, including laser tubes, reinforced tubes, oral RAE tubes, and nasal RAE tubes, are widely available in pediatric sizes in both cuffed and uncuffed versions (Figure 1.9).

Clinical Applications

Endotracheal Tube Size Selection

Selection of an appropriately sized ETT is based on age years for healthy patients older than 2. In general, the Cole formula [(age/4) + 4] is used for uncuffed tubes (Table 1.2), and the Khine formula [(age/4) + 3] is used for cuffed tubes. Some clinicians make the Cole formula

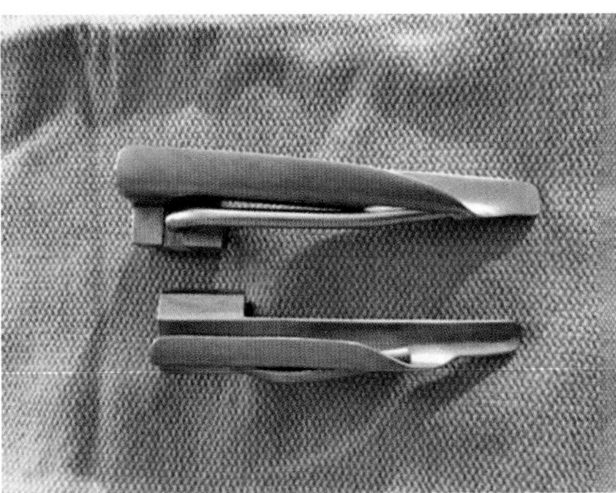

Figure 1.7 Size 1.5 Wis-Hipple laryngoscope blade (*top*) compared with size 1 Miller blade (*bottom*).

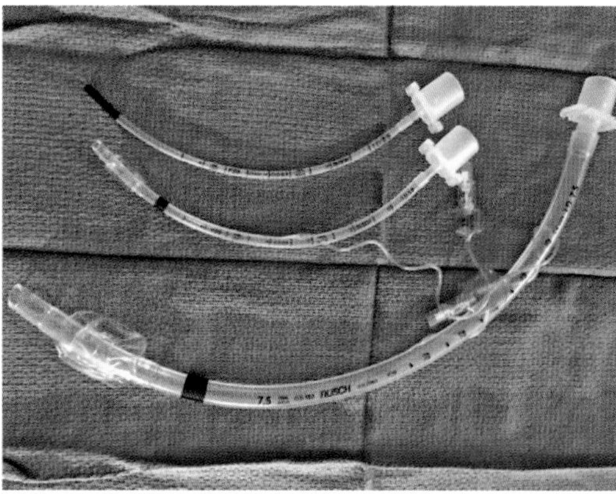

Figure 1.8 *Top to bottom:* 2.5-mm uncuffed endotracheal tube (ETT), 3-mm cuffed ETT, 7.5-mm cuffed ETT.

work for cuffed ETTs as well by simply subtracting 0.5 to "downsize," so [(age/4) + 4) – 0.5]. The results of the Cole and Khine formulas are within one size of each other and should only be used as estimates. Using an ETT that is too large can lead to subglottic edema causing postoperative complications such as croup or even, in rare cases, complete airway obstruction.

Choosing Cuffed versus Uncuffed Endotracheal Tubes

Historically, uncuffed tubes were recommended for patients younger than 8 years. Poorly designed ETTs and misunderstood pediatric airway anatomy fueled this recommendation. Bulky cuffs required using smaller diameter tubes to allow room for the cuff, even when the cuff was not inflated. Smaller diameter tubes can be problematic, owing to the associated increased resistance and work of breathing. Moreover, mucus and secretions may more easily obstruct a smaller tube. A conventional cuff resting in the infant trachea can cause uneven pressure on the tracheal wall with its bulky edges. This could lead to ischemia and mucosal damage and subsequent airway inflammation, scarring, and subglottic stenosis. Manufacturing of ETTs is not standardized, and the design is not always appropriate for pediatric laryngotracheal dimensions.[9] Cuff length and distance from the tip of the tube vary. This means that in some cases if the tip is placed above the carina, the cuff could be within the glottic opening, leading to potential VC edema or VC damage.

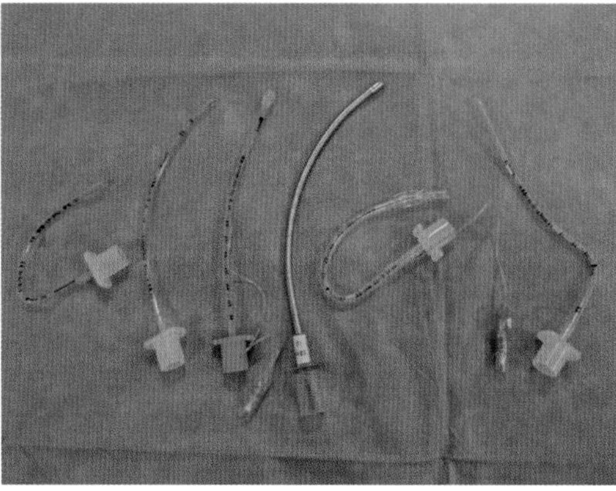

Figure 1.9 *Left to right:* 3-mm uncuffed oral RAE endotracheal tube (ETT), 3-mm uncuffed ETT, 3-mm Microcuff ETT, 3-mm laser ETT, 3.5-mm cuffed oral RAE ETT, 3.5-mm uncuffed nasal RAE ETT.

Table 1.2 Endotracheal Tube Sizing*

Age (years)	ETT (internal diameter in mm)
Premature	2.5–3
Newborn	3
3–12 months	3.5
1–2	4.0–4.5
2–4	4.5–5.0
4–6	5.0–5.5
6–8	5.5–6.0
8–10	6.0 cuffed
10–12	6.5 cuffed

*For patients older than 2 years, sizing in this table is based on the Cole formula.

The design of the low-pressure high-volume Microcuff ETT, introduced in 2004, solves many flaws of conventional cuffed ETTs. The micro-thin polyurethane balloon is very pliable and only adds 10 microns to the outer radius of the ETT when deflated, making downsizing typically unnecessary. Additonally, the Murphy eye is absent, which allows the cuff to be placed more distally on the ETT. The cuff can then be positioned below the glottic opening but above the carina (Figure 1.10).

In one study, the use of a cuffed ETT led to a lower incidence of microaspiration.[10] Even with careful attention to sizing, however, every patient is different, and when an uncuffed tube is used, sometimes the first ETT placed will be too big (no leak at <20 mmHg) or too small (insufficient seal to achieve adequate TVs), necessitating a second intubation with a different-sized ETT. This problem is minimized or eliminated with a cuffed ETT because a slightly smaller tube can be chosen for the first intubation attempt and the cuff can be inflated to achieve an adequate seal. Therefore, use of a cuffed ETT (and the resultant adequate seal) requires a lower fresh gas flow, thereby decreasing the consumption of anesthetic gases. An adequate seal will also result in less contamination of the operating room by inhalation agents. Compared with an uncuffed ETT, a properly sized and placed cuffed ETT will not lead to an increased risk for respiratory or airway complications.[11]

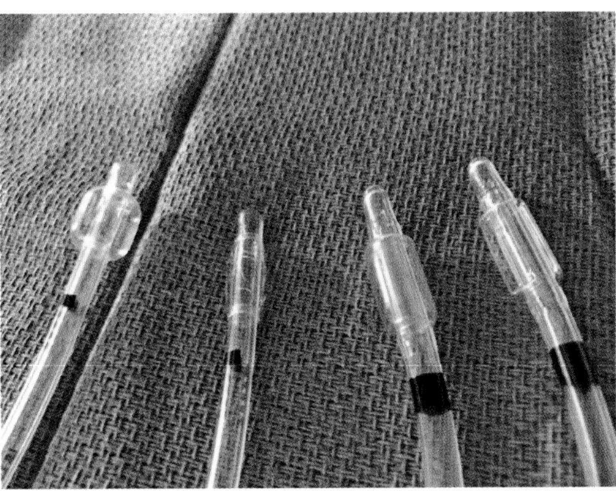

Figure 1.10 *Left to right:* 3.5-mm Microcuff endotracheal tube (ETT) (cuff inflated), 3.5-mm Microcuff ETT (cuff deflated), 3.5-mm conventional cuffed ETT (cuff inflated), 3.5-mm conventional cuffed ETT (cuff deflated).

The younger the child, the more advantageous it is to use a Microcuff tube, and we recommend these tubes in children younger than 8 years. If one is not available, the clinician must consider the risks and benefits of using a conventional cuffed tube or an uncuffed tube. The risks of using an uncuffed ETT include multiple direct laryngoscopies to place an ETT that has an adequate seal without a high leak pressure. If a conventional cuffed ETT is used, the clinician must ensure that when bilateral breath sounds are heard indicating tracheal placement without a mainstem intubation, the cuff is not positioned between the VCs. If the cuff is between the VCs, the ETT should be replaced.

Pearl: The cuff on a Microcuff ETT is only 10 microns thick. When deflated, the cuff completely conforms to the ETT. Therefore, its diameter mimics that of an uncuffed ETT. Hence, the Cole formula can be used when selecting the size of a Microcuff tube.

Caution! Cuffs should not be overinflated. ETT cuff inflation pressures should be kept at less than 20 mmHg to avoid tracheal mucosal damage in children (of note, some literature suggests that this number may be somewhat higher in adults).[12] Studies support the use of manometers to measure cuff pressures in children,[13] although unfortunately, use of intraoperative cuff manometry is not widely practiced, and no practice guidelines are in place requiring its use. In the absence of a manometer, inflating the cuff with the minimal amount of volume to a leak of less than 20 mmHg is the safest practice.[14]

Caution! Use of nitrous oxide (N_2O) can cause a gradual increase in cuff pressure. If N_2O is being used, periodic cuff pressure testing should be performed throughout the procedure.[13]

Supraglottic Airways and Best Uses

Almost all first- and second-generation SGAs are available in pediatric sizes and are smaller versions of the adult equivalent (Figures 1.11a and 1.11b). Both first- and second-generation SGAs have an elliptical mask that is attached to a ventilation shaft. When properly placed, an SGA will sit within the posterior pharynx, with the opening of the ventilation shaft directly above the glottis. Second-generation devices have an additional port that allows for the egress of stomach contents or placement of a suction tube for gastric decompression (see Figure 1.11b). Size selection varies by manufacturer but is generally weight based (Tables 1.3–1.5).

The Laryngeal Mask Airway (LMA) Classic (Teleflex Incorporated, Wayne, PA) is a reusable device with a cuff made of silicone. There is also a disposable version made of polyvinylchloride called the LMA Unique (see Figure 1.11a) The LMA Flexible, with a long wire-reinforced air tube, is commonly used in pediatric procedures, especially ocular or otolaryngology procedures (Table 1.3). Research regarding the risks and benefits of using an SGA for tonsillectomies is inconsistent;[15,16] although an SGA may be more convenient, the lack of a secured airway is a risk, especially in cases with larger amounts of bleeding.

The reusable LMA ProSeal (Teleflex Incorporated, Wayne, PA) (see Figure 1.11b) was the first second-generation device introduced into the market. The adult version has a dorsal cuff that, owing to size limitations, is not present on sizes smaller than 3. However, other features, such as the bite block and shorter reinforced ventilation shaft, are present.

(a)

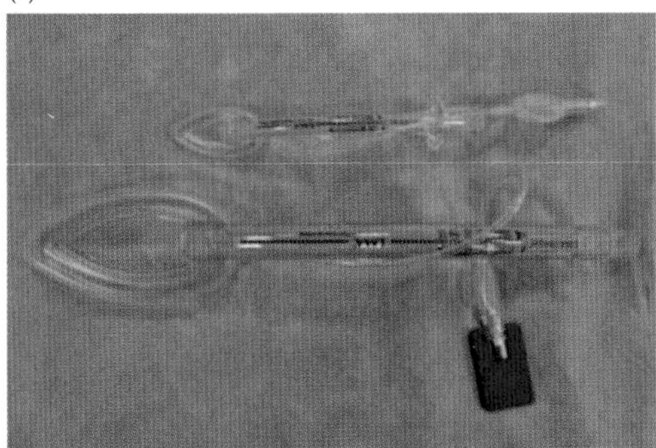

Figure 1.11a LMA Unique: adult and pediatric sizes.

The LMA Supreme (Teleflex Incorporated, Wayne, PA) (see Figure 1.11b) was introduced in 2007 as a hybrid of the LMA ProSeal (Teleflex Incorporated, Wayne, PA) and the LMA Fastrach (Teleflex Incorporated, Wayne, PA). It is a disposable device with a rigid angled shaft and built-in bite block.

The i-gel (Intersurgical Incorporated, East Syracuse, NY) is an SGA designed without an inflatable cuff (Table 1.4). The device is made from a gel-like thermoplastic elastomer, which enables it to conform its shape to the pharynx. The ventilation shaft allows for passage of an ETT and also has a parallel port to accommodate an orogastric tube.

The air-Q (Cookgas, St. Louis, MO) (Figure 1.11c) is a disposable SGA with a shorter, wider air tube and a detachable connector (Table 1.5). It does not have epiglottic bars within the mask. These features facilitate using the device as a conduit for tracheal intubation. The wider ventilation shaft more easily accommodates passage of the cuff of the ETT.

For intubation through any SGA, optimally, a fiberoptic bronchoscope should be used to guide the ETT through the VCs to decrease the likelihood of damage to the laryngeal structures. In an emergency situation, blind advancement of the ETT may be necessary.

Clinical Applications

An SGA can be used as a primary airway, rescue airway, or conduit for intubation. It can be placed quickly after induction without use of muscle relaxant. When using an SGA, side effects of reversal agents and potential trauma caused by laryngoscopy can be avoided. Contraindications to the use of an SGA as a primary airway in a child are similar to those for an adult and include a full stomach, active gastric reflux, need for a secured airway, an intrapharyngeal mass, and need

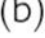

(b)

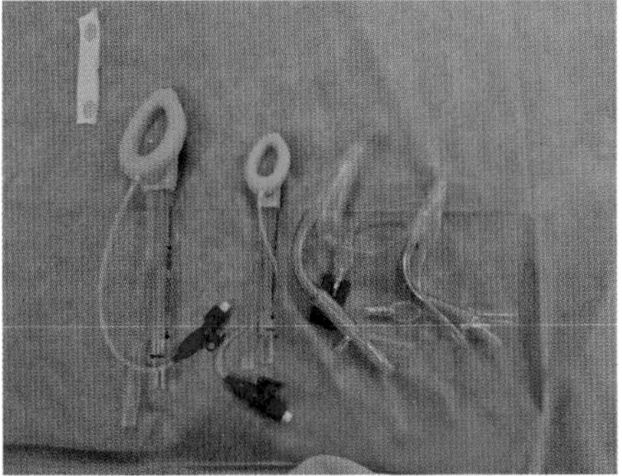

Figure 1.11b LMA ProSeal (*left*) and LMA Supreme (*right*): adult and pediatric sizes.

(c)

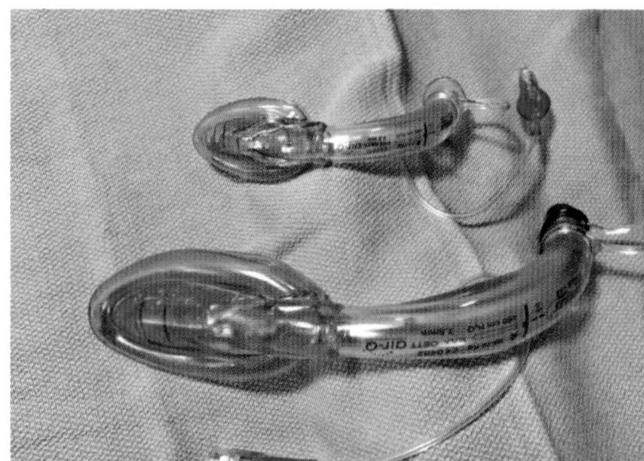

Figure 1.11c air-Q: adult and pediatric sizes.

Table 1.3 Laryngeal Mask Airway Sizes Based on Patient Weight

LMA (Classic, Unique, Flexible, Supreme, and ProSeal)	
Patient Weight (kg)	**LMA Size**
<5	1
5–10	1.5
10–20	2
20–30	2.5
30–50	3

Table 1.4 i-gel Sizes Based on Patient Weight

i-gel	
Patient Weight (kg)	**Supraglottic Airway Size**
2–5	1
5–12	1.5
10–25	2
25–35	2.5
30–60	3

Table 1.5 air-Q Size Based on Patient Weight

air-Q	
Patient Weight (kg)	**Supraglottic Airway Size**
<7	1
7–17	1.5
17–30	2
30–50	2.5
50–70	3.5

for high inspiratory ventilation pressures. Use of muscle relaxation with an SGA designed to accommodate higher ventilation pressures (e.g., the LMA ProSeal) is controversial. Advantages of using an SGA over an ETT include the possibility of less stimulation with insertion leading to fewer hemodynamic changes as well as less airway irritation, potentially leading to a decreased chance of laryngospasm, bronchospasm, and coughing after removal.

Caution! Similar to an ETT, the amount of air inserted into the SGA cuff should not exceed the manufacturer recommendation (often displayed on the shaft of the device). The amount of air injected into the cuff should be the minimal amount needed, with a leak pressure of less than 20 mmHg. Cuff pressures should not exceed the manufacturer's recommendation when measured by a manometer.[17]

!! **Potential Complications**: Stomach insufflation from excessive inspiratory pressures or a malpositioned device can increase the chance of gastric distension or aspiration. Gastric distension can make ventilation more difficult, especially in infants and young children. Minor manipulation of the patient or SGA can unintentionally dislodge the device. This unintentional dislodgment can easily occur in infants and therefore SGAs should be used cautiously in this population. Excessive cuff pressures can impede capillary perfusion to the pharyngeal mucosa and cause ischemia. Pressure against the hypoglossal or recurrent laryngeal nerves from an SGA can cause a nerve palsy.

References

1. Harless J, Ramaiah R, Bananker SM. Pediatric airway management. *Int J Crit Illn Inj Sci*. 2014;4(1):65–70.
2. Santillanes G, Gausche-Hill M. Pediatric airway management. *Emerg Med Clin North Am*. 2008;26(4):961–975.
3. Wani TM, Bissonnette B, Rafiq Malik M, et al. Age-based analysis of pediatric upper airway dimensions using computed tomography imaging. *Pediatr Pulmonol*. 2016;51(3):267–271.
4. Tobias JD. Pediatric airway anatomy may not be what we thought: implications for clinical practice and the use of cuffed endotracheal tubes. *Paediatr Anaesth*. 2015;25(1):9–19.
5. Andropoulos DB. Pediatric physiology: how does it differ from adults? In: Mason K, ed. *Pediatric Sedation Outside of the Operating Room*. 2nd ed. New York: Springer-Verlag; 2015:77–91.
6. Hislop AA, Wigglesworth JS, Desai R. Alveolar development in the human fetus and infant. *Early Hum Dev*. 1986;13(1):1–11.
7. Moss DR. Pediatric anesthesia. In: Matthes K, Urman R, Ehrenfeld J, eds. *Anesthesiology: A Comprehensive Board Review for Primary and Maintenance of Certification*. New York: Oxford University Press; 2013:143.
8. Berry F, Castro B. Neonatal anesthesia. In: Barash PG, Cullen B, Stoelting R, eds. *Clinical Anesthesia*. 4th ed. Philadelphia: Wolters Kluwer Health/Lippincott Williams & Wilkins; 2001:1176–1177.
9. Weiss M, Dullenkopf A, Gysin C, Dillier CM, Gerber AC. Shortcomings of cuffed paediatric tracheal tubes. *Br J Anaesth*. 2004;92(1):78–88.
10. Gopalareddy V, He Z, Soundar S, et al. Assessment of the prevalence of microaspiration by gastric pepsin in the airway of ventilated children. *Acta Paediatr*. 2008;97(1):55–60.

11. Taylor C, Subaiya L, Corsino D. Pediatric cuffed endotracheal tubes: an evolution of care. *Ochsner J*. 2011;11(1):52–56.
12. Lewis FR, Schlobohm RM, Thomas AN. Prevention of complications from prolonged tracheal intubation. *Am J Surg*. 1978;135:452–457.
13. Ong M, Chambers NA, Hullet B, Erb TO, Ungern-Sternberg V. Laryngeal mask airway and tracheal tube cuff pressures in children: are clinical endpoints valuable for guiding inflation? *Anaesthesia*. 2008;63(7):738–744.
14. Sultan P, Carvalho B, Rose BO, Cregg R. Endotracheal tube cuff pressure monitoring: a review of the evidence. *J Periop Pract*. 2011;21(11): 379.
15. Sierpina DI, Chaudhary H, Walner DL, et al. Laryngeal mask airway versus endotracheal tube in pediatric adenotonsillectomy. *Laryngoscope*. 2012;122(2):429–435.
16. Lalwani K, Richins S, Aliason I, Milczuk H, Fu R. The laryngeal mask airway for pediatric adenotonsillectomy: predictors of failure and complications. *Int J Pediatr Otorhinolaryngol*. 2013;77(1): 25–28.
17. Hernandez MR, Klock PA, Ovassapian A. Evolution of the extraglottic airway: a review of its history, applications, and practical tips for success. *Anesth Analg*. 2012;114(2):349–368.

Chapter 2

Mask Ventilation, Direct Laryngoscopy, and Supraglottic Airway Placement Procedures

Jennifer Anderson

Bag Mask Ventilation

Introduction

Bag mask ventilation is used extensively in the operating room, emergency department, and intensive care unit. Effective bag mask ventilation can save a child's life in emergent situations.[1] Respiratory assistance is provided to the patient through a mask on the patient's face, held in a specialized way to maximize airway patency (described later), that is attached to a device capable of delivering positive pressure manually or automatically. Oxygenation is achieved by compressing air/oxygen through the delivery device into the lungs, and ventilation is ensured by maintaining airway patency as the patient exhales with chest wall recoil.

Clinical Applications

Bag mask ventilation is used when hypopnea or apnea is induced by anesthetics or when patients are hypoventilating or in respiratory distress.

Contraindications

There are no absolute contraindications to bag mask ventilation. In patients with increased gastric contents, recent esophageal surgery, craniofacial trauma, or recent facial surgery, it is often desirable secure the airway with an endotracheal tube as soon as possible. Nevertheless, ventilating the patient is always the first priority, and sometimes bag mask ventilation may be required even in those situations.

Critical Anatomy

The clinician must have knowledge of the anatomy and physiology of the nasal and oral passages, tongue, pharynx, larynx, glottis, trachea, and cervical spine specific to pediatric patients to be able maintain a patent airway and troubleshoot obstruction or other complications in this population (see Chapter 1, Pediatric Airway Fundamentals).

Setup

Equipment

- Face mask (Figure 2.1)
- Self-inflating bag valve resuscitator (Figure 2.2) (e.g., Ambu Bag) or flow-inflating bag (Mapleson circuit or Jackson-Rees circuit—both flow-inflating bags require an O_2 supply)
- Adjunct equipment: oral airway (Figure 2.3), nasal trumpet, suction

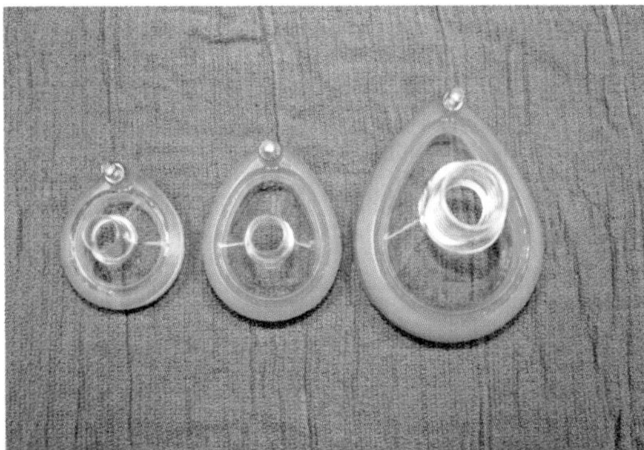

Figure 2.1 Face masks of varying sizes: neonate, infant, child.

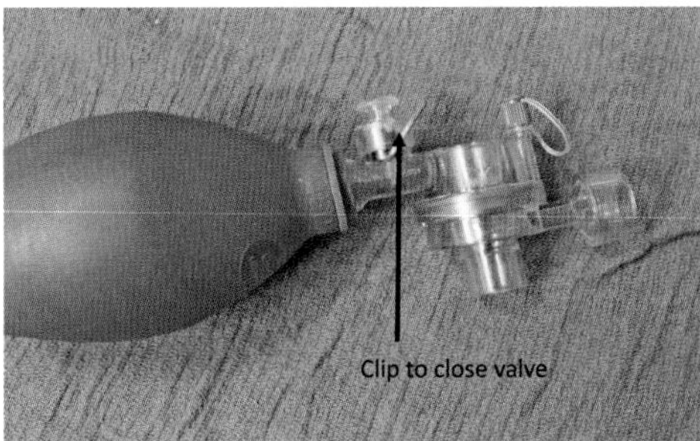

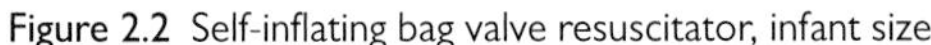

Figure 2.2 Self-inflating bag valve resuscitator, infant size.

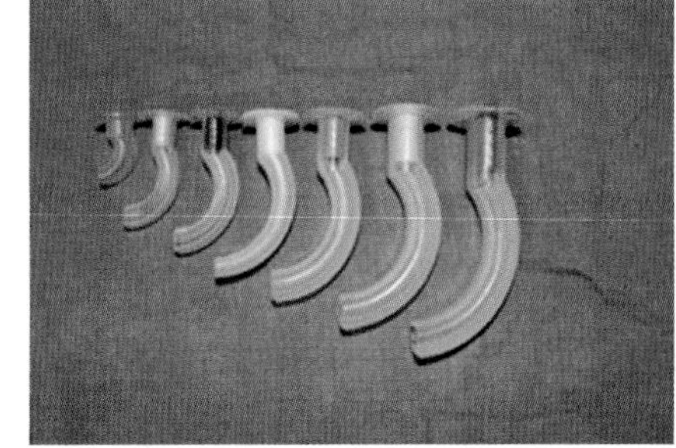

Figure 2.3 Oral pharyngeal airways: sizes 30 to 100 mm.

Most face masks are teardrop-shaped devices with an inflatable cuff and a standard 22-mm connector. They are made of clear plastic, allowing for prompt detection of secretions or vomitus. The teardrop shape and ability to add or remove air from the balloon allow creation of an even seal around the patient's nose and mouth. Several different manufacturers make masks appropriate for patients of all sizes.

Manual delivery devices include the self-inflating bag valve resuscitator (see Figure 2.2) and the flow-inflating bag (Mapleson circuit or Jackson-Rees circuit). Mechanical ventilators with an associated circuit can also be used. Each system attaches to a mask through the 22-mm connector. Bag valve resuscitators are available in infant, child, and adult sizes. Reservoir bags for flow-inflating systems are available in 0.5- to 3-liter sizes.

If positioning alone does not provide airway patency, then a properly sized and placed oral or nasal airway can alleviate obstruction caused by the tongue, adenoidal tissue, or soft palate. An oral airway similar in length to the distance between the mouth and earlobe should be selected. To place an oral airway, gently push the chin down with one hand and insert the oral airway into the mouth until the front edge is just anterior to the lips or mandible (Figure 2.4).

>> **Tip on Technique:** If difficulty placing an oral airway is encountered because the tongue is falling posteriorly, turn the oral airway upside down and rotate it 180 degrees during insertion. Care should be taken to avoid scraping the palate with the oral airway during this method of insertion.

If the clinician chooses to use a nasal trumpet, then a device similar in length to the distance between the naris and the earlobe should be selected. Lubricate the nasal trumpet and then gently insert it into the nasal passage. Keep in mind that the nasal passage runs straight back (e.g., parallel to the chin, and NOT up toward the forehead). If resistance is met during advancement, a smaller nasal trumpet may be needed to avoid trauma and bleeding from adenoidal tissue, but placement should never be forced. In some patients (e.g., with healed nasal fractures), passage of a nasal trumpet may not be possible.

>> **Tip on Technique:** It may be easier to place a nasal trumpet than an oral airway if the patient is biting down. Alternatively, airway patency can be attempted by providing continuous positive airway pressure of 5 to 20 mmHg.

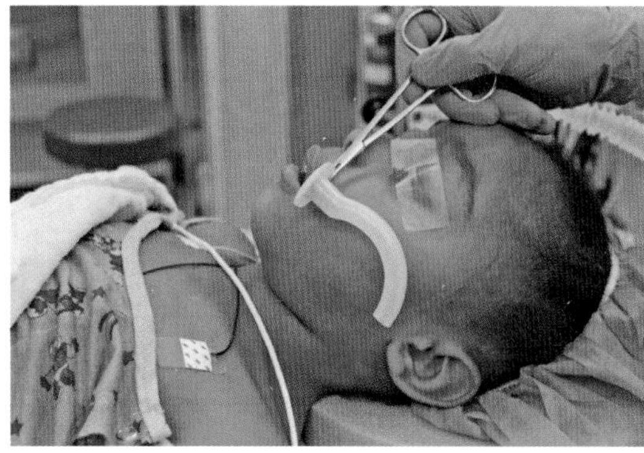

Figure 2.4 Proper size selection of oral airway. The oral airway is similar in length to the distance between the mouth and earlobe.

WARNING!! Severe bleeding can occur from inserting any device, including a nasal trumpet, into the nose. Consider avoiding or proceeding with caution in patients with a coagulation disorder, on anticoagulant medications, or with liver disease causing a bleeding diathesis. A nasal airway can also cause severe damage to a repaired cleft palate.

Step-by-Step

1. **Position the patient in the "sniffing position."** The patient should be placed in the "sniffing position" to optimize airway opening (Figure 2.5).[2] Obtaining a combination of lower cervical spine flexion and head extension for mask ventilation is different for infants and children because the occiput is relatively larger than in an adult. For a neonate or infant, a shoulder roll may bring the child into proper position (see Chapter 1, Pediatric Airway Fundamentals). For a child younger than 6 years, resting the head on the operating room bed will often optimize positioning. For a child older than 6 years, a small pillow can be placed under the head.

   The horizontal alignment of the earlobe with the sternal notch is one marker of proper positioning. The neck is extended, and the chin is lifted away from the chest. This position is historically advocated as the optimal position to align the oral, pharyngeal, and

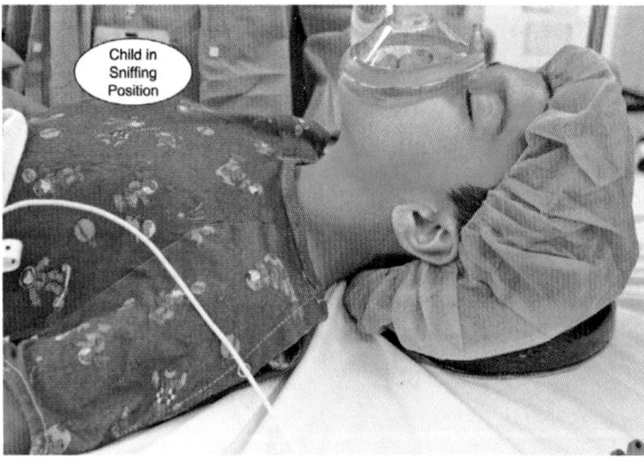

Figure 2.5 Child in "sniffing position." The earlobe is horizontal to the sternal notch.

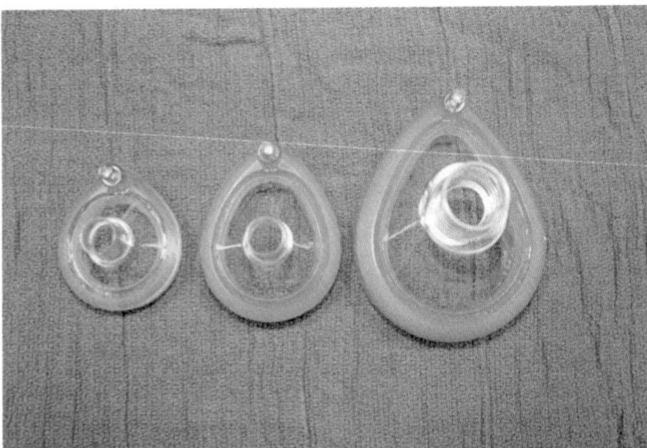

Figure 2.6 Appropriately sized mask fits around the nose and mouth.

laryngeal axes and maintain airway patency and to provide favorable conditions for mask ventilation and direct laryngoscopy. This position may not be optimal for all patients. The clinician must assess airway patency and adjust positioning based on individual patient characteristics.

2. **Choose an appropriately sized mask.** The mask should fit easily over the bridge of the nose and under the mouth (Figure 2.6).

   !! **Potential Complications:** Choosing a mask of an inappropriate size can inhibit the ability to create a good seal and deliver effective ventilation. Use of excessive pressure to overcome this inadequacy can cause bruising of the mandible or face.

   >> **Tip on Technique:** If the patient is between mask sizes, it may be easier to create a good seal using a slightly larger mask than a mask that is too small. When the mask is slightly too large, the curved end of the mask can be placed under the chin, and the mask itself can often be gently squeezed to achieve a good seal (Figure 2.7). Having several different sizes of masks immediately available is also essential so that the best-fitting mask can be chosen.

3. **Create a good seal between the mask and face.** Place the mask over the mouth and nose gently, but firmly. An E-C grip can be used. With the E-C grip, the thumb and forefinger of the left hand hold the mask to the face while the distal three fingers gently grip the

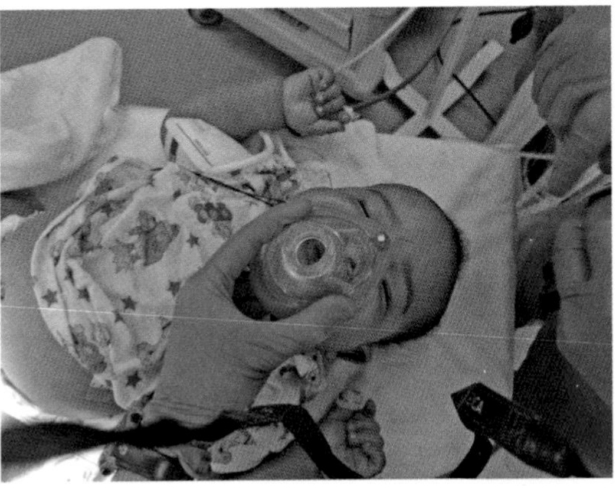

Figure 2.7 A larger mask placed partially under the chin can create a good seal.

(a)

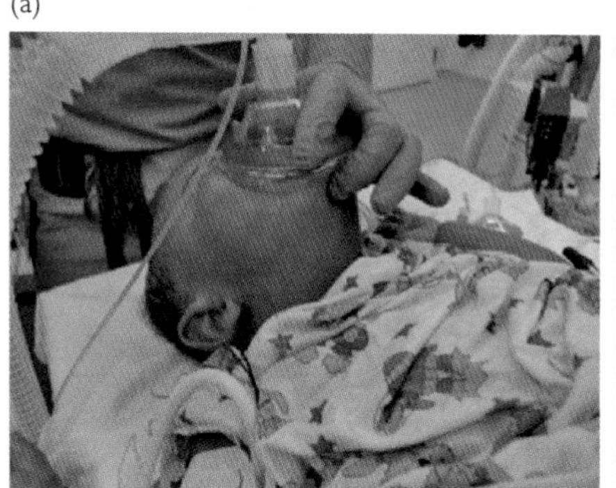

(b)

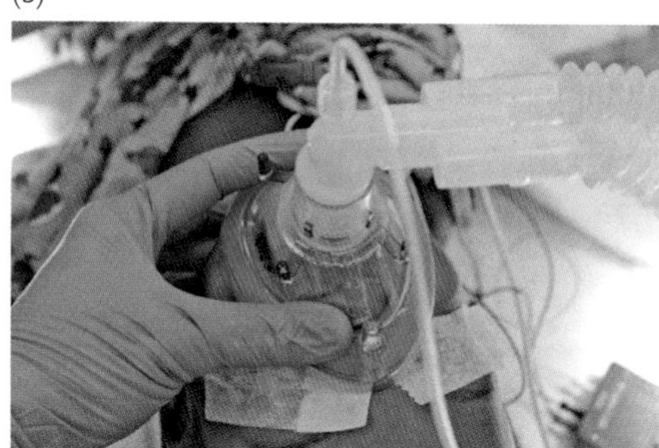

Figure 2.8a and b E-C Grip.

mandible and pull it up toward the mask. In small children and infants, only the third finger may be needed to pull up the mandible (Figure 2.8a and 2.8b).

>> **Tip on Technique:** Be very careful to keep your distal three fingers on the mandible (Figure 2.9) and to avoid letting your fingers slip toward the soft submandibular tissues because severe airway obstruction can be caused by compression of the submandibular tissues with your fingers. The mandible should be brought up to the mask rather than pressing the mask on the face.

>> **Tip on Technique:** If difficulty with mask ventilation occurs, a two-handed technique can be used. Both thumbs press the mask on either side while the first and second fingers grip under the rami of the mandible, lifting it upward in the temporomandibular joint and achieving a jaw thrust (Figure 2.10).

4. **Provide positive pressure ventilation.** While one hand holds the mask, squeeze the bag with the other hand at a rate appropriate for the age and size of the patient. The bag should be squeezed for a full 1 to 2 seconds and then released for twice as long, to achieve an inhale-to-exhale (I:E) ratio of 1:2. Chest rise that correlates with

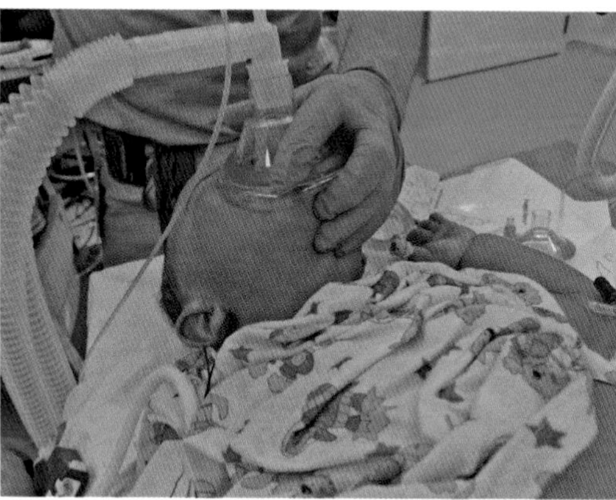

Figure 2.9 Incorrect placement of last three fingers. The last three fingers are compressing the soft submandibular tissue, which may cause airway obstruction.

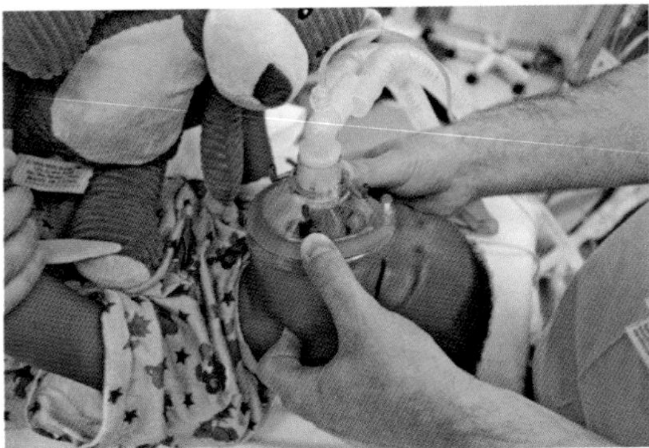

Figure 2.10 Two-handed mask grip with jaw thrust.

adequate tidal volumes of approximately 4 to 6 mL/kg should be seen. Pressure should be released between breaths because exhalation occurs by the passive egress of air out of the lungs due to chest wall recoil. Successful mask ventilation is indicated by appropriate chest rise and misting on exhalation into the clear mask. Adequacy of ventilation should be corroborated by auscultation, pulse oximetry, and end-tidal carbon dioxide measurements.

Caution! Use of excessive positive pressure can cause air to insufflate the stomach. This can lead to emesis and aspiration. Especially in younger children, air in the stomach may also press the diaphragm into the thorax, decreasing your ability to ventilate the patient. If air has been insufflated into the stomach, insert a lubricated red rubber catheter or orogastric tube and then suction this catheter or tube to remove air from the stomach.

>> **Tip on Technique:** Most pediatric-sized bag valve resuscitators have a pop-off valve to prevent barotrauma caused by use of high ventilating pressures. If high pressures are needed to deliver adequate breaths, flipping the metal or plastic clip over the spring closes the valve, although this technique must be used with great caution and clinical judgment of the risks and benefits. Always make sure that adequate exhalation occurs between breaths to avoid auto–positive end-expiratory pressure (auto-PEEP), which can quickly lead to hemodynamic collapse and possibly pneumothorax.

Postoperative Management Considerations

There are no special postoperative management considerations associated with this procedure.

Direct Laryngoscopy and Endotracheal Intubation

Introduction

Endotracheal intubation is the placement of an endotracheal tube into the mouth or nose, then through the glottis and into the trachea, in order to provide controlled oxygenation and ventilation. Use of direct laryngoscopy is often the most straightforward and expeditious method for intubation. A laryngoscope is used to displace the tongue and lift the epiglottis to create a direct line of sight to the glottis. The practitioner can then visualize the placement of the endotracheal tube through the vocal cords.

Clinical Applications

Intubation is indicated in any patient who is unable to maintain adequate spontaneous respiration or who is at risk for aspiration. Examples are patients in respiratory arrest, those in cardiac arrest, or sometimes those experiencing neurologic issues such as seizures. Patients undergoing surgical procedures will often require intubation because of the apnea and risk for aspiration caused by the anesthetics and the surgical procedure itself.

Contraindications

1. Advanced airway procedures (see Chapter 3, Fiberoptic, Video Laryngoscope, and Nasal Airway Procedures) and/or consultation with a pediatric otolaryngology surgeon should be considered for airways that are potentially difficult or in children with congenital disorders affecting the airway.

Critical Anatomy

To achieve successful direct laryngoscopy, the tongue must be laterally displaced and pressed into the submandibular space and the epiglottis lifted directly or indirectly off the glottis. The oral, pharyngeal, and laryngeal axes need to be aligned for direct visualization to occur.

Setup

Equipment

- Appropriately sized laryngoscope and endotracheal tubes (see Chapter 1, Pediatric Airway Fundamentals)
- Oxygen source
- Syringe
- Stylet
- Intravenous (IV) access
- Suction
- Standard monitors, including pulse oximeter, CO_2 detector, electrocardiogram, blood pressure cuff
- Stethoscope
- Tape

>> **Tip on Technique:** If deemed necessary, in preparation for intubation, a lightly lubricated stylet may be placed into the lumen of the endotracheal tube. The endotracheal tube can then be molded into a hockey-stick form, which can promote easier passage of the endotracheal tube.

Drugs, Dosages, Administration

Intubation can be completed under general anesthesia or using a local anesthetic with or without sedation. The latter technique is also known as "awake intubation," although in children, general anesthesia is usually necessary. For general anesthesia, the following medications are often used:

- **Mask induction:** sevoflurane, with or without nitrous oxide

- **IV induction:** propofol 1 to 2 mg/kg IV
- **Muscle relaxant:** rocuronium 0.6 to 1 mg/kg IV or succinylcholine 1 to 2 mg/kg IV

> **Caution!** Atropine 0.01 to 0.02 mg/kg IV is **ALWAYS** given before succinylcholine in infants and young children to decrease the risk of severe bradycardia.
>
> **Caution!** Succinylcholine is avoided in children in nonemergency situations because of the risk for life-threatening anesthetic-induced hyperkalemia in children with (sometimes previously undiagnosed) muscular dystrophy.

- **Have available:** Atropine or glycopyrrolate 0.01 to 0.02 mg/kg IV can be given at the discretion of the anesthesiologist before intubation to decrease the likelihood of bradycardia caused by volatile agents and vagal stimulation.

  Pearl: Muscle relaxant may not be needed for intubation in young patients who are apneic and deeply anesthetized.

Step-by-Step

1. **Place the patient in the "sniffing position."** The patient should be placed in the "sniffing position" (see Figure 2.5).

> **Caution!** If the cervical spine is not stable, then the neck should remain in a neutral position throughout the induction and intubation. This neutral position can be maintained by keeping a protective cervical collar on the patient or by in-line stabilization provided by an assistant. Backup methods for airway management (e.g., a supraglottic airway) and intubation (video laryngoscopy and/or fiberoptic laryngoscopy) should be immediately available because it may be difficult to obtain a view of the glottis with the neck in the neutral position during direct laryngoscopy. Keep in mind that a typical supraglottic airway will NOT provide airway protection from aspiration.

2. **Preoxygenate the patient and induce anesthesia.** Preoxygenation is the delivery of forced inspiratory oxygen (a FiO_2 of 1) by face mask before the induction of anesthesia to increase oxygen reserves. This extends the period of apnea that can occur before desaturation (after the induction of anesthesia), allowing additional time for intubation attempts. An end-tidal oxygen saturation of greater than 90%, indicating an adequate oxygen reserve, can be achieved in most children within 60 to 100 seconds.[3,4]

   Oxygenation is dependent on alveolar ventilation, distribution of the ventilation/perfusion ratio, and oxygen consumption.[5] Oxygen consumption in neonates and infants is two to three times that in adults (infants: 7–9 mL/kg/min; adults: 3–4 mL/kg/min). In infants, closing capacity occurs within tidal volume breathing, causing a ventilation/perfusion mismatch. These physiologic characteristics lead to rapid desaturation in the apneic neonate or infant.

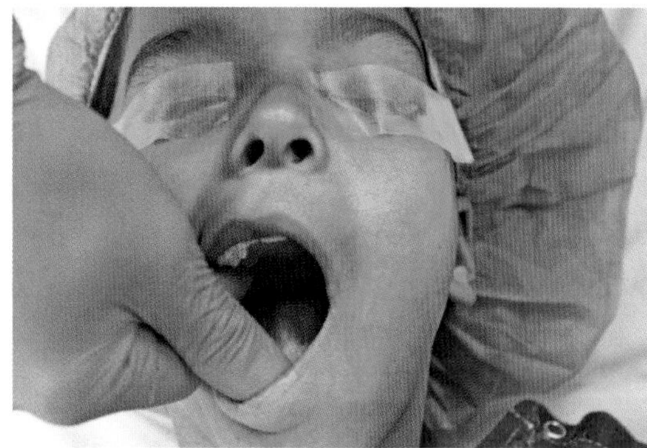

Figure 2.11 Opening the mouth with scissor technique.

Note: Obtaining a good seal with the mask is important; otherwise, inspired oxygen can be diluted up to 40%. However, placing a mask on the child's face may cause agitation. The practitioner must balance these opposing realities and act accordingly based on risks and benefits to the patient.

After adequate preoxygenation, anesthesia is induced.

3. **Open the patient's mouth maximally.** After the patient is fully anesthetized, open the mouth as wide as possible to allow for easy placement of the laryngoscope. In older children, the standard scissor technique can be used. The right thumb presses on the lower teeth while the index finger presses on the upper right molars, and the mouth is opened (Figure 2.11). In younger children and infants, this technique is often not possible because of limited space. Open the jaw by simply pressing down on the mandible, lower incisors, or alveolar ridge.

   >> Tip on Technique: Place the fingers of the right hand as far laterally in the mouth as possible to allow room for the laryngoscope.

4. **Perform direct laryngoscopy.** When there is enough room between the teeth or gums for the laryngoscope blade, slide the laryngoscope blade into the mouth until it rests on the base of the tongue and gently use it to open the jaw even further.[6]

   Macintosh 'Mac' blade: Place the blade on the right side of the mouth, with the base of the handle angled toward the right side of the patient, and slide medially to sweep the tongue out of the way. The tongue should be pressed into the submandibular space. Advance the tip of the blade until it lies in the vallecula. The angle of lift of the blade is roughly at 45 degrees to the bed. The epiglottis is indirectly lifted upward as the tip of the blade presses on the median glossoepiglottic fold in the vallecula (Figure 2.12). Avoid the teeth and lips.

   Miller blade: Slide the blade into the mouth just to the right of midline, with the base of the handle angled toward the left side of the patient. Advance the blade to the base of the tongue and toward the larynx, and slide the tip under the epiglottis. Lift the epiglottis directly up off of the glottis with the tip of the blade. Avoid the teeth and lips.

Caution! Care should be taken to avoid advancing the blade through the glottis because this can cause damage to the vocal cords. Inserting the blade into the esophagus and pulling back until the glottis comes into view is NOT recommended; doing so can cause trauma to the arytenoids and aryepiglottic folds.

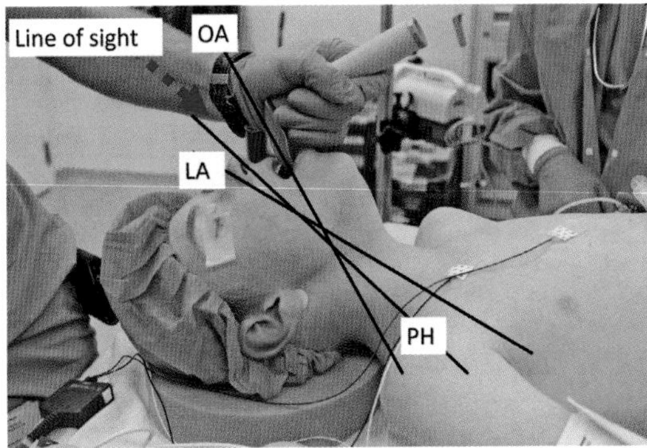

Figure 2.12 Patient positioned to optimize alignment of the oral, pharyngeal, and laryngeal axes. Macintosh blade inserted with force directed at a 45-degree angle to the bed. LA = laryngeal axis; OA = oral axis; PH = pharyngeal axis.

>> **Tip on Technique:** When using the Miller blade: The epiglottis can be "floppy" and difficult to control in small children. If so, focus on gently pressing the epiglottis into the soft tissue. This helps the epiglottis remain under the blade and not slip out from under the tip.

>> **Tip on Technique:** If positioning does not allow for a view of the glottis, an assistant can gently lift the head or remove the pillow to aid the clinician. Sometimes placing external pressure on the larynx can bring the glottis into view. This can be done by an assistant; in infants, the clinician can use the fifth finger of the left hand to press on the glottis. Care should be taken not to apply too much pressure because this can cause distortion of the very malleable infant larynx, making visualization more difficult.

WARNING!! Even in children who do not yet have their first set of teeth, trauma to the gums from laryngoscopy can cause later dental abnormalities. In children with their first set of teeth, damage or knocking out a tooth can cause abnormalities in the growth of the second set of teeth.

5. **Intubate the patient.** Intubation is the passing of an appropriately sized endotracheal tube through the glottis into the trachea. After a view of the glottis is obtained with the aid of a laryngoscope, hold the endotracheal tube with your right hand and gently advance it through the glottis into the trachea. The depth of insertion depends on the size of the child and the type of tube used (see Chapter 1, Pediatric Airway Fundamentals). If a cuffed endotracheal tube is used, the cuff should be inserted past the vocal cords to ensure that damage does not occur to the vocal cords after the cuff is inflated. After the endotracheal tube is in the appropriate position, remove the laryngoscope from the mouth and connect the endotracheal tube to the anesthesia circuit or bag mask resuscitator. Make sure to hold the endotracheal tube in place while the tube location is verified.

>> **Tip on Technique:** If the vocal cords are closed (Figure 2.13) or there is resistance to advancing the endotracheal tube, increasing the depth of anesthesia or paralysis can resolve this issue. If the vocal cords are open and resistance occurs more distally, then the endotracheal tube may be hitting the anterior tracheal wall. If this is suspected, decrease the angle of the hockey-stick form of the endotracheal tube or rotate the

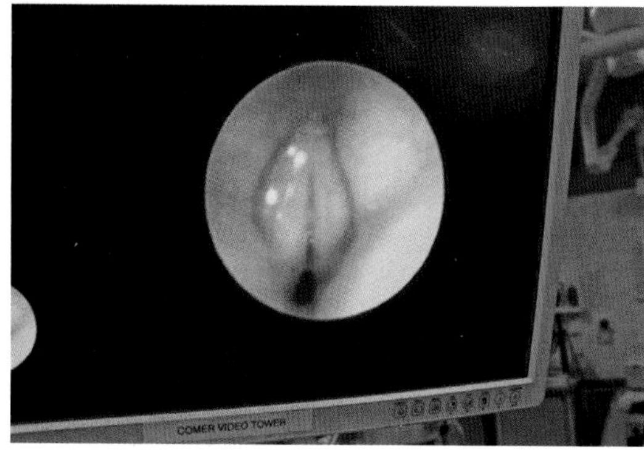

Figure 2.13 Closed infant vocal cords.

endotracheal tube during advancement. If this does not alleviate the difficulty, use a smaller endotracheal tube.

!! **Potential Complications:** Possible complications of intubation include trauma, bleeding, and swelling of the surrounding tissue.

WARNING!! Continued attempts at intubation after failure can be catastrophic. With each unsuccessful attempt, more inflammation of the laryngeal structures will occur, leading to narrowing of the glottis opening. Severe edema can lead to a complete inability to mask-ventilate. The Difficult Airway Society of the UK recommends limiting laryngoscopy to four attempts before trying other methods to secure the airway[7]; in many cases, even fewer attempts are warranted before waking the patient up and canceling an elective surgery.

>> **Tip on Technique:** When placing the endotracheal tube, "keep your eye on the tube" until the tube and cuff are safely through the glottis. Looking away or removing the blade prematurely can lead to error or trauma.

6. **Verify correct endotracheal tube placement.** Confirm proper placement of the endotracheal tube with multiple methods. (A) Confirm presence of end-tidal carbon dioxide with either a disposable CO_2 detector (for five breaths) or capnometry; capnometry is the gold standard for verifying endotracheal tube placement. (B) Auscultate the chest and stomach to confirm absence of ventilation of the stomach. (C) Confirm bilateral breath sounds and visualize bilateral chest rise. (D) Lung ultrasound can also be used in many cases to determine whether a mainstem intubation exists. (see Chapter 2, 'Lung Ultrasound' in Book 2 in this series, Ultrasound Guided Procedures and Radiologic Imaging for Pediatric Anesthesiologists) (E) Normal peak airway pressures are also typically an indicator of the ventilation of both lungs.

Caution! In small children, auscultation can be deceptive: auscultated sounds are transmitted easily, and sounds from insufflation of the stomach or a single lung can sometimes be auscultated in other parts of the thorax. Therefore, it is prudent to use multiple methods of detection for verification of tracheal intubation and bilateral lung insufflation.

Caution! Rarely, absence of breath sounds and end-tidal carbon dioxide in a patient with reactive airway disease can indicate severe bronchospasm caused by intubation. If the practitioner is certain the endotracheal tube was placed properly, bronchodilators (such as albuterol, ketamine, and if needed, low-dose epinephrine), attempting to deepen the anesthetic, and increasing delivered airway pressure may be indicated. It is important to keep in mind, however, that the endotracheal tube can easily slip out of the trachea because of small movements or patient coughing, and a low threshold should exist for quickly returning to mask ventilation.

7. **Check the endotracheal tube cuff.** Because excessive pressure on the mucosa of the trachea can lead to ischemic injury, perform a leak test for both cuffed and uncuffed endotracheal tubes. If an anesthesia machine is in use, set flows at approximately 6 to 7 L and slowly increase pressure using the adjustable pressure limiting (APL) valve. Stop when an audible leak is heard in the mouth. This point corresponds to the leak pressure. If a cuffed endotracheal tube is used, inflate the cuff until the leak is at less than 20 to 25 mmHg, with the ability to provide adequate tidal volumes. If an uncuffed endotracheal tube is used and the leak is at a slightly greater pressure than 20 mmHg, consider the risks and benefits of leaving the tube in place versus removing it and performing a second laryngoscopy. Ability to ventilate, expected length of intubation, and difficulty with masking or intubation should be considered when making this decision.
8. **Secure the endotracheal tube with tape.** Apply tape above and below the lip and wrapped around the endotracheal tube to keep it in place (Figure 2.14). Retaining precise endotracheal tube placement in infants is important because small changes in tube depth can lead to endobronchial intubation or unwanted extubation. Many different types of tape can

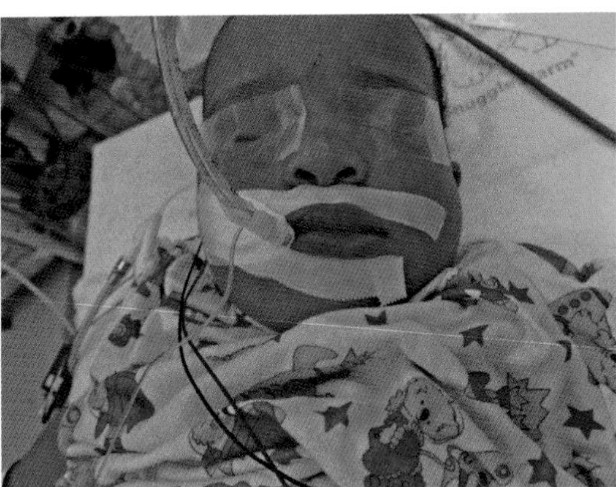

Figure 2.14 Silk tape above and below the lip, wrapped around the endotracheal tube, to keep the endotracheal tube in place.

be used. Consider using liquid adhesives to secure the tape when concern for proper placement is high; however, keep in mind that there is a risk for abrasions when liquid adhesives are used.

Caution! After the procedure, remove the tape carefully to avoid tearing fragile skin.

WARNING!! If the patient was initially difficult to intubate, and risks for laryngeal swelling and inflammation are high, extubation should only occur with extreme caution. Consider having advanced airway equipment and an otolaryngology surgeon present.

Postoperative Management Considerations

Laryngoscopy and intubation can cause inflammation and swelling of the larynx. Procedures near the larynx and multiple laryngoscopy attempts increase this risk. After extubation, if laryngeal edema is present, it can lead to stridor, increased work of breathing, and respiratory distress. If there is a high suspicion of laryngeal edema, consider using IV steroids and keeping the patient intubated until the swelling has resolved. If stridor occurs after extubation, monitor the patient closely for airway obstruction and the need for reintubation. For stridor after extubation, give inhaled racemic epinephrine and steroids. If respiratory compromise continues, consider reintubation. For severe respiratory compromise, immediately call pediatric otolaryngology because a rigid bronchoscope or even a surgical airway may be needed to re-establish ventilation.

Supraglottic Airway Placement

Introduction

The term *supraglottic airway* refers to a device that can be inserted into the mouth and pharynx with a ventilation orifice that rests above the glottis. Its final position should enable oxygenation and ventilation and delivery of volatile anesthetics. Second-generation devices have esophageal ports, which allow for suctioning of the stomach and egress of secretions or vomitus (see Chapter 1, Pediatric Airway Fundamentals). Each type of supraglottic airway has individual nuances associated with its placement. However, the method of the placement depicted in this chapter is applicable to supraglottic airways in general.

Clinical Applications

A supraglottic airway is useful to maintain an airway in patients undergoing general anesthesia. A supraglottic airway may also be useful as an airway rescue device when difficulty with mask ventilation or intubation is encountered or as a conduit for intubation for patients with a known difficult airway or high risk for desaturation.

Contraindications

Use of a supraglottic airway is contraindicated when there is a high risk for aspiration or (in general) a need for muscle relaxation during the case. A supraglottic airway should also not be used when a patient's oral aperture is too small to accommodate the device or if the patient has suspected or known anatomic abnormalities of the oral cavity or pharynx (relative

(a)

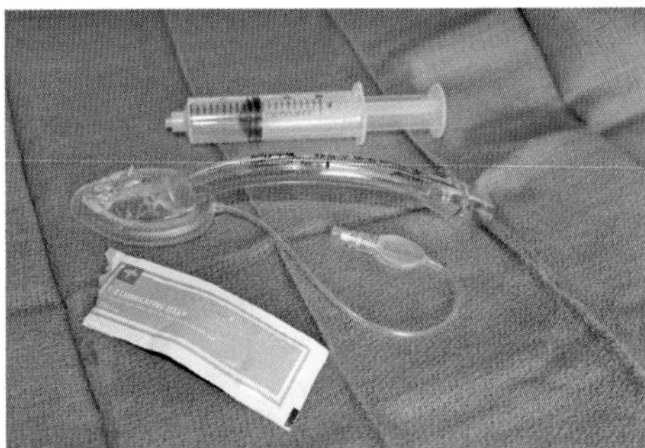

Figure 2.15a Supraglottic airway setup with the cuff kept inflated.

contraindication). Use of a supraglottic airway is also contraindicated when the patient will be placed in a prone position for a procedure.

Critical Anatomy

Proper placement of a supraglottic airway results in the ventilation tube resting over the glottis. The tip of the cuff or the esophageal port of second-generation devices lies just above the upper esophageal sphincter.

Setup

Equipment

- Appropriate type of supraglottic airway (Figures 2.15a and b). Choosing a supraglottic airway is based on availability, indication for use, and patient characteristics. For a routine anesthetic in an otherwise healthy patient, a first-generation supraglottic airway is appropriate (see Chapter 1, Pediatric Airway Fundamentals). For a longer procedure in which it is desirable to suction the stomach through a gastric port, a second-generation device may be the best choice.
- Appropriately sized supraglottic airway. The device is usually chosen based on the patient's weight. The corresponding weight is usually printed on the ventilating tube of the supraglottic airway.
- Water-based lubricant

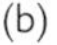

(b)

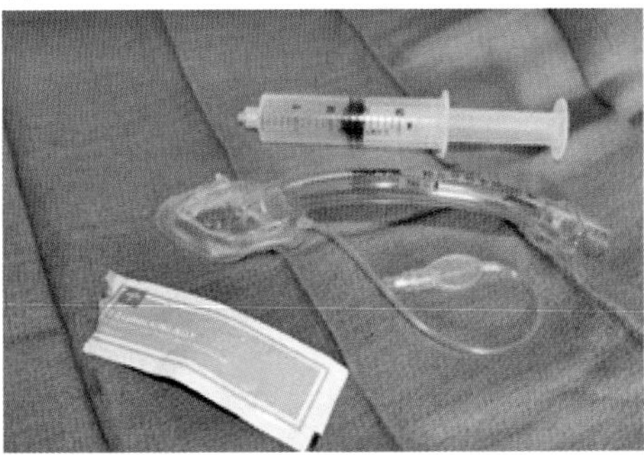

Figure 2.15b Supraglottic airway set up with the cuff partially deflated. The tip is pointing downward to help prevent upward folding on insertion.

- Syringe
- Suction
- Oxygen source and delivery device

Step-by-Step

1. **Prepare the device for use.** Spread lubricant on the posterior aspect of the portion of the supraglottic airway that will be placed into the mouth. The cuff should be either partially inflated (Figure 2.15a) or completely deflated and flattened (Figure 2.15b) at the discretion of the clinician. Both techniques have been used with a good success rate.

   Pearl: A larger supraglottic airway, filled with less air, will provide a better seal than a smaller supraglottic airway filled with more air. The more inflated the cuff, the more rigid the device becomes. A more inflated device is then less able to conform to the curves of the soft tissues in the hypopharynx.

2. **Position the patient in the "sniffing position."** The patient should be placed in the "sniffing" position (see Figure 2.5). Adjustments to positioning can be performed as needed during insertion of the supraglottic airway.

> **Caution!** If there is concern for cervical spine instability, the head should remain in a neutral position during the procedure.

3. **Assess airway reflexes.** Supraglottic airways are placed most easily in patients after the induction of anesthesia owing to the blunting of the glossopharyngeal and laryngeal reflexes that occurs under general anesthesia. If airway reflexes are present, deepening the anesthetic, if possible, is indicated.

   >> Tip on Technique: If the patient is easy to mask or jaw thrust does not elicit a response, then the patient is most likely adequately anesthetized for supraglottic airway insertion.

   Note: Avoid supraglottic airway placement during stage 2 of anesthesia. There is increased risk for coughing, laryngospasm, and bronchospasm if supraglottic airway insertion is attempted during this stage. Also, it may be difficult to create a good seal with the device during stage 2 of anesthesia because of residual muscle tone.

4. **Optimize the patient's mouth opening.** Hold the supraglottic airway in one hand, and with the thumb of the other hand open the patient's mouth by pressing on the bottom incisors or mandible. During insertion, use the nondominant hand to hold the crown of the head and gently press the crown of the head caudally. This will maximize mouth opening.[8]
5. **Insert the device and inflate the balloon.** There are two basic insertion methods, direct and rotational.

   Direct: Hold the device like a pen with the tip of the index finger at the base of the airtube. (Right-handed clinicians usually hold the device in their right hand.) Insert the supraglottic airway into the mouth with the tip pointing toward the hard palate. Advance the supraglottic airway while placing pressure against the hard palate in the direction of the occiput (Figure 2.16). Continue advancing the device until you meet mild resistance and the device is felt to rest in place. The path of the supraglottic airway is often compared with swallowing a bolus of food.

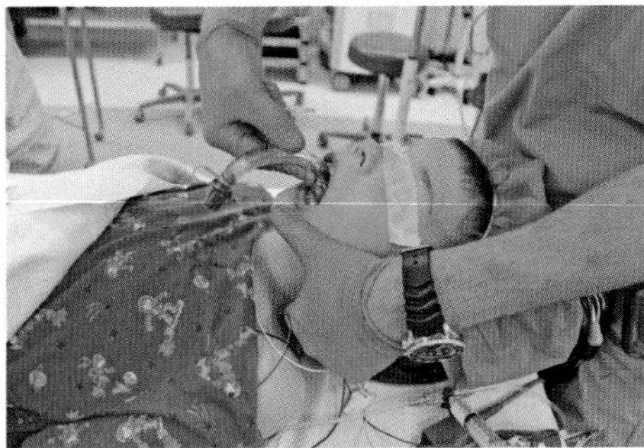

Figure 2.16 Direct insertion of a supraglottic airway.

Rotational: Hold the device upside down, and as you advance the supraglottic airway, corkscrew or rotate it 180 degrees into position (Figure 2.17). This technique can be useful if the tongue is obstructing insertion. Some studies indicate that the rotational technique with a partially inflated cuff has a better insertion success rate in children than the direct technique.[9,10]

After insertion, inflate the balloon until the device is stable. Do not inflate the balloon with more than the maximum recommended amount of air. This amount in milliliters may be written on the device itself or can be found with manufacturer guidelines. The exact amount of inflation is adjusted in the next step.

!! **Potential Complications:** Potential complications during insertion include aspiration of gastric contents, pressure-induced lesions, nerve palsies, trauma to soft tissues, laryngospasm, and causing a sore throat.

>> **Tip on Technique:** If the tongue keeps falling posteriorly during supraglottic airway insertion, use a tongue blade or laryngoscope to lift or press the tongue into the submandibular space.

>> **Tip on Technique:** If supraglottic airway placement is difficult, jaw thrust from an assistant may be helpful. Alternatively, grasp the mandible with one hand and gently lift upward while inserting the supraglottic airway with the other hand.

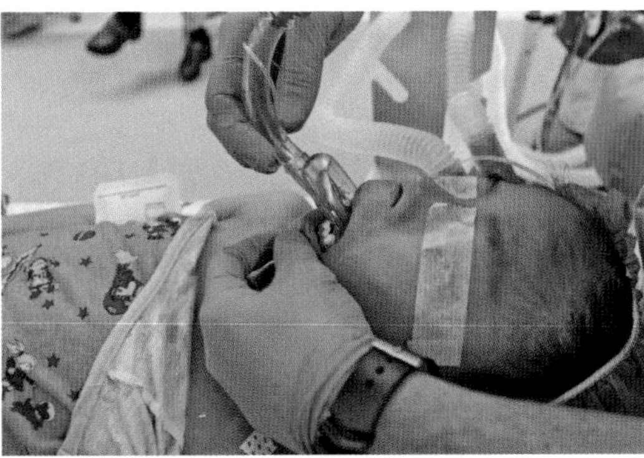

Figure 2.17 Rotational insertion of a supraglottic airway.

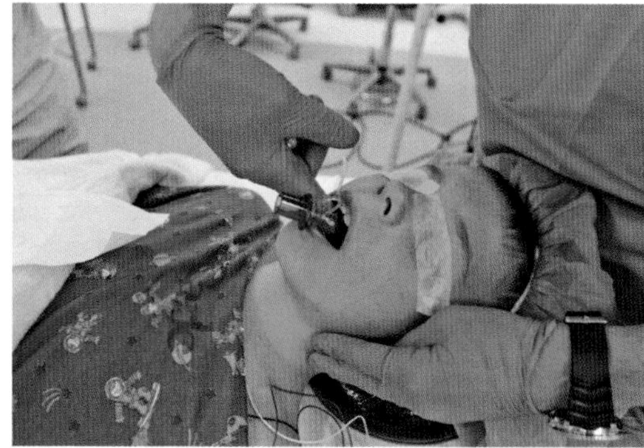

Figure 2.18 Manually checking proper placement of the supraglottic airway.

6. **Ensure proper seal/placement.** After the supraglottic airway is placed, perform a leak test. If gurgling or a large air leak is present with gentle manual ventilation, the supraglottic airway is not seated correctly. Some maneuvers that may resolve incorrect placement include the following: (A) add air to the balloon up to the maximum amount per the manufacturer guidelines (most supraglottic airways have a maximum inflation amount written on the device), (B) remove air from the balloon, (C) manually ensure the tip is not folded upward (Figure 2.18), (D) deepen the anesthetic, and (E) advance the device.

Caution! Overinflation of the cuff should be avoided. A hyperinflated cuff can lead to a sore throat, ischemia of the mucosa, or even nerve injury. Cuff pressures are specified for each device by the manufacturer, and are measured using a specialized device called a manometer.[11,12]

The following are signs of proper supraglottic airway placement:

All devices:

- Adequate chest rise with manual ventilation
- Adequate expired tidal volume
- Absence of sternal retractions during spontaneous ventilation
- Square wave on end-tidal carbon dioxide ($EtCO_2$) tracing
- No audible leak with peak airway pressures of up to 20 mmHg

Second-generation devices:

- Gel displacement test: place 1 mL of water-soluble gel at the proximal end of the esophageal tube. Deliver gentle positive pressure breaths to the patient. If the gel is ejected, a leak is present, and the supraglottic airway should be repositioned. If positive pressure ventilation causes minimal movement of the gel, the supraglottic airway is seated correctly.
- Evidence of gastric contents suctioned from the stomach through a suction tube placed through the gastric port

>> **Tip on Technique:** If placement continues to be tenuous, insert a fiberoptic bronchoscope through the ventilating tube to check the relation of the orifice of the supraglottic airway to the glottis. If there is poor alignment, the amount of cuff inflation and depth of the device can be altered under direct visualization.

>> **Tip on Technique:** Not all supraglottic airways have the same shape. If one type cannot be seated properly, consider switching to a different type before converting to intubation.

7. **Secure the supraglottic airway.** Similar to an endotracheal tube, a supraglottic airway should be secured with tape to prevent inadvertent removal.

Caution! Some devices, such as the classic laryngeal mask airway (LMA), do not have a built-in bite block. It is highly recommended to place a soft bite block in the mouth next to the ventilating tube. If a bite block is absent and the patient bites down, the tube may become totally occluded, leading to an inability to ventilate the patient.

Postoperative Management Considerations

There are no special postoperative management considerations associated with this procedure.

References

1. Valois-Gómez T, Oofuvong M, Auer G, et al. Incidence of difficult bag-mask ventilation in children: a prospective observational study. *Pediatr Anesth.* 2013;23(10):920–926.
2. Bannister FB, Macbeth RG. Direct laryngoscopy and tracheal intubation. *Lancet.* 1944;244(6325):651–654.
3. Butler PJ, Munro HM, Kenny MB. Preoxygenation in children using expired oxygraphy. *Br J Anaesth.* 1996;77(3):333–334.
4. Morrison JE, Collier E, Friesen RH, Logan L. Preoxygenation before laryngoscopy in children: how long is enough? *Paediatr Anaesth.* 1998;8(4):293–298.
5. Bouroche G, Bourgain JL. Pre-oxygenation and general anesthesia: a review. *Minerva Anestesiol.* 2015;81(8):910–920.
6. Santillanes G, Gausche-Hill M. Pediatric airway management. *Emerg Med Clin North Am.* 2008;26(4):961–75.
7. Difficult Airway Society. Unanticipate difficult tracheal intubation—during routine induction of anaesthesia in a child aged 1 to 8 years. Available at: https://www.das.uk.com/files/APA2-UnantDiffTracInt-FINAL.
8. Verghese C, Mena G, Ferson DZ, Brain AIJ. Laryngeal mask airway. In: Hagberg CA, ed. *Benumof and Hagberg's Airway Management.* 3rd ed. Philadelphia: Elsevier Saunders; 2013:443–465.
9. Ghai B, Makkar JK, Bhardwaj N, Wig J. Laryngeal mask airway insertion in children: comparison between rotational, lateral and standard technique. *Pediatr Anesth.* 2008;18(4):308–312.
10. Nakayama S, Osaka Y, Yamashita M. The rotational technique with a partially inflated laryngeal mask airway improves the ease of insertion in children. *Pediatr Anesth.* 2002;12(5):416–419.
11. Wong JGL, Heaney M, Chambers NA, Erb TO, von Ungern-Sternberg BS. Impact of laryngeal mask airway cuff pressures on the incidence of sore throat in children. *Pediatr Anesth.* 2009;19(5):464–469.
12. Schloss, B, Julie R, Joseph D. Tobias. The laryngeal mask in infants and children: what is the cuff pressure? *Int J Pediatr Otorhinolaryngol.* 2012;76(2):284–286.

Chapter 3

Fiberoptic, Video Laryngoscope, and Nasal Airway Procedures

Heather Ballard, Michelle Tsao, and Narasimhan Jagannathan

Fiberoptic Laryngoscopy Fundamentals

Introduction

Flexible fiberoptic laryngoscopy is a means of indirectly visualizing airway structures by threading a fiberoptic scope with a camera at the end of the scope into the airway. The goal of fiberoptic laryngoscopy is endotracheal intubation using a Seldinger technique, whereby an endotracheal tube is guided into the trachea over the fiberoptic bronchoscope. Fiberoptic endotracheal intubation may be performed through the mouth or nose, or through a supraglottic airway (SGA). The use of the fiberoptic scope through an SGA is an especially useful technique in infants who suffer from airway obstruction at rest (e.g., infants with Pierre Robin syndrome).

Clinical Applications

Fiberoptic laryngoscopy is invaluable in performing endotracheal intubation in patients with a known or suspected difficult airway. The small size of the fiberoptic scope, compared with a direct or video laryngoscope, allows it to be used in patients with limited mouth opening. Its flexibility facilitates its use in patients with reduced cervical spine mobility. An fiberoptic intubation can be performed in a patient who is awake, sedated, or under general anesthesia. Keep in mind, however, that an awake intubation can be very difficult in the pediatric population because of limited cooperation. Fiberoptic bronchoscopy can also be used to confirm proper endotracheal tube placement after intubation or to assist with lung isolation techniques (see Chapter 4, Lung Isolation Procedures).

!! **Potential Complications**: Esophageal intubation, laryngospasm, and pharyngeal and laryngeal trauma are all possible complications of fiberoptic laryngoscopy.

Contraindications

Bleeding or secretions in the airway may occlude the small camera on a fiberoptic scope, leading to a partial or complete inability to see airway structures. Fiberoptic laryngoscopy is often more time-consuming than direct or video laryngoscopy. Therefore, its use may not be desired for rapid sequence induction because additional time between induction (with resultant loss of airway reflexes) and securing of the airway will increase the risk for aspiration.

Critical Anatomy

Whether the nose, mouth, or SGA is used as an entrance, the fiberoptic bronchoscope is first advanced through this conduit, then past the base of the tongue and hypopharynx to visualize the epiglottis and vocal cords. The scope is directed at the apex of the vocal cords (located anteriorly) to avoid inadvertent esophageal intubation and is then advanced to immediately above the carina. Visualizing the tracheal rings allows the clinician to further confirm the correct intratracheal location.

Setup

Equipment

- Fiberoptic scope of an appropriate size
- Appropriately sized endotracheal tube
- Silicone spray or gel

Table 3.1 Common Fiberoptic Bronchoscope Sizes

Type of Fiberoptic Bronchoscope	Outer Diameter (mm)	Smallest ETT Inner Diameter (mm)
Olympus LF-P	2.2	3.0 (2.5 is a snug fit, ETT adapter must be removed and scope well lubricated with silicone)
Olympus LF-DP	3.1	4.0 (3.5 if ETT adapter removed)
Olympus LF-V	4.1	5.5
Olympus LF-GP	4.1	5.0
Olympus LF-TP	5.2	6.0
Storz AA1	2.8	3.5
Storz BD2	3.7	4.0
Storz BN1	5.2	5.5

ETT = endotracheal tube.

- Epidural catheter for an intubation in which the patient is awake or spontaneously breathing. For larger bronchoscopes an epidural catheter can be threaded through channel to spray local anesthetic.
- Topical and local anesthetic for intubations in which the patient is awake or spontaneously breathing
- Glycopyrrolate, sedation medications for awake intubations, if desired.

The fiberoptic scope comes in a variety of sizes to accommodate children of all ages. The smallest size currently available has a 2.2-mm outer diameter, which accommodates a 2.5 mm endotracheal tube. Table 3.1 contains common fiberoptic bronchoscope sizes and corresponding endotracheal tube sizes, and Figure 3.1 shows various sizes of fiberoptic bronchoscopes.

>> **Tip on Technique:** Lubricate the scope and the inside of the endotracheal tube with silicone spray or gel; it is very slippery so spray over a garbage can and avoid spilling on the floor! Soaking the endotracheal tube in hot water will also make it more pliable and easier to advance over the bronchoscope.

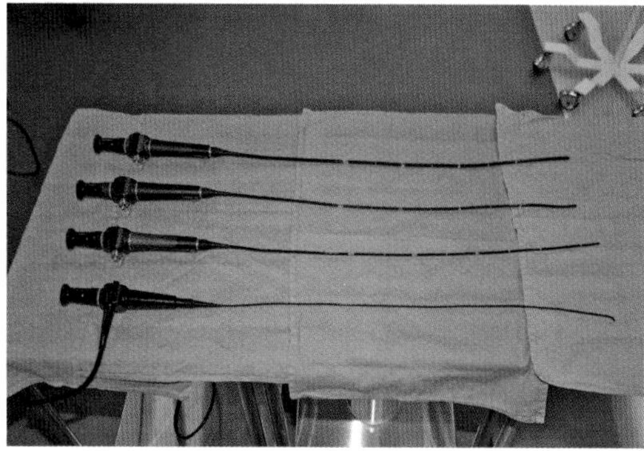

Figure 3.1 Various sizes of fiberoptic bronchoscopes.

>> **Tip on Technique:** On many larger fiberoptic bronchoscopes, a channel exists through which an epidural catheter can be placed. This catheter can be used to spray topical anesthetic as the endotracheal tube is advanced.

Drugs, Dosages, Administration

Glycopyrrolate may be helpful to dry airway secretions to improve the fiberoptic view; however, it is most beneficial when given ahead of time (ideally 15 minutes before the airway procedure). For awake intubations, the desiccation of secretions from glycopyrrolate will subsequently help the local anesthetic to work better because the local anesthetic will then be less likely to be washed away from secretions. For an awake infant, one can inject lidocaine jelly into a pacifier, create several perforations in the pacifier, and then insert the pacifier into the infant's mouth. Judicious administration of ketamine or dexmedetomidine may preserve spontaneous ventilation when mask induction with a volatile anesthetic is contraindicated. Topical local anesthetic can be applied by manual application, atomizer and/or nebulizer as appropriate.

Note: If not already given, consider an anticholinergic to prevent reflex bradycardia from vagal stimulation or hypoxemia during induction and intubation, especially in young infants.

> **WARNING!!** When using a local anesthetic, be vigilant to not exceed the maximum allowable dose. Carefully calculate the total dose to avoid local anesthetic systemic toxicity (LAST). Even at submaximal doses, dysrhythmias and toxicity can occur. Use the local anesthetic concentration that allows a sufficient volume to be given (e.g., lidocaine 1% for infants). Information on Local Anesthetic Systemic Toxicity Treatment is provided in Chapter 15.

Fiberoptic Laryngoscopy under General Anesthesia

Readers should refer to the previous Fiberoptic Laryngoscopy Fundamentals section for an overview of fiberoptic laryngoscopy, including clinical applications, contraindications, critical anatomy, equipment, and drugs used in the procedure.

Step-by-Step

1. **Position the patient.** Position the patient supine, with the head of the bed angled up slightly. Neck extension is helpful in aligning the axes for an optimized view of the vocal cords.

> **Caution!** In infants with upper airway obstruction at rest, the supine position may lead to significant hypoxia. Consider maintaining infants with upper airway obstruction at rest in the prone position until an SGA can be placed to relieve the airway obstruction.

>> **Tip on Technique:** Performing bronchoscopy from a standing position in front of the patient may be easier than standing at the head of the bed (e.g., if the patient is sitting upright). This position may be especially suitable in conditions in which the airway is compressed in the supine position (e.g., a patient with an anterior mediastinal mass).

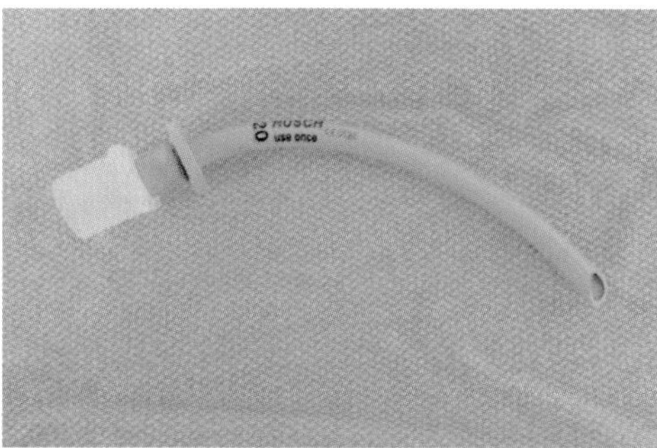

Figure 3.2 An endotracheal tube connector attached to a nasal trumpet.

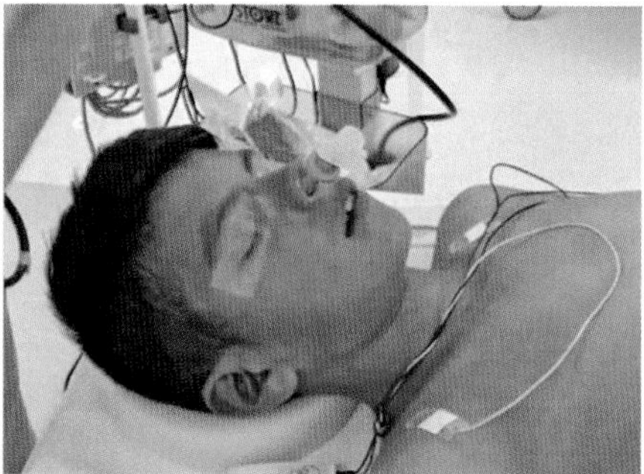

Figure 3.3 An endotracheal tube connector attached to a nasal trumpet, in situ.

2. **Preoxygenate the patient.** Preoxygenate when possible, then induce general anesthesia. During the fiberoptic intubation itself, if desired, supplemental oxygen can be delivered through a nasal cannula, or through a nasal trumpet that has been altered by attaching an endotracheal tube connector, then attaching the anesthesia circuit to this endotracheal tube connector to deliver oxygen, continuous positive airway pressure, and/or volatile anesthetics (Figures 3.2, 3.3, and 3.4).
3. **Prepare the airway for the fiberoptic bronchoscope.** Airway maneuvers can ease placement of the bronchoscope. A jaw thrust can be used to increase the amount of pharyngeal and laryngeal space. If intubating orally, for children older than 12 years and adults, the tongue can be displaced by a specialized oral airway, such as the Ovassapian oral airway, for fiberoptic intubation. Care must be taken, and a jaw lift is suggested when placing the Ovassapian oral airway to avoid scraping the hard palate during placement. A suction catheter can be applied to the tip of the tongue to draw the tongue out of the mouth, or the tongue can be gently grasped with gauze using either your fingers or a Magill forceps (Figure 3.5).

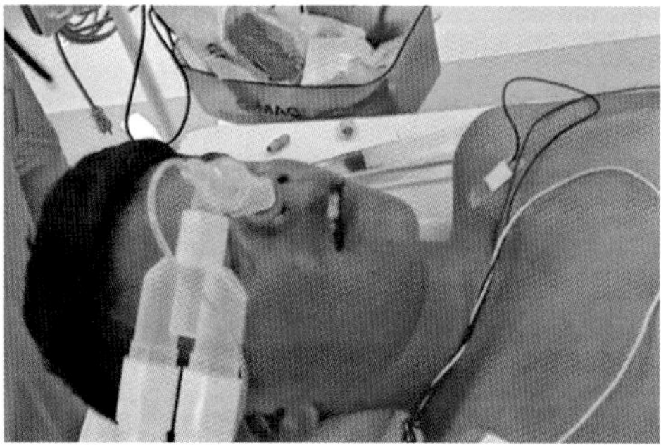

Figure 3.4 An endotracheal tube connector attached to a nasal trumpet attached to the anesthesia machine circuit, in situ.

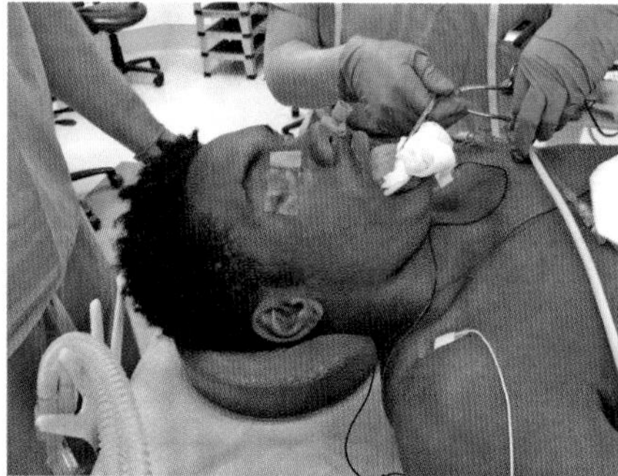

Figure 3.5 Magill forceps and gauze used to safely hold the tongue out of the way during a fiberoptic intubation.

>> **Tip on Technique:** In young children and infants, the tight curvature of the oropharynx and larynx may make directing the flexible bronchoscope challenging. Use of an additional laryngoscope, video laryngoscope, or SGA conduit with the fiberoptic bronchoscope can help bring the mouth and the pharyngeal and tracheal axes into closer alignment. Additionally, extension of the neck, anterior laryngeal pressure, and jaw thrust can be helpful.

4. **Advance the fiberoptic bronchoscope.** Advance the flexible bronchoscope into the airway, guiding it to the vocal cords (Figure 3.6). (If the intubation is being performed "awake" or with the patient spontaneously breathing, spray local anesthetic onto the vocal cords, then wait at least 5–10 seconds for the local anesthetic to take effect before advancing the bronchoscope.)
5. **Advance the fiberoptic bronchoscope past the vocal cords.** Advance the fiberoptic scope until endotracheal placement is verified by visualization of the carina and tracheal rings (Figure 3.7).

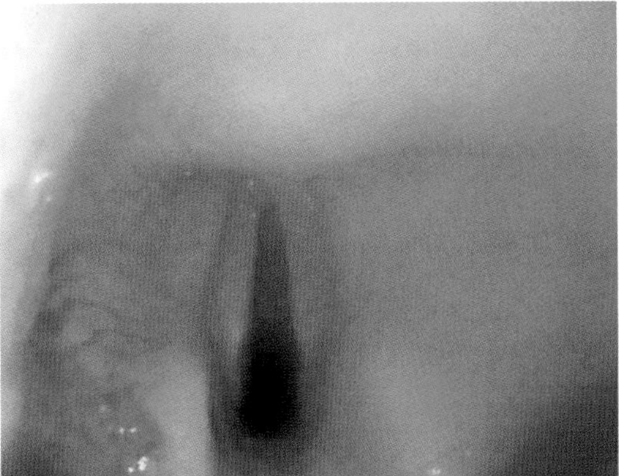

Figure 3.6 View of the vocal cords with a fiberoptic bronchoscope.

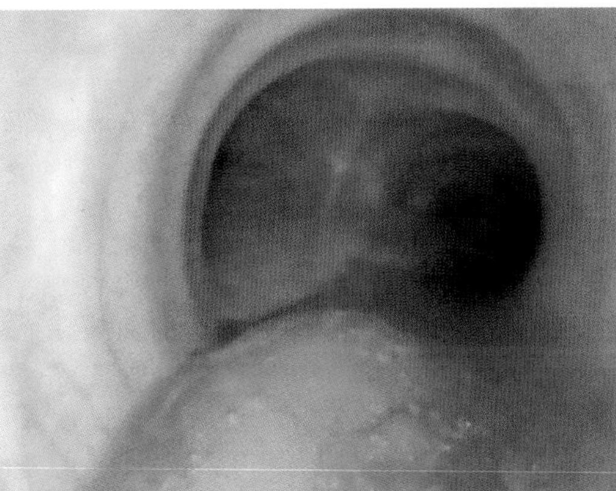

Figure 3.7 Tracheal rings, anteriorly, and the carina as the trachea divides into the left and right main bronchi.

6. **Advance the endotracheal tube into trachea.** Turn the endotracheal tube so that the numbers face away from you, which will allow for ideal positioning of the bevel of the endotracheal tube to pass easily through the glottis. Advance the endotracheal tube off of the fiberoptic scope while gently rotating the endotracheal tube in a counterclockwise direction and keeping your scope immobile. Once you see the endotracheal tube appear at the tip of the scope, remove the scope while leaving the endotracheal tube in place. The proper position for your endotracheal tube can be confirmed by seeing the carina with your fiberoptic bronchoscope (Figure 3.8). The tube position can also be confirmed by auscultating bilateral breath sounds, capnography, and lung ultrasound if needed.

   >> **Tip on Technique:** If the endotracheal tube does not advance easily, it may have become "stuck" on the arytenoid cartilage. Rather than forcefully advancing the endotracheal tube and risking airway injury, try withdrawing a few centimeters and rotating the tube counterclockwise 90 to 180 degrees before readvancing. This rotates the bevel of the endotracheal tube away from the arytenoid cartilage.

Postoperative Management Considerations

There are no special postoperative management considerations associated with this procedure.

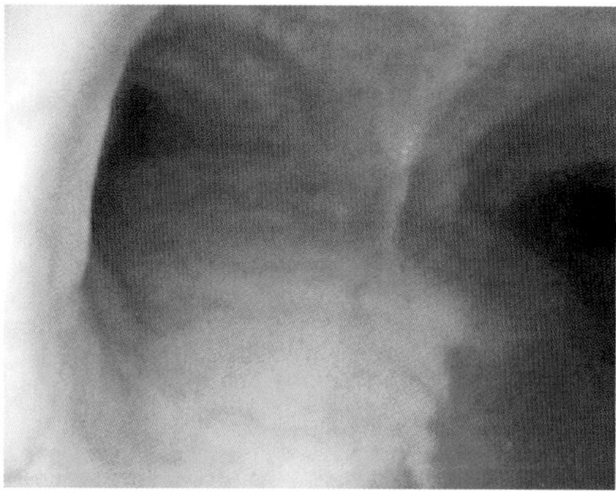

Figure 3.8 Carina as seen through a fiberoptic bronchoscope.

Fiberoptic Laryngoscopy through a Supraglottic Airway under General Anesthesia

Step-by-Step

The following steps are in addition to steps listed previously in the 'Fiberoptic Laryngoscopy under General Anesthesia' section.

1. **Place the SGA and advance the endotracheal tube.** Before the procedure begins, remove the airway connector from the endotracheal tube and keep it in a readily accessible place (e.g. tape it to the anesthesia machine). Next, prepare the fiberoptic bronchoscope by

threading this endotracheal tube over the scope. Place the SGA with your usual technique (see Chapter 2, Mask Ventilation, Direct Laryngoscopy, and Supraglottic Airway Placement Procedures). Advance the flexible bronchoscope through the SGA (Figure 3.9). Advance the ETT over the flexible bronchoscope into the trachea. Reattach the airway connector to the endotracheal tube. Confirm endotracheal tube placement using the technique described in the previous section. Ventilate the patient through the ETT.

>> **Tip on Technique:** SGA placement can affect the laryngeal view. When the SGA is placed correctly, it can fix the epiglottis out of the way to allow a clear path to the vocal cords. (Figures 3.10a–c) show views of the vocal cords as the SGA is being correctly placed. Figure 3.10d shows the SGA on its way to being incorrectly placed, and Figure 3.10e shows the epiglottis in a downward facing position, blocking the vocal cords. If the epiglottis is downfolded, one can improve the laryngeal view by performing a jaw thrust, applying anterior laryngeal pressure, or by gently withdrawing and then advancing the SGA under visualization with the fiberoptic bronchoscope.

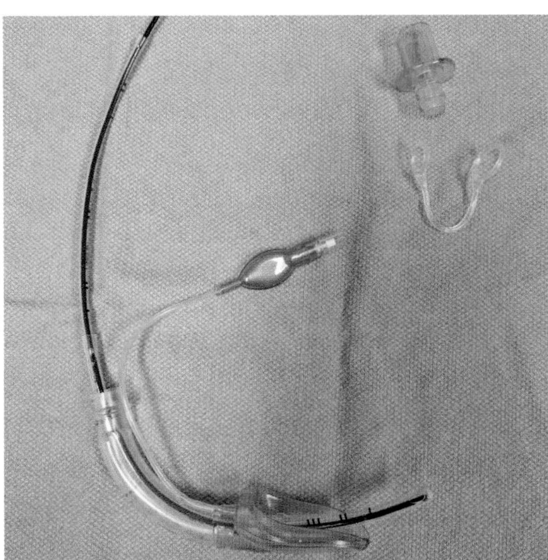

Figure 3.9 The fiberoptic bronchoscope with the endotracheal tube loaded through the supraglottic airway. Note that the supraglottic airway circuit connector has been removed to allow advancement of the endotracheal tube.

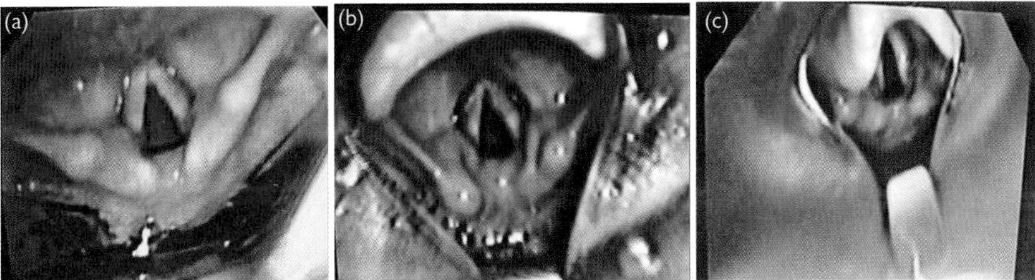

Figure 3.10a–c Views of vocal cords as the supraglottic airway is being placed.

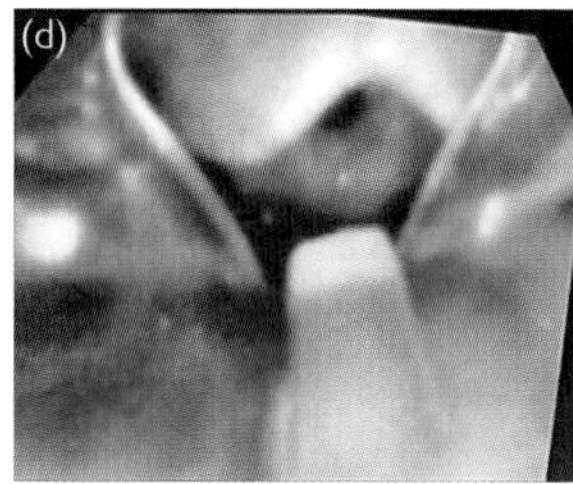

Figure 3.10d The supraglottic airway on its way to being incorrectly placed.

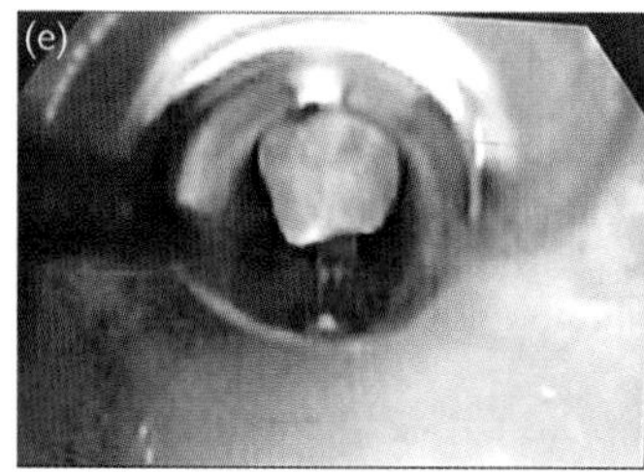

Figure 3.10e Supraglottic airway placed incorrectly forcing the epiglottis into a downward-facing position.

Pearl: The air-Q SGA (Cookgas, St. Louis, MO) is designed as an "intubating" SGA to facilitate tracheal intubation because it has a wider, shorter inner lumen with a detachable circuit connector. If the connector is not removed, the endotracheal tube will NOT advance through the air-Q SGA.

2. **Remove the SGA.** After the endotracheal tube is advanced through the SGA and into the trachea, and adequacy of placement and ventilation is confirmed (see earlier), remove the SGA, if desired. There are two main techniques for removing the SGA: the two-endotracheal tube technique (Figures 3.11a and 3.11b) and the pusher method (Figure 3.12). Both these methods use the Seldinger technique, in which the SGA is withdrawn from the pharynx by using the additional endotracheal tube or pusher as a conduit. The endotracheal tube circuit connector must be taken off before removing the SGA because the endotracheal tube circuit connector will not fit through the SGA. If the SGA is left in place for more than a short period of time, the risk for airway swelling may be increased.

(a)

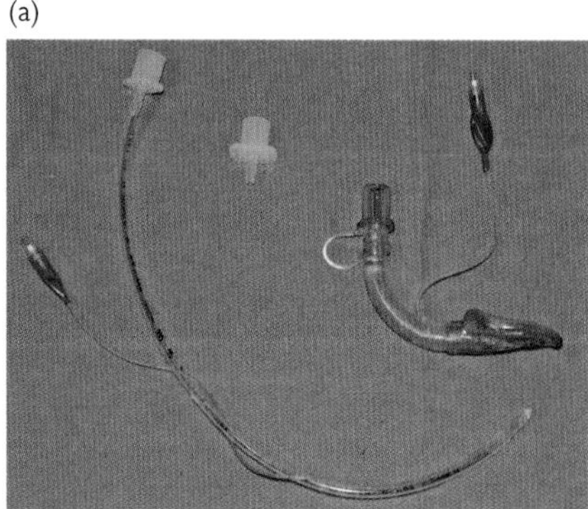

Figure 3.11a The two–endotracheal tube technique in which two endotracheal tubes are joined together to facilitate removal of the supraglottic airway. The second endotracheal tube acts as a "pusher" to help advance the desired endotracheal tube into position.

(b)

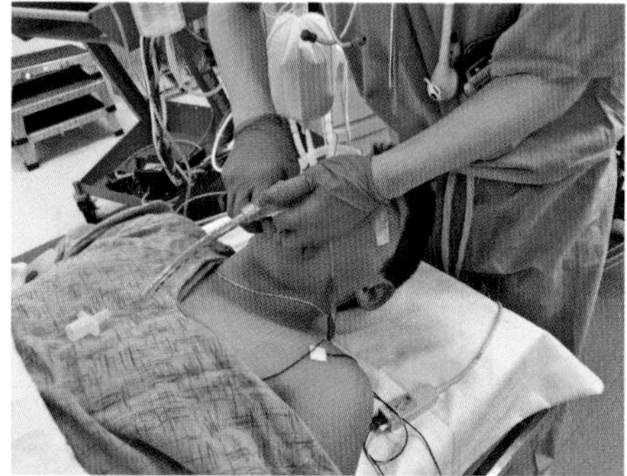

Figure 3.11b The second endotracheal tube being pushed through the supraglottic airway by the first endotracheal tube. The first endotracheal tube extends only a few centimeters past the supraglottic airway.

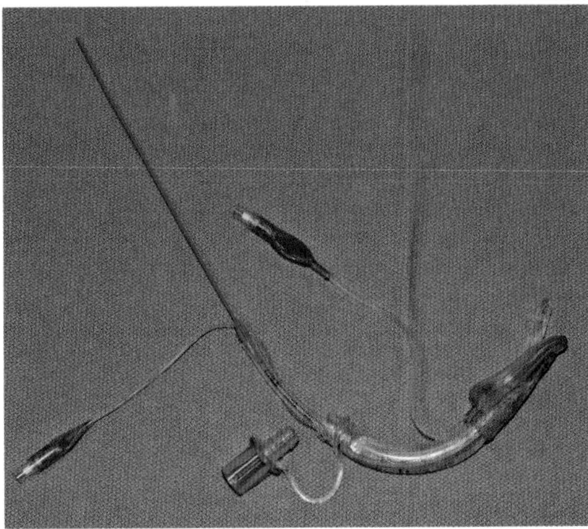

Figure 3.12 The pusher inserted into the top of the endotracheal tube and the endotracheal tube inserted into the supraglottic airway.

>> **Tip on Technique:** All airway equipment (SGA, endotracheal tube, bronchoscope) should be lubricated before induction. Ideally, the second "pusher" endotracheal tube should not have a cuff, for ease of movement. Keep a tight grip on the endotracheal tube so that it does not dislodge while removing the SGA. In patients with limited cardiopulmonary reserve, continuous oxygenation can be performed by temporarily attaching the circuit to the pusher endotracheal tube during SGA removal (when that technique is used).

3. **Salvage the pilot balloon.** One of the most challenging parts of advancing the endotracheal tube is passing the pilot balloon through the SGA opening. If the pilot balloon is inadvertently cut during the process, there are a few techniques you can employ to reinflate the endotracheal tube cuff. A 22-gauge angiocatheter (Figure 3.13) or epidural catheter clip (Figure 3.14) can be attached to the pilot balloon tubing. Using the Luer-Lok™ connection, a syringe can be used to reinflate the endotracheal tube cuff. An insidious cuff leak may still occur, so these techniques should be a temporizing measure only.

Note: A blue and black epidural catheter connector should not be used because it is NOT compatible with the pilot balloon tubing.

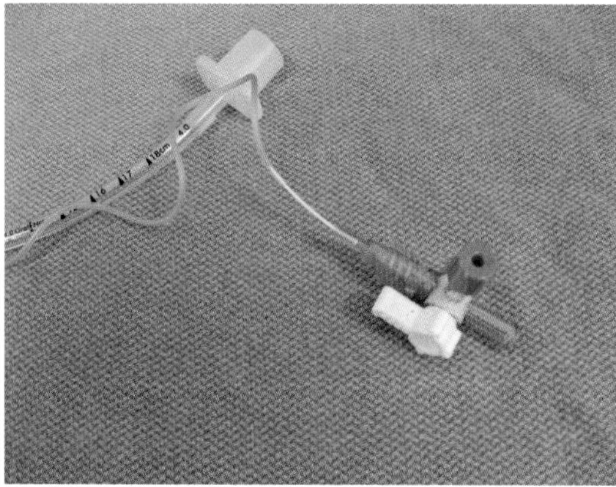

Figure 3.13 A 22-gauge Angiocath inserted into the pilot balloon tubing.

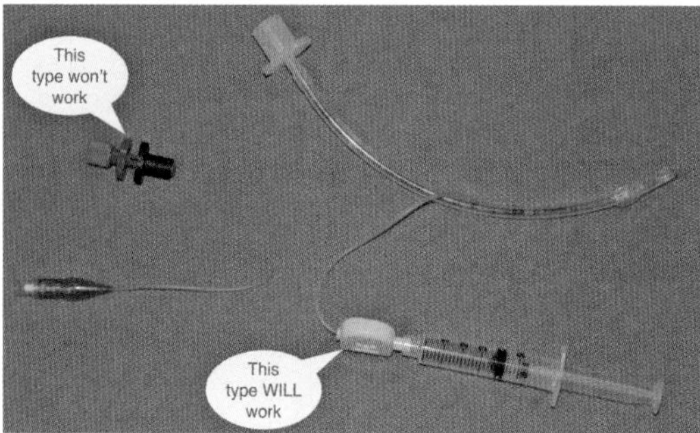

Figure 3.14 An epidural catheter clip connected to the pilot balloon tubing.

Awake Fiberoptic Laryngoscopy

Additional Contraindications

An awake fiberoptic laryngoscopy is rarely performed in children but has been described in the literature and is sometimes performed in a newborn or in a teenager with a very difficult airway. It is contraindicated if the patient is uncooperative or if the patient or parent refuses the procedure.

Step-by-Step

The following steps are in addition to steps listed previously in the 'Fiberoptic Laryngoscopy under General Anesthesia' section.

1. **Administer glycopyrrolate.** Glycopyrrolate should be administered at least 15 minutes before topicalization is started. This will greatly assist with drying secretions, so that the local anesthetic will "stick" better. If glycopyrrolate is contraindicated, dexmedetomidine may be considered to dry secretions.
2. **Preoxygenate and topicalize the patient.** Preoxygenate and administer sedative doses of medications for the procedure if appropriate. During the fiberoptic intubation itself, if

desired, supplemental oxygen can be delivered through a nasal cannula. When topicalizing, be very careful to stay under the maximum dose of local anesthetic to decrease the possibility of local anesthetic systemic toxicity (LAST; see Chapter 15, Local Anesthetic Systemic Toxicity)

>> **Tip on Technique:** If sedation is administered for an awake intubation, it is recommended to only use one or two agents to avoid polypharmacy and resultant unpredictable effects. One popular regimen for older children and teenagers is to administer small amounts of midazolam alternating with fentanyl, until conditions are achieved in which the patient is sleepy but breathing well spontaneously and opening his or her eyes to simulation. An advantage to this regimen is the fact that midazolam may help with amnesia and fentanyl helps abate the cough reflex. If midazolam and fentanyl are used for this purpose, have naloxone and flumazenil readily available. Another popular regimen for an awake sedated intubation is to use remifentanil and dexmedetomidine infusions.

3. **Anesthetize the vocal cords and place the endotracheal tube through the glottis.** Once a view of the glottis is achieved, reflexes must be abated by either (1) spraying local anesthetic onto the vocal cords, then waiting 5 to 10 seconds for the local anesthetic to take effect; or (2) administering induction agents with or without a muscle relaxant. Administering induction agents with or without a muscle relaxant has the advantage of a decreased risk for laryngospasm and bronchospasm; however, it also increases the risk for a potential "cannot intubate, cannot ventilate" situation. Additionally, there remains a risk for aspiration from the time when these induction medications are administered until the airway is secured. If uncertain, err on the side of preserving spontaneous ventilation until the airway is secured. Next, place the endotracheal tube through the vocal cords and confirm position as described previously.
4. **Induce general anesthesia.** When the endotracheal tube position is confirmed, general anesthesia (or intensive care unit sedation) should be started.

>> **Tip on Technique:** Inducing general anesthesia with 8 atm% sevoflurane (instead of propofol) after the endotracheal tube position is confirmed will initially keep the patient breathing spontaneously and therefore may be a safer anesthetic until the endotracheal tube is secured and its position confirmed. Do not forget to decrease the sevoflurane level after the patient is asleep and before manually or mechanically ventilating the patient!

Video Laryngoscopy

Introduction

Video laryngoscopy employs a laryngoscope with a camera at the end of the blade to enable the user to indirectly visualize airway structures. Direct laryngoscopy requires being able to see along the blade directly to the glottic opening. The angle of viewing will be 15 degrees. A video laryngoscope typically has a blade with an angle greater than 15 degrees, with a camera at the inflection point giving a view of the larynx that is more anterior, to improve glottic views without requiring a complete alignment of the oral, pharyngeal, and tracheal axes.

Clinical Applications

Video laryngoscopy is useful as a tool for endotracheal intubation in difficult airway management. This may be especially true in patients with limited cervical spine mobility because less neck extension may be required. It is also useful in teaching airway management because the video screen allows for multiple observers at the same time. The video laryngoscope view is less susceptible to degradation from secretions or blood in the airway than the fiberoptic bronchoscope technique. Because this technique typically takes less time than fiberoptic laryngoscopy, it can be used during a rapid-sequence induction for experienced practitioners.

Contraindications

The use of video laryngoscopy is limited in children who have restricted mouth openings.

Critical Anatomy

The video laryngoscope blade is placed carefully in the back of the mouth, sweeping the tongue to the side, with direct vision to avoid a pharyngeal laceration. When the blade is at the tongue base, the blade is placed in the vallecula and lifted (with either a direct or a video screen view) to view the glottic structures.

Setup

Equipment

- Appropriate video laryngoscope blades
- Appropriately sized endotracheal tube

  Available C-MAC© (Karl Storz GmbH & Co. KG, Tuttlingen, Germany) and GlideScope® (Verathon, Bothell, WA) blade sizes (Figures 3.15 and 3.16) are comparable to conventional Miller and Macintosh blades (Table 3.2).

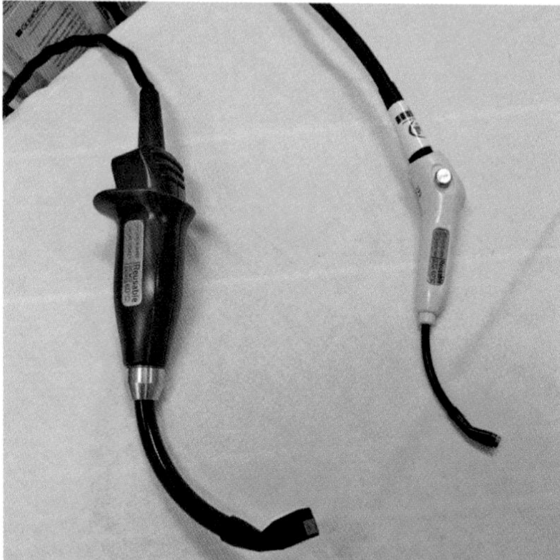

Figure 3.15 Pediatric and adult batons for the GlideScope video laryngoscope. GlideScope manufacturers four pediatric blades (GVL 0, 1, 2, 2.5) and two adult blades (GVL 3, 4) to cover these batons.

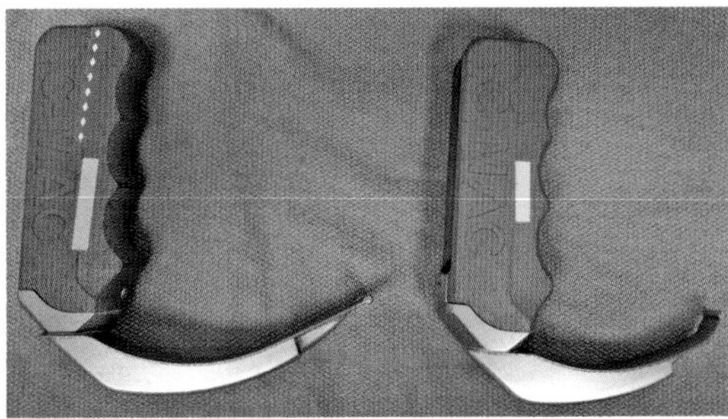

Figure 3.16 C-MAC pediatric blades.

Table 3.2 **C-MAC and GlideScope Sizes**

Patient Size	C-MAC	GlideScope
Neonate	MIL0, MAC0	GVL0
Infant	MIL1	GVL1
Small Child	MIL1, MAC2	GVL2
Large Child	MAC2, MAC3	GVL2.5
Adult	MAC3, MAC4	GVL3, GVL4

>> **Tip on Technique:** A stylet is almost always necessary when using a video laryngoscope. The GlideScope manufacturer, because of the unique shape of the blade, has designed a rigid stylet for use with this device. This stylet, however, may not be advantageous because it becomes deformed from its original shape with repeated sterilizations. Many practitioners instead shape a conventional stylet to match the curvature of the GlideScope blade to improve success. Another option is to use the Cohn technique (created by Stephen Cohn) with a video laryngoscope, which involves bending a conventional styletted endotracheal tube into a shape resembling a three-dimensional question mark (Figures 3.17, 3.18, and 3.19). The Cohn technique provides the advantage of a more manipulatable endotracheal tube, where the distal end will not bump into the patient when it is inserted at various angles.

Pearl: Intubation with a C-MAC is comparable to direct laryngoscopy in terms of the view attained and the curvature of the stylet. An intubation with the GlideScope can be more challenging because the camera is mounted further anterior compared with a C-MAC. Therefore, while the glottic view appears better, advancement of the tube into the trachea is more challenging and requires a greater curvature of the endotracheal tube stylet.

Drugs, Dosages, Administration

Drugs are the same as those used during conventional direct laryngoscopy; there are no special considerations.

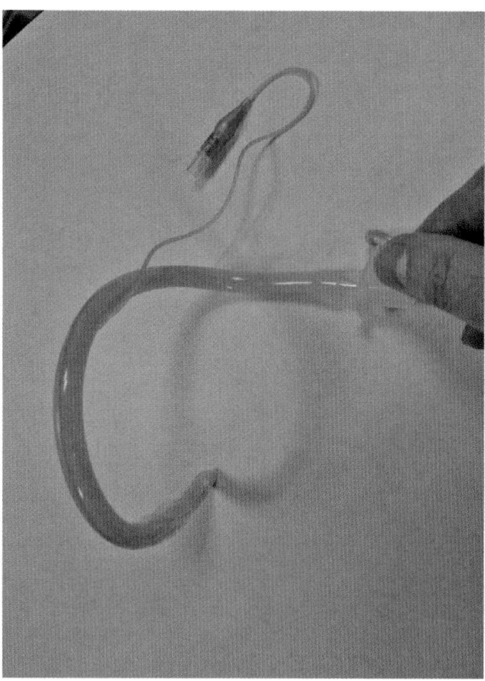

Figure 3.17 Step 1 of forming a styletted endotracheal tube into the three-dimensional question mark shape for the Cohn technique.

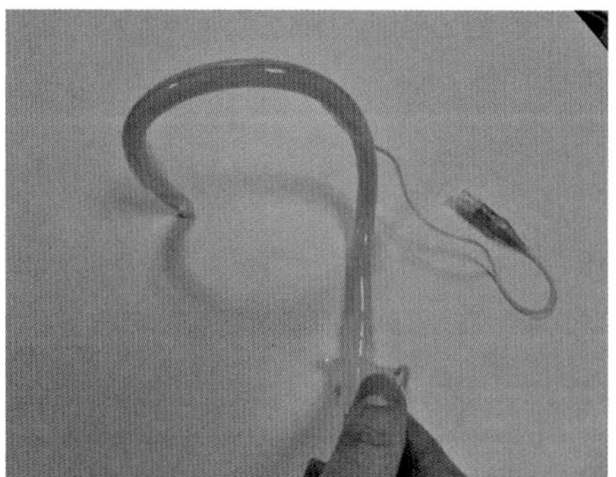

Figure 3.18 Step 2 of forming a styletted endotracheal tube into the three-dimensional question mark shape for the Cohn technique.

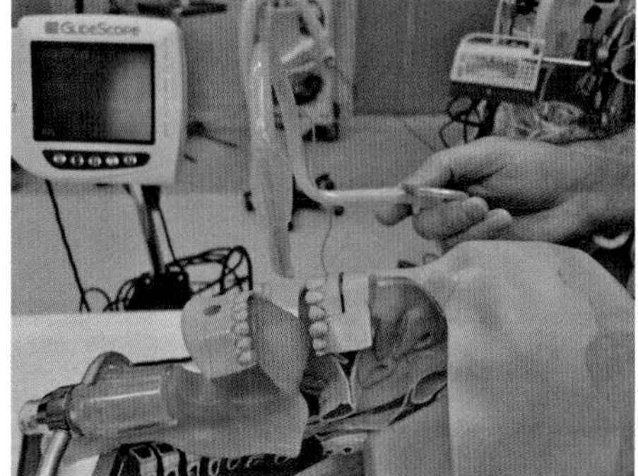

Figure 3.19 Three-dimensional question mark–shaped styletted endotracheal tube inserted into the mouth.

Step-by-Step

1. **Position the patient.** Position the patient supine, with the head of the bed angled up slightly. Similar to direct laryngoscopy, neck extension is helpful in aligning the axes for an optimized view of the vocal cords. Jaw thrust may be useful, especially in patients with macroglossia, small submandibular spaces, or copious pharyngeal tissue (e.g., mucopolysaccharide disorders).

> **Caution!** In infants with upper airway obstruction at rest, the supine position may lead to significant hypoxia. Consider maintaining infants with upper airway obstruction at rest in the prone position until an SGA can be placed to relieve the airway obstruction.

2. **Preoxygenate the patient.** Preoxygenate the patient fully and then induce general anesthesia.
3. **Insert the video laryngoscope blade.** Open the mouth under direct vision, similarly to conventional laryngoscopy. Insert the video laryngoscope into the oral cavity. Because the C-MAC can be used for both direct and video laryngoscopy, the tongue can be swept to the left to ensure there is enough room for the endotracheal tube (Figures 3.20 and 3.21).

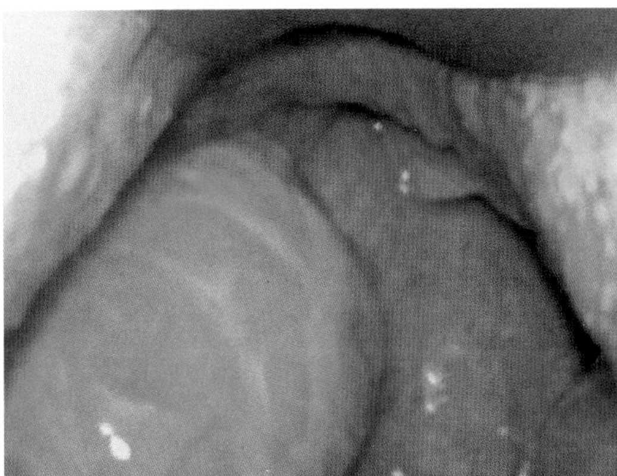

Figure 3.20 Illustration of a video laryngoscope blade that has not been inserted deeply enough. The tongue is seen herniating over the right side of the blade. Incidentally, this patient also has large tonsils.

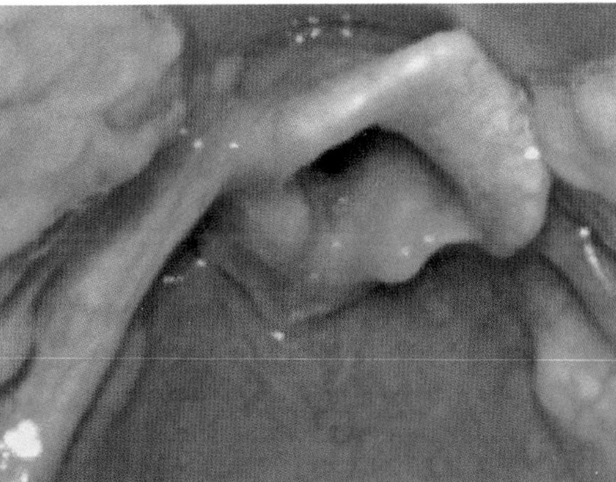

Figure 3.21 A grade III view that may be improved with inserting the blade more firmly into the vallecula, upward lift of the blade, and/or cricoid pressure.

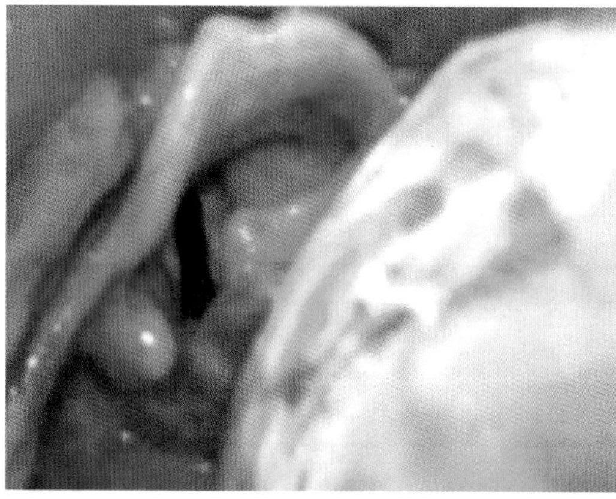

Figure 3.22 The endotracheal tube advanced into view. The grade III view in Figure 3.21 is improved to a grade II view here, with small adjustments in laryngoscope positioning.

Caution! Be vigilant when placing the blade in the mouth, especially with the sharper curvature of the GlideScope blade. Soft tissue injury can occur. **Do NOT look at the video screen** before the blade is completely in the mouth.

>> **Tip on Technique:** Some practitioners prefer to insert the GlideScope into the mouth with the blade rotated 90 degrees. This technique bypasses the acute angle needed for blade insertion, avoids the handle pressing on the patient's chest, and can be especially helpful if the patient has a short neck or large chest.

4. **Expose the glottis.** Obtain your view of the vocal cords. This can be accomplished by placing the tip of the laryngoscope blade either in the vallecula or under the epiglottis. Placing the blade in the vallecula may enable easier passage of the endotracheal tube because of limited space for manipulation. Lifting the laryngoscope blade upward or applying cricoid pressure, using the video screen as a guide, may also improve the view (Figure 3.22).
5. **Insert the endotracheal tube into the pharynx.** Gently place the endotracheal tube in the mouth while looking down into the mouth to avoid dissecting the palate or tonsils with the endotracheal tube during insertion. Advance the endotracheal tube to the posterior pharynx until it can be visualized by the video laryngoscope camera.
6. **Pass the endotracheal tube into the trachea.** Advance the endotracheal tube through the vocal cords while watching the video laryngoscope screen. When the endotracheal tube is at the level of the arytenoids, some practitioners prefer to slightly withdraw the stylet. Next, slide the endotracheal tube off of the stylet past the glottic opening. The endotracheal tube's passage into the trachea is obstructed by the arytenoid cartilage in Figure 3.23. To successfully pass the endotracheal tube through the vocal cords, you may need to adjust the laryngoscope by advancing or withdrawing the blade slightly, or decreasing or gently increasing the upward force on the laryngoscope. You may also need to adjust the stylet curvature to successfully pass the endotracheal tube. Figure 3.24 shows the endotracheal tube in the correct position.

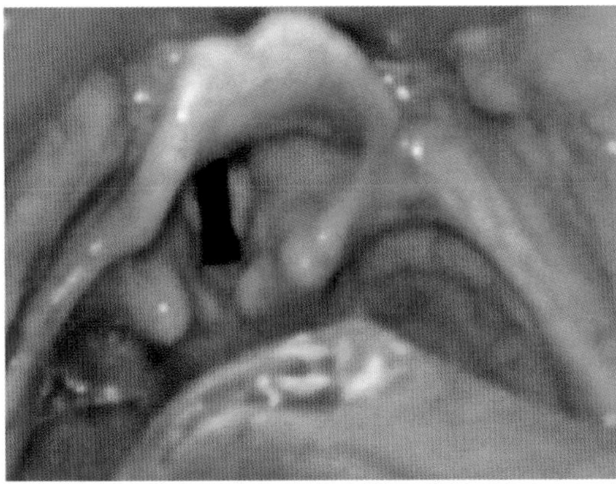

Figure 3.23 Arytenoid cartilage obstructing the endotracheal tube's passage into the trachea.

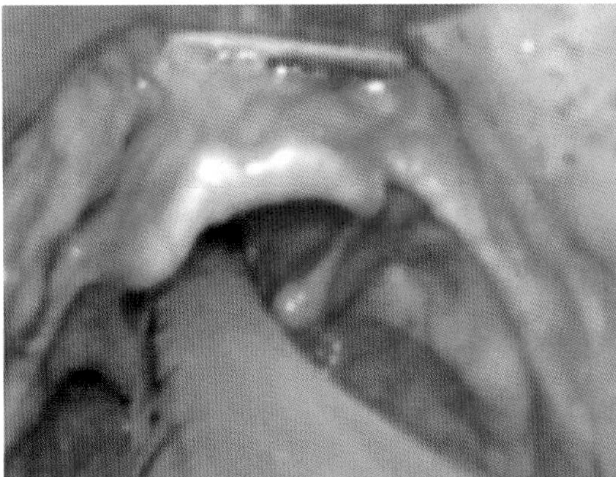

Figure 3.24 Correct position of the endotracheal tube.

>> **Tip on Technique:** If you are able to see the vocal cords well, but it is difficult to achieve endotracheal tube passage through the vocal cords, you may need to decrease the upward force on the laryngoscope (e.g., relax your view slightly), which will lead to a poorer view of the vocal cords but a straighter angle of the larynx for endotracheal tube passage. With this "relaxed" view, move the endotracheal tube forward toward and through the vocal cords, then gently increase the upward force on the laryngoscope blade again, to achieve your original view of the vocal cords and to confirm that the endotracheal tube has passed through the vocal cords.

>> **Tip on Technique:** If your endotracheal tube tip is at the level of the vocal cords, but it is difficult to pass the endotracheal tube through the glottis, it may be necessary to rotate the endotracheal tube in a twisting counterclockwise "corkscrew" motion to help it pass through the vocal cords.

Postoperative Management Considerations

There are no special postoperative management considerations associated with this procedure.

Nasotracheal Intubation

Introduction

Nasotracheal intubation is the placement of an endotracheal tube through the nares into the trachea. It can be performed with direct laryngoscopy and a Magill forceps, with a fiberoptic bronchoscope, or with no view of the vocal cords, also known as a "blind" intubation. Intubation under direct visualization is the standard of care, and blind nasotracheal intubation should be performed ONLY under extenuating circumstances where direct visualization is unachievable.

Clinical Applications

Nasotracheal intubation is commonly used in oropharyngeal surgery (plastics, oromaxillofacial, dental) to keep the endotracheal tube away from the surgical site. It is also used for patient comfort when prolonged postoperative intubation is expected or when oropharyngeal intubation is unsuccessful or cannot be attempted.

Contraindications

Placing an endotracheal tube into the nose can result in severe epistaxis, so nasal instrumentation should be avoided in patients with coagulopathy or increased central venous pressure (e.g., after a Glenn or Fontan procedure, superior vena cava syndrome, liver or heart disease). The nasal route should not be used in patients with skull base fractures because of the risk for trauma to surrounding structures and risk for entry of the endotracheal tube into the brain. Additionally, nasal instrumentation should be avoided after a cleft palate repair, even if the repair was completed many years ago, because nasal instrumentation will destroy the surgical repair.

WARNING!! If the endotracheal tube does not pass easily through the nose, do not apply force because doing so can result in severe epistaxis or damage to nasopharyngeal structures.

>> **Tip on Technique:** If a nasal route is required by the surgical team, but relative contraindications exist, or if there is resistance to passing the tube, if the surgical team has expertise with the nasopharynx (e.g., otolaryngologists, oral surgeons), consider having the surgical team pass the tube from the nose into the hypopharynx, with the anesthesiology team taking over for the passage of the tube from the hypopharynx through the vocal cords and into the trachea. If this is decided before the patient is brought into the operating room, the surgical team can add this part of the procedure to the surgical consent.

Critical Anatomy

The endotracheal tube is gently guided into the nares, past the nasopharynx. Take care as large inferior turbinates or adenoid tissue can obstruct passage of the endotracheal tube through the nasal passageway. Pharyngeal and laryngeal anatomy was described previously in the 'Fiberoptic Laryngoscopy Fundamentals' section.

Setup

Equipment

- A nasal vasoconstrictor, such as oxymetazoline
- Nasal trumpets
- Surgical lubricant
- Magill forceps
- A fiberoptic bronchoscope
- Warmed fluid bottles

>> **Tip on Technique:** Placing the endotracheal tube in hot saline or water makes it more pliable and eases passage through the naris.

>> **Tip on Technique:** Either an oral endotracheal tube or a nasal RAE tube can be used for nasal intubation. Nasal RAE tubes are longer and are particularly useful if the lower half of the face is in the operative field because the pre-formed bend directs the distal end of the endotracheal tube over the forehead.

Caution! In patients requiring a smaller diameter endotracheal tube than otherwise indicated (e.g., a patient with subglottic stenosis), the smaller tube may not be long enough to reach the trachea from the nasal cavity. Additionally, if using a smaller diameter nasal RAE tube, the pre-formed bend may not be in the correct position.

Pearl: It may be more difficult to manipulate the fiberoptic bronchoscope when using a nasal RAE tube because of the tube's longer length compared with a traditional endotracheal tube.

Drugs, Dosages, Administration

Administer oxymetazoline spray or phenylephrine spray to vasoconstrict nasal blood vessels and minimize the risk for bleeding. Administer topical local anesthetic (e.g. lidocaine, benzocaine, or prilocaine) if performing an awake intubation. Local anesthetics can be applied by manual application, atomizer, and/or nebulizer as appropriate.

WARNING!! When using a local anesthetic, be vigilant that one does not exceed the maximum allowable dose. Carefully calculate the total dose to decrease the possibility of local anesthetic systemic toxicity (LAST). Information on Local Anesthetic Systemic Toxicity Treatment is provided in Chapter 15. Additionally, even at submaximal doses, dysrhythmias can occur.

Note: Consider an anticholinergic to prevent reflex bradycardia from vagal stimulation or hypoxemia, especially in young infants.

>> **Tip on Technique:** Vasoconstrictors can be placed on cotton applicators or mixed with surgical lube or lidocaine jelly to reduce the total amount used. This is especially important in infants and small children.

!! **Potential Complications:** Phenylephrine nasal spray is typically supplied as a 0.25% formulation, equal to 2.5 mg/mL. Systemic absorption of excessive phenylephrine can cause severe hypertension, leading to cardiac side effects and potential stroke.

Step-by-Step

1. **Position the patient.** There are no special considerations regarding patient positioning other than that the patient should be lying supine as well as slightly head up, if desired, or if an aspiration risk exists.
2. **Prepare the nares.** Apply vasoconstricting agents (e.g., phenylephrine, oxymetazoline) to the nares, either by spraying directly into the nose or placing soaked cotton pledgets gently into the nose. Gently dilate the naris that will be used by placing an appropriately sized, well-lubricated nasal trumpet (optional). Keep in mind that the nasal passage runs straight back (e.g., parallel to the chin, and NOT up toward the forehead). Therefore, your nasal trumpet and endotracheal tube will need to be angled accordingly.

> **WARNING!!** Manipulating the naris by spraying a vasoconstrictor and/or placing a nasal trumpet may cause laryngospasm. It is prudent to obtain intravenous access before instrumentation of the nose.

3. **Insert the endotracheal tube into the naris.** When the nares are appropriately prepared, remove the nasal trumpet (if used), and guide the lubricated endotracheal tube into the desired naris.
4. **Guide the endotracheal tube into the trachea.** Either fiberoptic or direct laryngoscopy can be used for tracheal intubation by the nasal route. Fiberoptic laryngoscopy was described in detail earlier in the 'Fiberoptic Laryngoscopy Fundamentals' section.

   If direct laryngoscopy is chosen, a laryngoscope is used to view the glottic opening directly. The endotracheal tube is manually advanced through the naris, and when it is close to the vocal cords, the Magill forceps are used to guide the endotracheal tube through the vocal cords. Another individual may be needed to advance the endotracheal tube at the nares, while the primary airway proceduralist stabilizes the laryngoscope in the left hand and uses the Magill forceps in the right hand to guide the endotracheal tube through the vocal cords (Figures 3.25 and 3.26).

   >> **Tip on Technique:** If the endotracheal tube is difficult to advance past the vocal cords because of obstruction from the cricoid cartilage, try withdrawing the endotracheal tube a few centimeters, rotate the endotracheal tube 90 or 180 degrees counterclockwise to change the orientation of the bevel, and readvance the tube. Another technique to improve endotracheal tube passage is to lift the shoulders or apply cricoid pressure to better align the axes.

Postoperative Management Considerations

There are no special postoperative management considerations associated with this procedure.

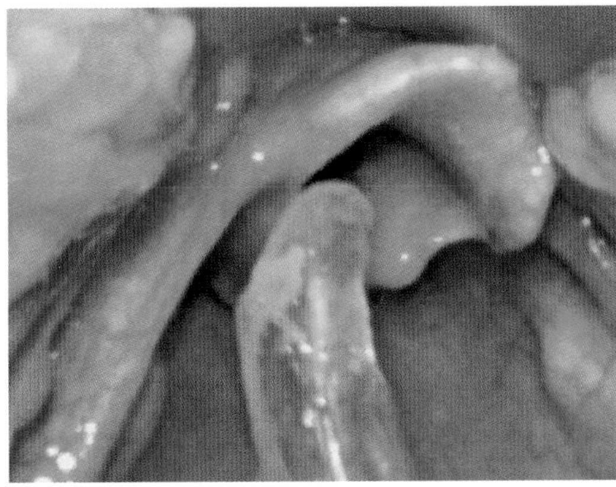

Figure 3.25 Laryngoscope in place and the endotracheal tube advanced to the level of the vocal cords.

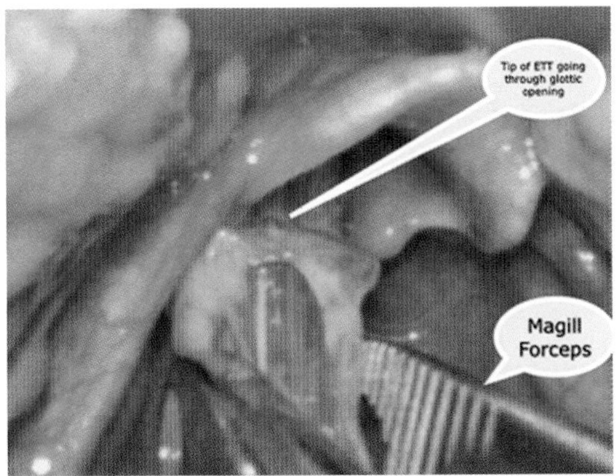

Figure 3.26 Magill forceps used to direct the endotracheal tube (ETT) past the glottic opening.

Further Reading

Asai T, Nagata A, Shingu K. Awake tracheal intubation through the laryngeal mask in neonates with upper airway obstruction. *Pediatr Anaesth*. 2008;18:77–80.

Black AE, Flynn PER, Smith HL, Thomas ML, Wilkinson KA. Development of a guideline for the management of the unanticipated difficult airway in pediatric practice. *Pediatr Anesth*. 2015;25(4):346–362.

Burjek NE, Nishisaki A, Fiadjoe JE, et al. Videolaryngoscopy versus fiber-optic intubation through a supraglottic airway in children with a difficult airway: an analysis from the Multicenter Pediatric Difficult Intubation Registry. *Anesthesiology*. 2017;127(3):432–440.

Fiadjoe JE, Nishisaki A, Jagannathan N, et al. Airway management complications in children with difficult tracheal intubation from the Pediatric Difficult Intubation (PeDI) registry: a prospective cohort analysis. *Lancet Respir Med*. 2016;4:37–48.

Holm-Knudsen R, Eriksen K, Rasmussen LS. Using a nasopharyngeal airway during fiberoptic intubation in small children with a difficult airway. *Pediatr Anesth*. 2005;15:839–845.

Jagannathan N, Sohn LE, Eidem JM. Use of the air-Q intubating laryngeal airway for rapid-sequence intubation in infants with severe airway obstruction: a case series. *Anaesthesia*. 2013;68; 636–638.

Jagannathan N, Sohn L, Fiadjoe JE. Paediatric difficult airway management: what every anaesthetist should know! *Br J Anaesth*. 2016;117(Suppl 1):i3–i5.

Jagannathan N, Sequera-Ramos L, Sohn L, et al. Elective use of supraglottic airway devices for primary airway management in children with difficult airways. *Br J Anaesth*. 2014;112:742–748.

Khattab A, Cohn S. The 3D question mark: Facilitating GlideScope intubation. Abstract: MARC Conference, 2016.

Kovatsis PG, Fiadjoe JE, Stricker PA. Simple, reliable replacement of pilot balloons for a variety of clinical situations. *Pediatr Anesth*. 2010;20(6):490–494.

Lee J-H, Park Y-H, Byon H-J, et al. A comparative trial of the GlideScope video laryngoscope to direct laryngoscope in children with difficult direct laryngoscopy and an evaluation of the effect of blade size. *Anesth Analg*. 2013;117(1):176–181.

Sunder RA, Haile DT, Farrell PT, Sharma A. Pediatric airway management: current practices and future directions. *Pediatr Anesth*. 2012;22(10):1008–1015.

Chapter 4

Lung Isolation Procedures

Renata Miketic and Vidya T. Raman

Lung Isolation Overview

Introduction

Lung isolation is used for many thoracic surgeries to provide exclusive ventilation of the nonoperative lung, allowing for the operative lung to be desufflated and improving surgical conditions and exposure. Additionally, in severe cases of unilateral lung infection or bleeding, ventilation of only the healthy lung can decrease the risk for contamination with blood and infected material from the diseased lung. Techniques used for achieving lung isolation include bronchial blocker placement, mainstem intubation, and use of a double-lumen tube. Although provider comfort and surgical preference often influence choice of technique, patient size and quality of lung isolation required are also guiding factors.

Double-lumen tubes are currently only available in size 26 (equivalent to a 6.0 endotracheal tube) and larger, limiting their use to older age groups. Bronchial blockers can be difficult to place in the appropriate bronchus, especially in infants and smaller children, and the smallest size available is a 2 French, which is appropriate for a 3.5 to 4.0 endotracheal tube. As an alternate technique, purposeful mainstem intubation is used in infants requiring a 3.0 endotracheal tube and may be the best choice in some infants requiring a 3.5 or 4.0 endotracheal tube as well as in children for whom a bronchial blocker or double-lumen tube cannot be easily placed or in whom perfect lung separation is not needed based on the nature of the operation.

Critical Anatomy

The trachea is composed of incomplete C-shaped cartilaginous rings and bifurcates into the right and left primary bronchi at the carina (Figures 4.1–4.3). For orientation purposes, it is important to note that tracheal rings are located anteriorly. The right lung has three lobes (superior, middle, and inferior), and the left lung has two lobes (superior and inferior)—each lobe with its own bronchi, known as the secondary bronchi. The secondary bronchi branch into smaller bronchi known as bronchioles. The right bronchus is typically shorter, wider, and more vertical than the left bronchus. These landmarks are used during fiberoptic bronchoscopy.

Bronchial Blocker Placement Fundamentals

Introduction

A bronchial blocker is one method that can be used when one-lung ventilation is required. The device is a catheter with a balloon at its tip. It is used with a single-lumen tube, placed into either the right or left mainstem bronchus, and inflated to occlude that bronchus. Bronchial blockers

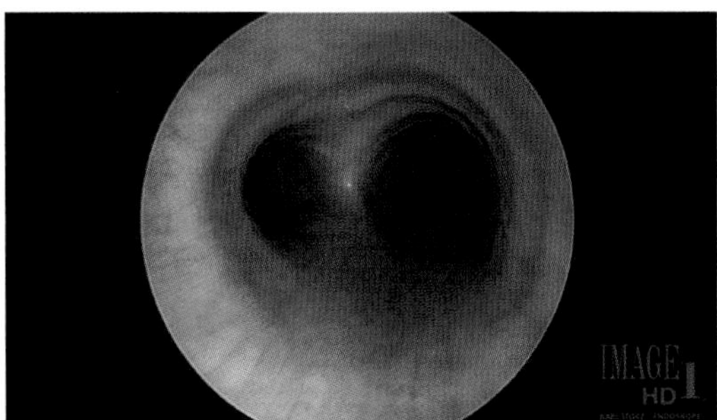

Figure 4.1 Fiberoptic view of the carina.

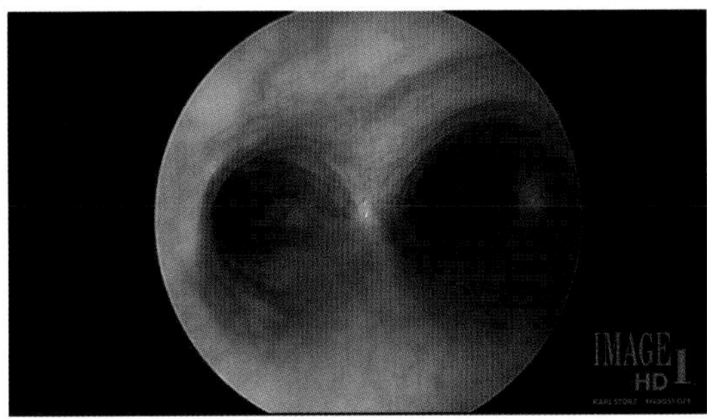

Figure 4.2 Fiberoptic view of the carina, left primary bronchi, and right primary bronchi with right upper lobe bronchi. Tracheal rings can be seen at the top of the picture.

can be placed within the lumen (intraluminal) or outside the lumen (extraluminal) of the endotracheal tube. Intraluminal bronchial blockers are placed inside of a single-lumen endotracheal tube and are typically used with larger endotracheal tubes in older children. Extraluminal bronchial blockers are placed through the vocal cords, outside of a single-lumen endotracheal tube, and are used more often with smaller endotracheal tubes in younger children. Modern bronchial blockers have the built-in safety feature of a relatively high-volume balloon that is inflated to a low pressure to decrease the risk for mucosal injury. Although both closed- and open-tipped bronchial blockers are available, the ability to suction the airway and apply continuous positive airway pressure makes the open-tipped bronchial blocker more clinically useful (in some cases, the surgeon may request suctioning of the bronchial blocker to assist with fully desufflating the operative lung). Placement can be time-consuming. However, in pediatric patients, bronchial blockers have gained popularity because of a larger number of sizes available. Inadvertent placement of the bronchial blocker in the wrong mainstem bronchus can arise from the inability to identify key anatomical structures.

Contraindications

No absolute contraindications exist for use of a bronchial blocker; however, placement of a bronchial blocker can be difficult.

!! **Potential Complications:** Damage to the tracheal mucosa and surrounding structures from using excessive force or an inappropriately sized bronchial blocker is a potential complication. Overdistension or overinflation of the balloon can damage the airway. Accidental dislodgment of an inflated bronchial blocker into the trachea can block ventilation to both lungs.

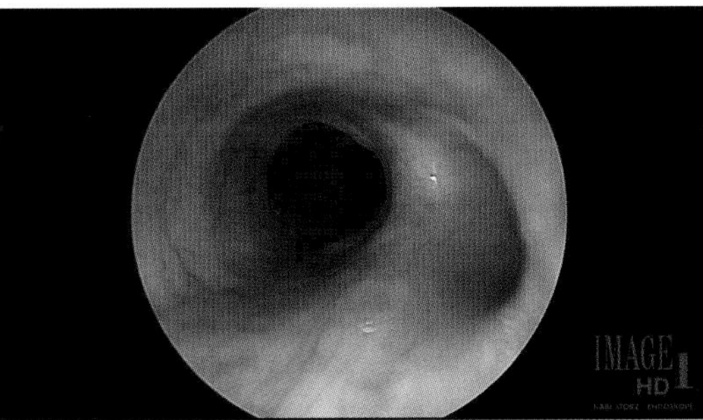

Figure 4.3 Fiberoptic view of the right primary bronchi with right upper lobe bronchi.

Setup

Equipment

Needed equipment includes the following in appropriate sizes for the patient's age:

- A variety of sizes of single-lumen endotracheal tubes (Table 4.1)
- Bronchial blocker (see Table 4.1)
- Laryngoscope blade (Table 4.2)
- Fiberoptic bronchoscope (Table 4.3)
- Stethoscope
- An extra set of experienced hands

>> **Tip on Technique:** Be familiar with your fiberoptic bronchoscope. Taking the time to understand how your fiberoptic bronchoscope works before starting the procedure can save you time and frustration.

>> **Tip on Technique:** Make sure that all equipment is working appropriately and have additional sizes of both endotracheal tubes and bronchial blockers available to avoid delays in gathering needed materials. Making sure that all equipment is functioning will also help avoid potential delays and frustrations. An experienced operator of the fiberoptic bronchoscope can help in identifying issues if problems arise.

Caution! Damage to the tracheal mucosa and surrounding structures can occur from using excessive force or an inappropriately sized endotracheal tube, bronchial blocker, or fiberoptic scope. Also, styletted bronchial blockers can lead to perforation of the trachea or bronchi if not used carefully. Overdistension or inflation of the balloon can damage the airway, and/or lead to incomplete lung isolation.

Table 4.1 Endotracheal Tube and Bronchial Blocker Selection for Single-Lung Ventilation in Children

Age	ETT (ID in mm)	BB (Fr)	Univent	DLT
Premature	2.5–3			
Newborn	3			
3–12 months	3.5	2	None	None
1–2 years	4.0–4.5	3	None	None
2–4 years	4.5–5.0	5	None	None
4–6 years	5.0–5.5	5	None	None
6–8 years	5.5–6.0	5	3.5	None
8–10 years	6.0 cuffed	5	3.5	26
10–12 years	6.5 cuffed	5	4.5	26–28
12–14 years	6.5–7.0 cuffed	5	4.5	32
14–16 years	7.0 cuffed	5, 7	6.0	35
16–18 years	7.0–8.0 cuffed	7, 9	7.0	35, 37

BB = bronchial blocker; DLT = double-lumen tube; ETT = endotracheal tube; Fr = French.

Table 4.2 **Suggested Laryngoscope Blade Types and Sizes Based on Patient Age**

Age	Miller	Wis-Hippel	Macintosh
Small premature infant	00		0
Premature infant	0		0
Term neonate	0–1		1
1–12 months	1		
1–2 years	1	1.5	2
2–6 years	2		2

ETT = endotracheal tube.

WARNING!! Always make sure that the patient is well oxygenated before the commencement of any intubation attempt. Remember that the decreased functional residual capacity-to-alveolar ventilation ratio in infants will result in quick desaturation. The clinician may need to stop the procedure to oxygenate.

Drugs, Dosages, Administration

The precise drugs used will depend on the need for spontaneous or controlled ventilation.

Patient Position

Place the patient in an optimal intubating position. This should include placing the operating room table at an optimal height for the practitioner as well as placing a shoulder roll and head support for the patient if needed.

Note: The height of the table to perform an endotracheal intubation is often higher than the height of the table that is needed to manipulate the fiberoptic bronchoscope comfortably. Adjust as necessary.

Table 4.3 **Common Fiberoptic Bronchoscope Sizes**

Type of Fiberoptic Bronchoscope	Outer Diameter (mm)	Smallest ETT inner diameter (mm)
Olympus LF-P	2.2	3.0 (2.5 is a snug fit, ETT adapter must be removed and scope well lubricated with silicone)
Olympus LF-DP	3.1	4.0 (3.5 if ETT adapter removed)
Olympus LF-V	4.1	5.5
Olympus LF-GP	4.1	5.0
Olympus LF-TP	5.2	6.0
Storz AA1	2.8	3.5
Storz BD2	3.7	4.0
Storz BN1	5.2	5.5

ETT = endotracheal tube.

Intraluminal Bronchial Blockers

Introduction

Readers should refer to the earlier 'Lung Isolation Overview' and 'Bronchial Blocker Placement Fundamentals' sections for information about critical anatomy, contraindications, equipment, drugs, preparation, and patient positioning for this procedure.

Step-by-Step

1. **Intubate the trachea with a single-lumen tube.** Check your equipment before intubation to ensure that the bronchial blocker attached to the fiberoptic scope fits easily through the selected endotracheal tube. Intubate the trachea with the appropriately sized single-lumen tube. Confirm endotracheal intubation with auscultation and end-tidal carbon dioxide ($EtCO_2$) capnography. Ventilate the patient with an FiO_2 of 100% to oxygenate fully before going to the next step.
2. **Place the bronchial blocker.** Prepare the bronchial blocker according to the manufacturer's instructions. Use the loop/lariat at the end of the bronchial blocker to attach the bronchial blocker to the fiberoptic bronchoscope. Ensure that the loop/lariat is attached to the very distal tip of the fiberoptic scope. Place the bronchial blocker (attached to the fiberoptic bronchoscope) (Figure 4.4) into the endotracheal tube and use the fiberoptic bronchoscope to guide placement to the appropriate primary bronchi using anatomical landmarks. Release the loop/lariat that is attaching the bronchial blocker to the fiberoptic bronchoscope and withdraw the fiberoptic bronchoscope to visualize the primary bronchi from a position slightly above the carina. While visualizing with the fiberoptic bronchoscope, inflate the balloon with the appropriate amount of air or saline indicated on the manufacturer's instructions (often on the package). Remove the fiberoptic bronchoscope and confirm correct placement by auscultation. Ensure that peak airway pressures are not excessive.

   Note: Specialized endotracheal tubes with a built-in channel for the bronchial blocker are also available (Figure 4.5).

Postoperative Management Considerations

At the end of the procedure, after two-lung ventilation is re-established, patients may initially need a higher positive end-expiratory pressure (PEEP) because the lung that was not ventilated during the procedure may be atelectatic. Before extubation, take care to maximize lung recruitment.

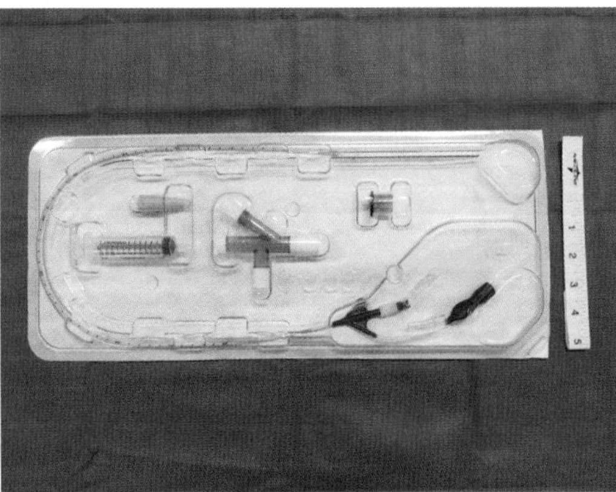

Figure 4.4 Bronchial blocker kit.

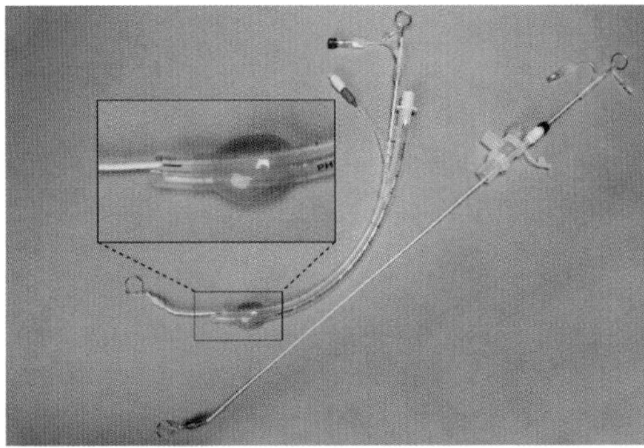

Figure 4.5 Endotracheal tube with specialized channel for a bronchial blocker.

Intentional Mainstem Intubation for Lung Isolation

Introduction

Mainstem intubation is also known as endobronchial intubation. When used for lung isolation, it is the intentional placement of a single-lumen endotracheal tube in either the right or left mainstem bronchus to facilitate one-lung ventilation.

Clinical Applications

> **WARNING!!** Sometimes listening to lung fields in very small infants can be deceiving. Fiberoptic confirmation of placement is always best. Lung ultrasound also has utility in confirming an intentional mainstem intubation.

This technique is used in a patient whose airway is too small to accommodate either a bronchial blocker or a double-lumen endotracheal tube.

Contraindications

Using purposeful mainstem intubation to achieve lung isolation is not ideal when the clinician needs to achieve true lung isolation or when lung isolation is being performed to prevent contamination of the ventilated lung.

!! **Potential Complications:** Potential complications of a purposeful mainstem intubation include inadvertent intubation of the inappropriate/wrong side, damage to the bronchus secondary to an aggressive technique or inappropriately sized single-lumen endotracheal tube, inadequate lung isolation especially if using an uncuffed endotracheal tube, and hypoxemia secondary to occlusion of the right upper lobe (during a right mainstem intubation for left lung isolation).

Setup

Equipment

Needed equipment includes the following in appropriate sizes for the patient's age:

- A variety of sizes of single-lumen endotracheal tubes (see Table 4.1)
- Laryngoscope blade (see Table 4.2)

- Fiberoptic bronchoscope (see Table 4.3)
- Stethoscope
- An extra set of experienced hands

>> **Tip on Technique:** Practice and know how to manipulate your fiberoptic scope before placing it in the endotracheal tube. Understanding how it works will save you time and effort. Make sure that all equipment is working appropriately to avoid potential delays and frustrations.

WARNING!! Always make sure that the patient is well oxygenated before the commencement of any intubation attempt. Remember that the increased oxygen consumption in infants will result in quick desaturation. The clinician may need to stop the procedure to oxygenate.

>> **Tip on Technique:** Have multiple sizes of single-lumen endotracheal tubes readily available to avoid delays in gathering appropriate tools.

Drugs, Dosages, Administration

The precise drugs used will depend on the need for spontaneous or controlled ventilation.

Patient Position

Place the patient in an optimal intubating position before commencement. This should include placing the operating room table at an optimal height for the practitioner as well as a shoulder roll and head support for the patient if needed.

Step-by-Step

1. **Intubate the trachea with a single-lumen tube.** Intubate the trachea as per usual with direct or video laryngoscopy, but with the bevel of the endotracheal tube facing upward.
2. **Place the endotracheal tube into a mainstem bronchus either with or without a fiberoptic bronchoscope**.

   Using the fiberoptic bronchoscope: Proceed to use the fiberoptic bronchoscope to identify the appropriate mainstem bronchus using anatomical landmarks, and then advance the single-lumen endotracheal tube over the bronchoscope.

   Without the fiberoptic bronchoscope: Rotate the endotracheal tube 45 degrees in the direction of the desired mainstem bronchus while simultaneously turning the head gently in the opposite direction. For example, for a left mainstem intubation, rotate the endotracheal tube 45 degrees to the left while simultaneously turning the head gently to the right. Next, advance the single-lumen tube into the desired mainstem bronchus.

   For either method, use auscultation, lung ultrasound, and/or a fiberoptic bronchoscope to confirm appropriate placement (Figure 4.6). (See Chapter 2, 'Lung Ultrasound' in Book 2 in this series, Ultrasound Guided Procedures and Radiologic Imaging for Pediatric Anesthesiologists, for more information.)

Postoperative Management Considerations

At the end of the procedure, after two-lung ventilation is re-established, patients may initially need a higher PEEP because the lung that was not ventilated during the procedure may be atelectatic. Before extubation, take care to maximize lung recruitment.

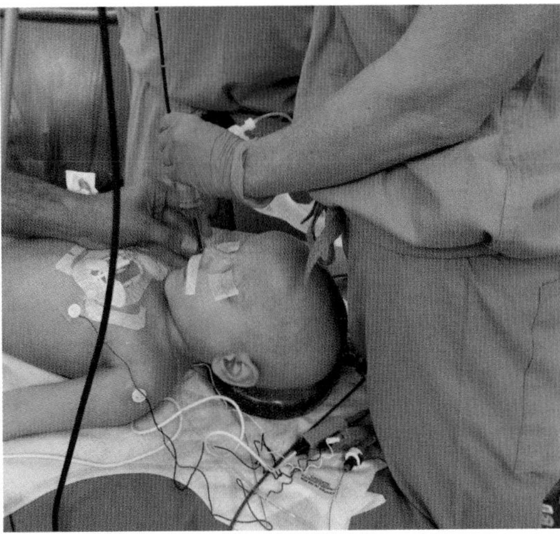

Figure 4.6 Fiberoptic scope through endotracheal tube in an infant.

Double-Lumen Tubes

Introduction

A double-lumen tube is a specially designed endotracheal tube that consists of two single endotracheal tubes molded together. These two endotracheal tubes are unequal in length and designed so that the shorter end is situated in the trachea while the longer end rests in the primary bronchus. Double-lumen tubes have a clear cuff on the tracheal lumen and a blue cuff on the bronchial lumen. Inflation of the tracheal cuff allows for ventilation of both lungs through the tracheal port if the bronchial cuff is deflated.

Double-lumen tubes are manufactured in two orientations: right and left. With a left double-lumen tube, the bronchial lumen is placed into the left mainstem bronchus, allowing the left lung to be ventilated by the bronchial lumen and the right lung to be ventilated by the tracheal lumen. With a right double-lumen tube, the bronchial lumen is placed into the right mainstem bronchus, allowing the right lung to be ventilated by the bronchial lumen and the left lung to be ventilated by the tracheal lumen.

Right double-lumen tubes can be more difficult to position because of the proximal orientation (and resultant ease of accidental occlusion) of the right upper lobe bronchus. To account for this issue, a right double-lumen tube has an extra ventilation hole close to the tip, on the side of the tube, to ventilate the right upper lobe. Exact placement of this ventilation hole, however, can be difficult, and the right upper lobe is easily obstructed. Left double-lumen tubes are also easier to place because of the longer length and more favorable angle of the left mainstem bronchus, and for these reasons they are generally preferred to right double-lumen tubes. A right double-lumen tube, however, may be required in those cases when the bronchus on the left side is compressed, injured, or missing. Examples may include but are not limited to a tumor in the left bronchus or trauma that has injured the left bronchus.

Readers should refer to the 'Lung Isolation Overview' section at the beginning of this chapter for more background and critical anatomy information associated with the use of double-lumen endotracheal tubes.

Clinical Applications

The use of a double-lumen tube is appropriate for any procedure in which lung isolation is needed. Reasons for requiring lung isolation are to optimize surgical exposure by collapsing the lung on the operative side or to minimize the risk for contamination of the nonoperative lung with blood and/or infected material. A double-lumen tube can only be used in larger pediatric patients (smallest available double-lumen size is a 26, corresponding to a 6.0 single-lumen ETT).

Setup

Equipment

Needed equipment includes the following in appropriate sizes for the patient's age and weight:

- A variety of sizes of double-lumen endotracheal tubes (see Table 4.1). These are typically packaged with all needed components, including a long stylette, an adapter to allow ventilation of both ports, an extension for each port, and a long suction catheter
- A hemostat to clamp the tube extension on the side that is not ventilated
- Laryngoscope blade (see Table 4.2)
- Fiberoptic bronchoscope (see Table 4.3)
- Stethoscope
- An extra set of experienced hands

>> **Tip on Technique:** Have multiple sizes of double-lumen tubes available to avoid delays in gathering appropriate materials. Age-appropriate sizes of both single-lumen endotracheal tubes and bronchial blockers should be available in case a double-lumen tube can not be successfully placed.

Drugs, Dosages, Administration

The precise drugs used will depend on the need for spontaneous or controlled ventilation.

Patient Position

Place the patient in an optimal intubating position before commencement. This should include placing the operating room table at an optimal height for the practitioner as well as a shoulder roll and head support for the patient, if needed.

Step-by-Step

1. **Prepare the double-lumen tube.** Double-lumen endotracheal tubes (Figure 4.7) are packaged with six separate components: the double-lumen tube itself, a long stylet, an adapter to allow ventilation of both ports, an extension for each port, and a long suction catheter. Before the case begins, lubricating the stylet and placing it into the double-lumen tube and connecting the adapter to both port extensions will save time during the case and decrease the likelihood that one of these components will be misplaced. Keep in mind that the stylet is always inserted into the bronchial lumen.
2. **Intubate with the double-lumen endotracheal tube.** For a left double-lumen tube: Perform a direct or video laryngoscopy. When the vocal cords are visualized, insert the double-lumen tube with the bronchial lumen facing anteriorly. Advance the double-lumen tube until the bronchial cuff is passed through the vocal cords. Rotate the double-lumen tube 90 degrees to the left. Continue to advance the double-lumen tube while having another clinician pull out the stylet. Attach the adapter/extension piece. Inflate the tracheal cuff as usual and the bronchial cuff with a smaller amount of air, taking care to avoid overinflation. Ventilate the patient with an FiO_2 of 100% to oxygenate the patient fully. Figure 4.8 shows a left double-lumen tube in situ.

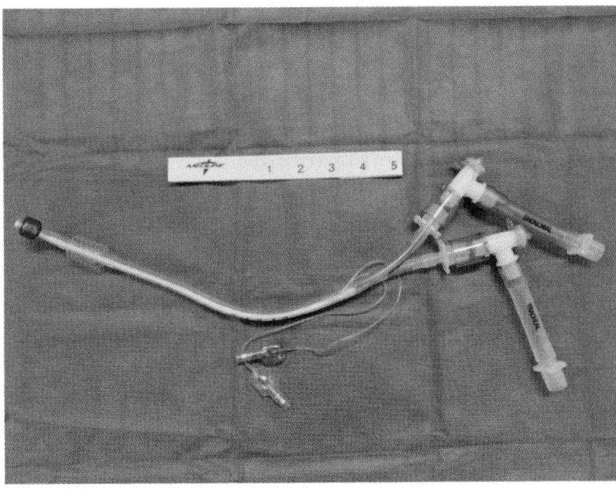

Figure 4.7 Double-lumen endotracheal tube.

>> **Tip on Technique:** When the fiberoptic scope is used for initial placement of the double-lumen tube, it should be placed through the bronchial lumen.

3. **Confirm placement of the double-lumen endotracheal tube** with a fiberoptic bronchoscope, with auscultation, and/or with lung ultrasound. (See Chapter 2, 'Lung Ultrasound' in Book 2 in this series, Ultrasound Guided Procedures and Radiologic Imaging for Pediatric Anesthesiologists, for more information.)

With a fiberoptic bronchoscope. *For a left double-lumen tube:* Place the fiberoptic scope into the tracheal lumen until you arrive at the level of the carina (Figure 4.9). For correct placement, verify that the blue bronchial cuff is barely visible as it occludes the left mainstem bronchus.

When clamping one lumen to achieve lung isolation, always clamp distal (further from the patient) to the cap, then open the cap to room air (see Figure 4.8).

With auscultation or lung ultrasound. *For a left double-lumen tube:* First, to isolate the right lung and ventilate the left lung only, clamp the tracheal lumen and open the cap on that lumen to room air. Auscultate or perform lung ultrasound to ensure breath sounds and/or lung sliding on the left side only. Unclamp, close the cap, and ventilate both lungs. Second, to isolate the left lung and ventilate the right side only, clamp the bronchial lumen and open the cap on that lumen to room air. Auscultate or perform lung ultrasound to ensure breath sounds and/or lung sliding on the right side only. Unclamp, close the cap, and ventilate both lungs. For a right double-lumen tube, these instructions will be reversed (Table 4.4).

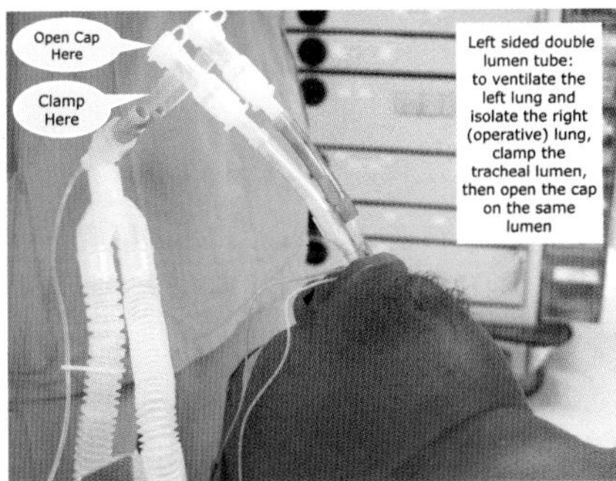

Figure 4.8 Double-lumen tube in situ.

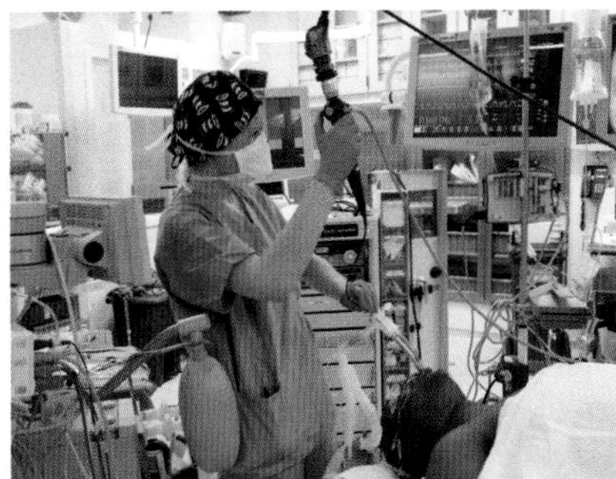

Figure 4.9 Fiberoptic scope being used to confirm correct placement of the double-lumen tube.

4. **Isolate the lung.** *For a left double-lumen tube:* to isolate the right lung and ventilate the left lung only, clamp distal (further from the patient) to the cap on the right side/tracheal lumen of the tube extension, then open the cap to the room air so that the lung can deflate. For other options, see Table 4.4.

   >> **Tip on Technique:** For quicker lung deflation, suction the relevant lumen and/or disconnect the tube extender (so that a larger port is then open to air).

WARNING!! Remove the suction promptly from the endotracheal tube after the lung is deflated to avoid atelectasis

Postoperative Management Considerations

At the end of the procedure, after two-lung ventilation is re-established, patients patients may initially need a higher PEEP because the lung that was not ventilated during the procedure may be atelectatic. Before extubation, take care to maximize lung recruitment. If postoperative ventilation is required, it may be necessary to change a double-lumen endotracheal tube to a

Table 4.4 Lung Isolation

Type of Double-Lumen Tube (Type Indicates the Bronchial Lumen)	Desired Lung to Isolate (Surgical Lung)	Desired Lung to Ventilate	Tracheal Lumen	Bronchial Lumen
Left	Right	Left	Clamped and cap open	Not clamped
	Left	Right	Not clamped	Clamped and cap open
Right	Right	Left	Not clamped	Clamped and cap open
	Left	Right	Clamped and cap open	Not clamped

single-lumen endotracheal tube owing to the lack of familiarity with management of double-lumen tubes in the intensive care unit. This may be more challenging in patients with significant fluid shifts, traumatic intubations, long procedures, or other causes of postoperative swelling. Keep in mind that using an exchange catheter for this procedure may be more challenging in a pediatric patient than in an adult patient.

Further Reading

1. Hammer GB. Anesthesia for thoracic surgery. In: Coté CJ, Lerman J, Anderson BJ, eds. *Coté and Lerman's A Practice of Anesthesia for Infants and Children*. 5th ed. New York: Elsevier; 2013:270–290.
2. Hammer, GB, Fitzmaurice, BG, Brodsky JB. Methods for single-lung ventilation in pediatric patients. *Anesth Analg*. 1999;89:1426–1429.
3. Hammer GB. Single-lung ventilation in infants and children. *Pediatr Anesth*. 2004;14:98–102.
4. Hammer GB, Harrison TK, Vricella LA, Black MD, Krane EJ. Single lung ventilation in children using a new paediatric bronchial blocker. *Paediatr Anesth*. 2002;12:69–72.
5. Hammer GB, Manos SJ, Smith BM, Skarsgard ED, Brodsky JB. Single-lung ventilation in pediatric patients. *Anesthesiology*. 1996;84(6):1503–1506.
6. Hammer GB, Brodsky JB, Redpath JH, Cannon WB. The Univent tube for single-lung ventilation in paediatric patients. *Paediatr Anaesth*. 1998;8:55–57.
7. Hammer GB, Hall S, Davis PJ. Anesthesia for general abdominal, thoracic, urologic, and bariatric surgery. In: Coté CJ, Lerman J, Anderson BJ, eds. *Coté and Lerman's Smith's Anesthesia for Infants and Children*. 8th ed. New York: Elsevier; 2011: 745–785.
8. Bordsky JB, Maracrio A, Mark JDB. Tracheal diameter predicts double-lumen tube size: a method for selecting left double-lumen tubes. *Anesth Analg*. 1996;82:861–864.

Chapter 5

Rigid Bronchoscopy and Surgical Airway Procedures, Foreign Body Aspiration, and Gastric Content Aspiration Management

Audra Webber and John Faria

Rigid Bronchoscopy

Introduction

Rigid bronchoscopy is a shared airway procedure, performed by the otolaryngologist, with ventilation and general anesthesia performed by the anesthesiologist. Rigid bronchoscopy is performed through suspension laryngoscopy. Spontaneous ventilation is frequently preferred in the initial stages, both to assess vocal cord function and to maintain airway patency when the specific pathology is unknown or when continued ventilation necessitates maintenance of airway tone. Spontaneous ventilation can often be achieved through an inhalation induction, switching to intravenous (IV) maintenance agents when IV access is acquired, or as a pure total intravenous anesthetic (TIVA), if IV access is already present. Figures 5.1 to 5.5 show a variety of airway pathologies on rigid bronchoscopy.

Clinical Applications

Rigid bronchoscopy is used for evaluation of stridor. It is also used to evaluate patients with hoarseness, airway trauma, or laryngeal and pharyngeal pathologies. Rigid bronchoscopy can also be used to remove a foreign body lodged in the airway or to evaluate and biopsy an airway mass.

Contraindications

Rigid bronchoscopy is contraindicated in a patient who has undergone a laryngectomy (very rare in pediatrics). Relative contraindications include a friable airway, bleeding diathesis, or a laryngeal or tracheal arteriovenous malformation.

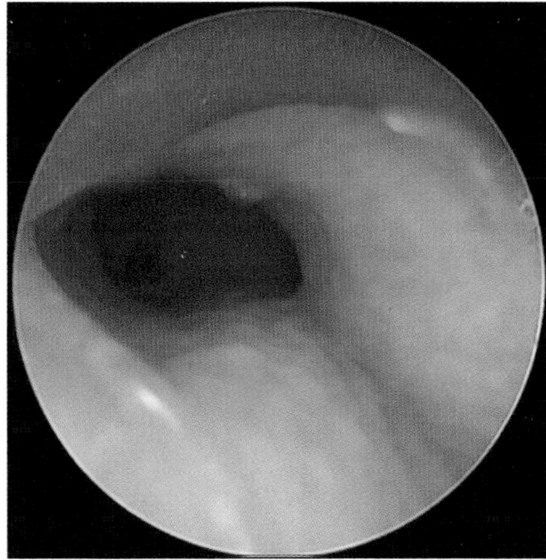

Figure 5.1 Double aortic arch.

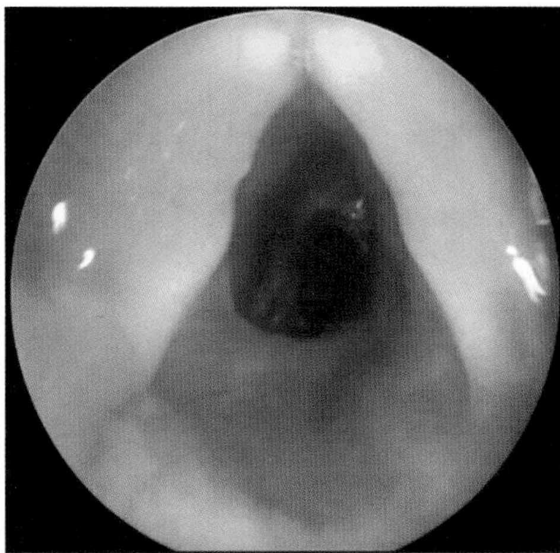

Figure 5.2 Subglottic stenosis.

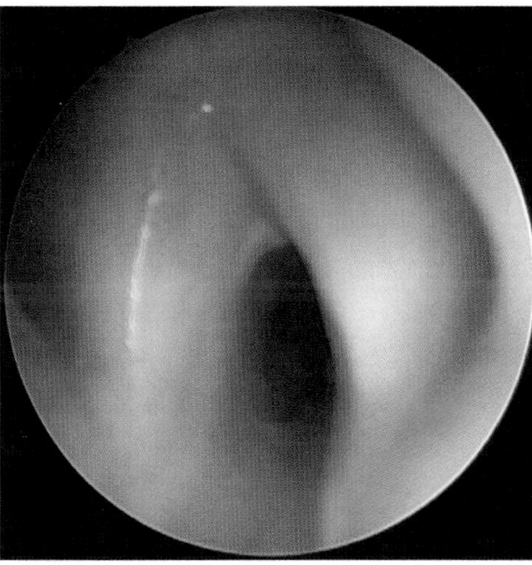

Figure 5.3 Glottic web.

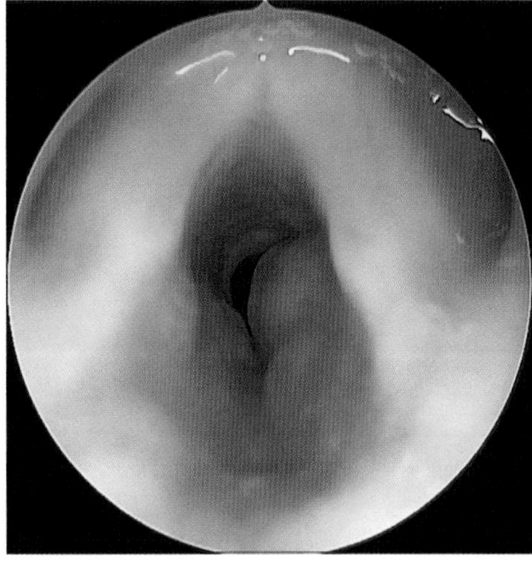

Figure 5.4 Subglottic cyst.

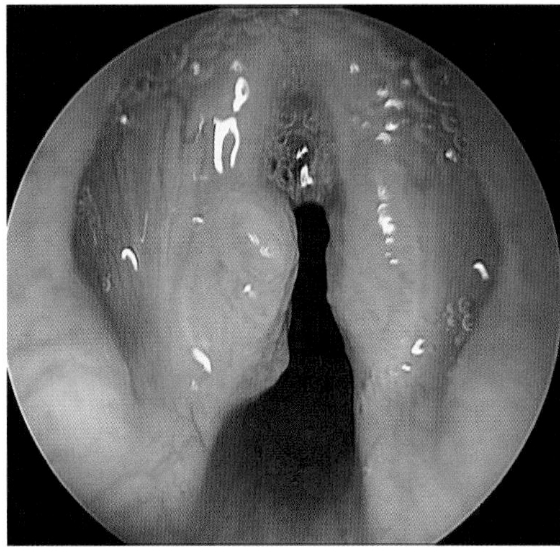

Figure 5.5 Respiratory papillomatosis.

Critical Anatomy

Performance of a rigid bronchoscopy involves all basic airway anatomy. You should review all available scans, images, and previous otolaryngology scopes before formulating your anesthetic plan. It is especially important to look for any signs of airway compression, either external (mediastinal mass, vascular ring) or internal (tracheomalacia or laryngomalacia; Figures 5.6 and 5.7). Be cognizant of the location of any airway masses (supraglottic, glottic, or subglottic) and formulate a plan in conjunction with the otolaryngologist.

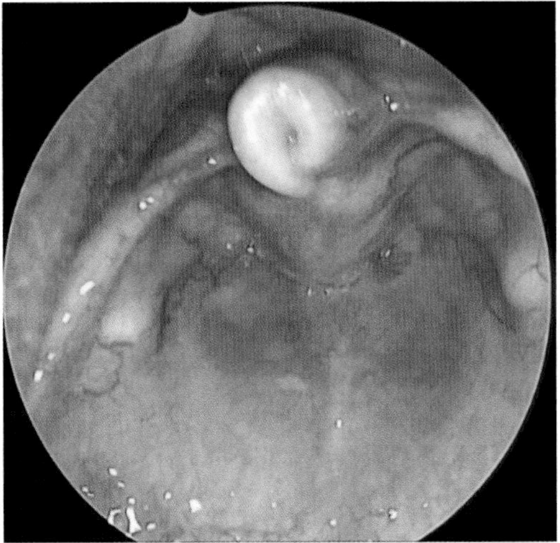

Figure 5.6 Laryngomalacia before surgical repair.

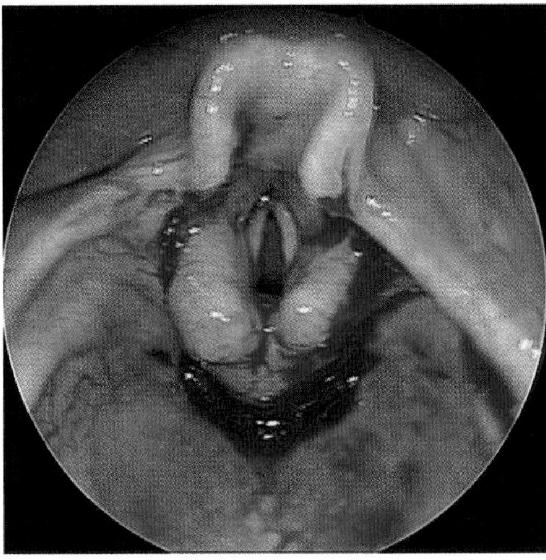

Figure 5.7 Laryngomalacia after surgical repair.

Setup

Equipment

- Endotracheal tubes—variety of sizes, cuffed and uncuffed
- Fiberoptic bronchoscope, appropriate size
- Equipment that the otolaryngology team typically has available is shown in figure 5.8

WARNING!! One should always have multiple airway devices in a variety of sizes immediately available for backup. These include supraglottic airways of several types (including intubating supraglottic airways, if available), oral airways, and nasal airways.

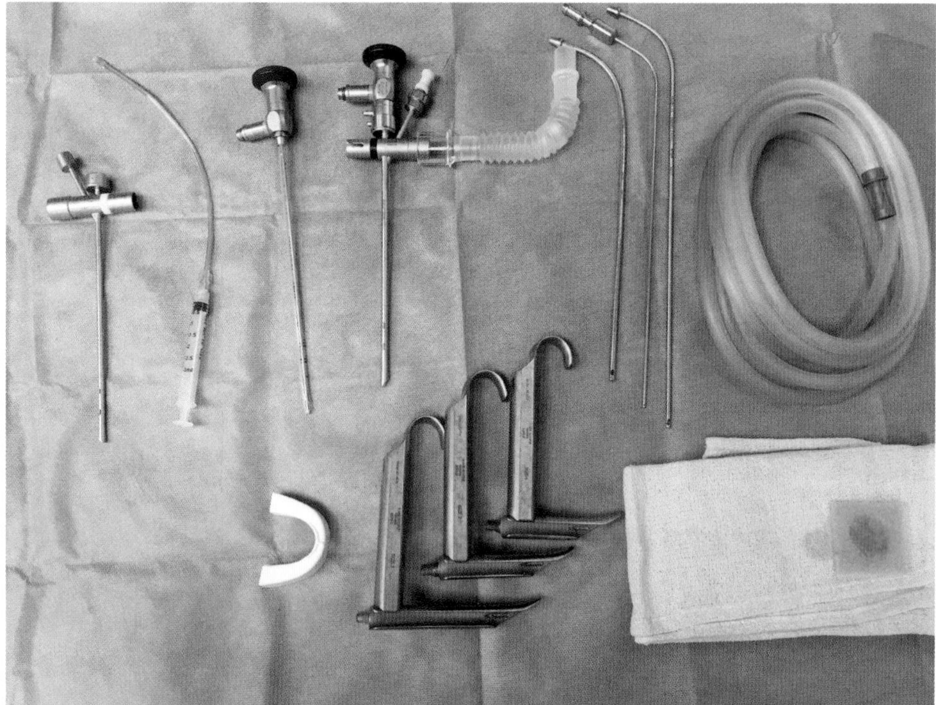

Figure 5.8 Instruments used for rigid bronchoscopy: The leftmost instrument is a rigid bronchoscope before it has been prepared for usage. It has an internal channel which can accommodate a rigid telescope (3rd instrument from left, 0 degree telescope). The fourth instrument from the left is a rigid bronchoscope assembled together with a rigid telescope and ready to be used for patient care. A "gooseneck" adapter is attached to the ventilation port. A bag-mask ventilator or anesthesia machine circuit is then attached to the "gooseneck" adapter to ventilate the patient after the rigid bronchoscope is placed through the vocal cords by the otolaryngologist. The second instrument from the left is a laryngeal atomizer which is used to spray the vocal cords and supraglottis with lidocaine. To intubate a child with subglottic airway obstruction under direct visualization, load an endotracheal tube over the rigid telescope (third instrument from the left). The fifth, sixth, and seventh instruments from the left are 3 sizes of laryngeal suction. In the bottom row is a soft plastic tooth protector that is used during laryngoscopy and 3 sizes of Parson's laryngoscopes. The bottom right is a towel prepared with a sponge soaked in defogger. Wiping the tip of the telescope on the sponge soaked in defogger prior to use decreases the chance of fogging.

Have at least two endotracheal tubes of an appropriate size styletted and ready to hand off to the otolaryngologist. Ensure that a fiberoptic bronchoscope is available and ready in the operating room. Most frequently, the otolaryngology service will have its own fiberoptic bronchoscope available; however, depending on the facility, it may be necessary for the anesthesiologist to ensure that a difficult airway cart with a flexible fiberoptic bronchoscope in the appropriate size is in the operating room before the start of the case. It is helpful for the otolaryngologist to have an endotracheal tube loaded onto the rigid bronchoscope before beginning the exam.

>> **Tip on Technique:** For IV induction techniques, as well as the IV maintenance of anesthesia, slow titration and patience are the key to maintaining spontaneous ventilation.

!! **Potential Complications**: Potential complications include loss of spontaneous ventilation leading to obstruction and hypoxia or complete airway collapse in extreme cases.

Drugs, Dosages, Administration

There are many IV agents that can be used safely in combination to maintain both spontaneous ventilation and airway tone. Your patient's individual characteristics, as well as your local resources and skill level, must be taken into account when deciding on a technique.

Example 1

A 19-month-old girl with a large obstructive supraglottic mass was given 0.2 mg/kg intranasal midazolam and taken to the operating room 15 minutes later. A 60/40 combination of nitrous oxide/oxygen was provided by mask with the patient spontaneously ventilating while IV access was obtained. Ketamine 2 mg/kg as an IV bolus was given along with 0.1 mg glycopyrrolate. Spontaneous ventilation was maintained, and a two-handed jaw thrust assisted in maintaining airway patency. One mcg/kg of dexmedetomidine was given over 5 minutes. One mg/kg of IV lidocaine was given by bolus just before insertion of the rigid bronchoscope. Anesthesia was maintained with further 0.5 mg/kg ketamine boluses as necessary. Supplemental oxygen was provided through the ventilating sideport of the bronchoscope until the airway was secured.

Example 2

A 4-year-old male with existing IV access presented for evaluation of suspected laryngotracheomalacia. He was given 0.1 mg/kg IV midazolam in the preoperative area for anxiolysis and was taken to the operating room 1 minute later. Induction was begun with an infusion of remifentanil 0.2 mcg/kg/min. A small propofol bolus (0.5 mg/kg) was given and its effect observed. Additional small boluses were given until the child was breathing spontaneously but no longer reactive to a significant jaw thrust. The rigid bronchoscope was then placed by the otolaryngologist. Anesthesia was maintained by incremental adjustments of the remifentanil infusion and/or additional small titrated boluses of propofol.

Alternative plan: A standard inhalation induction was performed with sevoflurane, with maintenance of anesthesia with sevoflurane and spontaneous ventilation maintained. After the rigid bronchoscope was placed and ventilation confirmed, total IV anesthesia was started.

!! **Potential Complications**: IV techniques are only as reliable as the IV line through which they are infusing. Ensure that the IV line is patent at the beginning of its use and check frequently for infiltration.

WARNING!!	If you are giving lidocaine intravenously to attenuate the airway reflex, ensure that the total dose of local anesthetic, including any topical lidocaine used by otolaryngology, does not exceed the maximum dose, to decrease the possibility of local anesthetic systemic toxicity (LAST); see Chapter 15: Local Anesthetic Systemic Toxicity Treatment. Because of their low body weight and decreased clearance of local anesthetics, it is important to be especially careful to avoid LAST in infants.

Pearl: Many anesthesiologists prefer to initially titrate small boluses of IV anesthetic agents rather than to use a continuous infusion because this allows more control when trying to maintain spontaneous ventilation.

!! **Potential Complications**: It is difficult to achieve a depth of anesthetic during which the patient is spontaneously breathing yet deep enough to tolerate the significant stimulus of rigid bronchoscopy.

Step-by-Step

1. **Conduct a preoperative evaluation and prepare for procedure.** Review the patient's airway evaluation, images, and pertinent past medical history. Oral, nasal, or IV midazolam may be desired in some patients. In an otherwise healthy patient, no special labs are necessary. If available, review the arterial blood gas. Maintain normothermia by prewarming the operating room. Use a heated bed pad or underbody forced-air warmer if available.
2. **Position the patient.** Place routine American Society of Anesthesiologists (ASA) monitors on the patient. For induction, place the patient supine with a shoulder roll unless the patient has a mass or an anomaly that will cause the patient to have better ventilation in the lateral position. For the procedure, the patient should be placed supine with a shoulder roll and his or her head in extension. Suspension laryngoscopy equipment and the surgeon will be at the head of the bed.
3. **Perform the induction.** There are multiple options for induction as described earlier under Drugs, Dosages, Administration. Often, the otolaryngologist will request that IV steroids be given at the beginning of the procedure to decrease airway swelling.
4. **Place the rigid bronchoscope (typically done by the surgeon).** Place a moist gauze or mouth guard is on the upper alveolar ridge. Insert an appropriately sized Parsons laryngoscope into the mouth and advance into the vallecula to allow for visualization of the glottic opening. Anesthetize the vocal folds are with topical lidocaine. Pass a zero-degree telescope between the vocal folds and into the airway, avoiding the mucosal walls and allowing visualization of the airways. Maintain spontaneous ventilation. Attach the anesthesia machine circuit is to the ventilating sideport of the scope, and manually assist spontaneous ventilation as needed. After the rigid bronchoscopy is performed by the surgeon, the surgeon may place an endotracheal tube.

WARNING!! In this case, you are sharing the airway with the surgeon. Ensure there is adequate communication regarding patient status (oxygenation and ventilation) throughout case and make adjustments accordingly.

Caution! Try to not wait until the patient desaturates completely before initiating assisted ventilation. Patient desaturation may result in atelectasis and a prolonged time to achieve adequate oxygenation after ventilation is re-established.

Postoperative Management Considerations

Caution! It is not uncommon for children to do well initially after extubation, but later to have respiratory failure due to fatigue or obstruction. That is why it is important to observe the patient after extubation in the operating room until you are sure that adequate ventilation will be maintained by the extubated patient. It is essential to have the otolaryngology surgeon remain at the bedside until this decision is made, especially if reintubation is likely to require use of a rigid bronchoscope.

Postoperative extubation is determined on a case-by-case basis with the input of both the anesthesiologist and otolaryngology surgeon. In many cases, the patient is left intubated. In some cases, it may be reasonable to extubate in the operating room, observe the patient for a set period of time, and, based on ventilation parameters (e.g., respiratory rate, tidal volume, work of breathing, obstruction, oxygen saturation), come to a mutual decision with the otolaryngologist as to whether the patient is likely to continue to maintain the airway and can remain extubated, or requires reintubation.

>> **Tip on Technique:** If a child with a difficult airway must be transported to a different location after surgery (especially across a significant distance or late at night with no backup), consider keeping the child intubated.

Tracheostomy, Planned

Introduction

A tracheostomy is a surgical airway and is best performed in an operating room by a pediatric otolaryngologist or pediatric general surgeon. Infant tracheostomies are technically difficult, even for skilled surgeons.(Figure 5.9) In difficult airway emergencies, a tracheostomy may be performed in the emergency department or at the bedside, typically by an otolaryngologist, pediatric surgeon, or trauma surgeon.

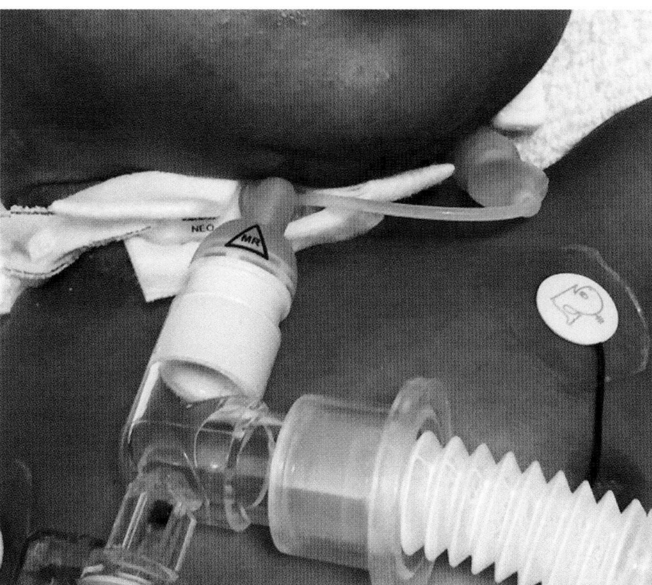

Figure 5.9 Tracheostomy in situ.

Clinical Applications

A tracheostomy is performed in some cases as a planned procedure in patients who are already intubated and are anticipated to need continued ventilatory support. The need for continued ventilatory support may be due to a hypoventilation syndrome, prolonged respiratory failure, or an airway abnormality. A tracheostomy is also performed in some children with an anatomic syndrome such as Pierre Robin if the child will need frequent anesthetics for facial and mandibular reconstruction. Finally, in emergency situations, performing a surgical airway (tracheostomy or cricothyroidotomy) is the last step in the difficult airway pathway when all other methods of securing an airway (often including rigid bronchoscopy) have failed.

Critical Anatomy

Critical anatomy for a tracheostomy includes basic laryngeal and tracheal anatomy (Figure 5.10).

Setup

Equipment

- Shoulder roll
- Accordion connector or extension
- Several endotracheal tubes available in an array of sizes (for reintubation or to place through the tracheostomy site)
- Supraglottic airway device
- Flexible fiberoptic scope (if available, to confirm placement)
- Rigid bronchoscope (if available, as an emergency airway device)
- Tracheostomy tube of the correct size and type (Figure 5.11)

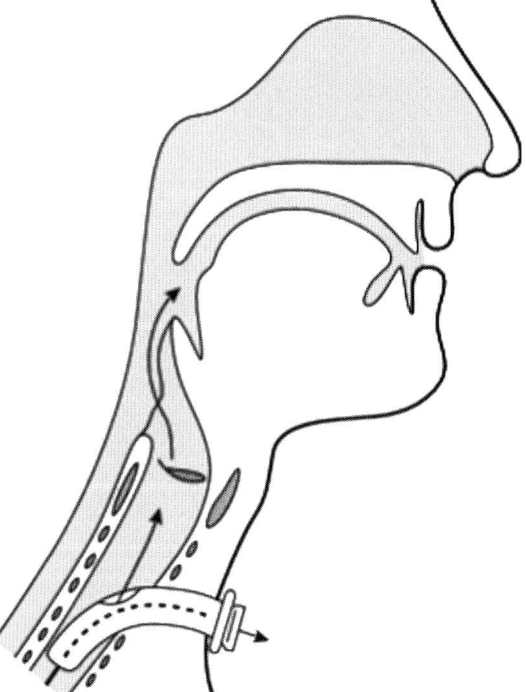

Figure 5.10 Diagram of tracheostomy tube position (note fenestration). Reproduced with permission from: The Oxford American Handbook of Otolaryngology—Blitzer A, Schwartz J, Song P, Young N. Oxford University Press 2008. Figure 8.14, page 189.

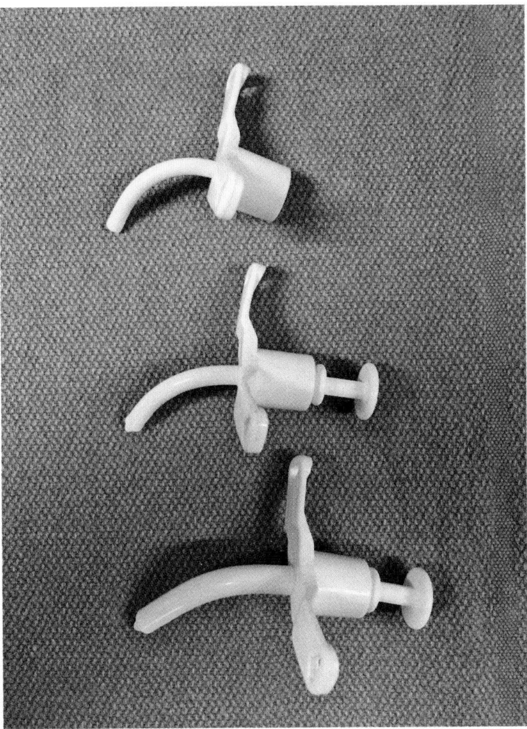

Figure 5.11 Tracheostomy Tubes: Neonatal uncuffed Bivona in three sizes. Top to bottom: 2.5, 3.0, 3.5. The top tracheostomy tube is pictured without an obturator in place. The bottom two tracheostomy tubes are pictured with an obturator in place. When replacing a tracheostomy tube, the obturator should be in place as it increases the rigidity of the tracheostomy tube, facilitating passage into the trachea. The otolaryngologic surgeon will decide on the type of tracheostomy tube. For children, many types and sizes or tracheostomy tubes are available, and are additionally classified as "Pediatric" (longer) or "Neonatal" (shorter) and "Cuffed" or "Uncuffed".

!! **Potential Complications**: For all airway surgeries, a risk of airway fire exists. Have saline or sterile water readily available.

Drugs, Dosages, Administration

This procedure is typically performed with a patient who is already intubated and under general anesthesia.

Step-by-Step

1. **Conduct a preoperative evaluation and prepare for the procedure.** Assess the patient's readiness for the tracheostomy. If the patient has had a recent deterioration of his or her respiratory status secondary to a newly acquired infection, it may be best to delay the tracheostomy until the patient is back to his or her respiratory baseline. Make sure you know the patient's current ventilator settings, positive end-expiratory pressure (PEEP), and FiO_2 requirements, as well as the frequency and necessity of suctioning, before bringing the patient to the operating room for a tracheostomy. This will ensure the smoothest transition from the intensive care unit to the operating room and will also assist in the assessment of the patient's overall respiratory status. Maintain normothermia by warming the room and placing an underbody warming device.
2. **Position the patient.** Place standard ASA monitors. Ensure working, noninfiltrated IV access. The patient should be positioned supine with a shoulder roll and significant head extension to maximize anatomic exposure.

   !! **Potential Complications**: Excessive head extension can result in the surgical ostomy inadvertently placed too low in the trachea.

3. **Induce the patient.** General anesthesia can be induced and maintained with inhalation and/or IV agents. After induction, protect the patient's eyes per your institution's routine (e.g., tape or cotton pads). Often, the otolaryngologist will request that IV steroids be given at the beginning of the procedure to decrease airway swelling. Typically, the patient will already be intubated. Sometimes, a supraglottic airway device will be used in patients with a known difficult airway, while spontaneous ventilation is maintained.
4. **Manage anesthesia during the tracheostomy procedure and entering of the airway.** The surgery will first consist of a skin incision and dissection down to the trachea itself. Next, the surgical team will perform the incision to enter the trachea. Close communication is needed so that the anesthesiologist will know when airway entry is occurring. If the trachea will be entered using electrocautery (e.g., Bovie), it is essential that the FiO_2 is below 30% at this point in order to decrease the risk for an airway fire. Immediately before the surgeons enter the trachea, the anesthesiology clinician will be asked to withdraw the endotracheal tube to rest above the anticipated incision and tracheostomy site. It is important to withdraw the endotracheal tube only the minimum amount needed. This is so that if the surgeons fail to enter the trachea quickly, the endotracheal tube can be readvanced, if possible, and ventilation through the endotracheal tube can be re-established. The endotracheal tube should be left in situ until tracheostomy placement is confirmed with chest rise, bilateral breath sounds, and end-tidal carbon dioxide ($EtCO_2$) monitoring.

Caution! If no $EtCO_2$ or chest rise is seen after the tracheostomy is placed, immediately reconnect your circuit to the endotracheal tube (which should have remained in situ). If this is not possible, quickly establish ventilation by reintubation or with a supraglottic airway or mask.

Caution! In premature infants and those with reactive airways, bronchospasm is common on initial placement of the tracheostomy. If bronchospasm is strongly suspected (i.e., no $EtCO_2$ or chest rise), quickly confirm tracheostomy placement by a flexible fiberoptic bronchoscope through the tracheostomy and simultaneously treat the bronchospasm.

Note: The surgeon will typically leave two stay sutures as anatomical markers to aid in replacing or changing the tracheostomy as necessary.

Postoperative Management Considerations

Postoperatively, almost all patients will be admitted to the intensive care unit. Take extreme care with the new tracheostomy during transport. It is frequently useful to have a "gooseneck" or "accordion" airway extension device between the tracheostomy and the ventilation tubing.

Caution! Sometimes, a newly placed "fresh" tracheostomy will become dislodged. Never blindly replace a newly placed tracheostomy because trying to do so can dissect tissue planes and make subsequent placement difficult or impossible. Use a flexible fiberoptic bronchoscopy as an obturator or guide. Have the surgeon perform the reinsertion of a newly placed tracheostomy if possible.

Surgical Airway, Unplanned or Urgent: Emergency Cricothryotomy and Emergency Percutaneous Needle Cricothyrotomy

Introduction

These procedures are best performed in an operating room by a pediatric otolaryngologist or pediatric general surgeon. Infant surgical airways are technically difficult, even for skilled surgeons. If no surgeon is immediately or imminently available in a "cannot ventilate (via mask or supraglottic airway), cannot oxygenate, cannot intubate" situation, then it is within the anesthesiologist's purview to attempt a surgical or percutaneous cricothyrotomy.

Clinical Applications

Emergent or urgent tracheostomy or cricothyrotomy is performed in a "cannot ventilate, cannot oxygenate, cannot intubate" situation. The incidence of "cannot ventilate, cannot oxygenate, cannot intubate" situations has decreased dramatically with the advent of pediatric supraglottic airway devices but does still occur, sometimes secondary to a traumatic airway or unexpected difficult airway. A cricothyrotomy is a temporizing measure until a tracheostomy can be performed.

Contraindications

There are no contraindications for performing a surgical airway, and this procedure is the last recourse before inevitable hypoxic brain injury and death.

Critical Anatomy

Critical anatomy for these procedures includes basic laryngeal and tracheal anatomy.(Figure 5.12)

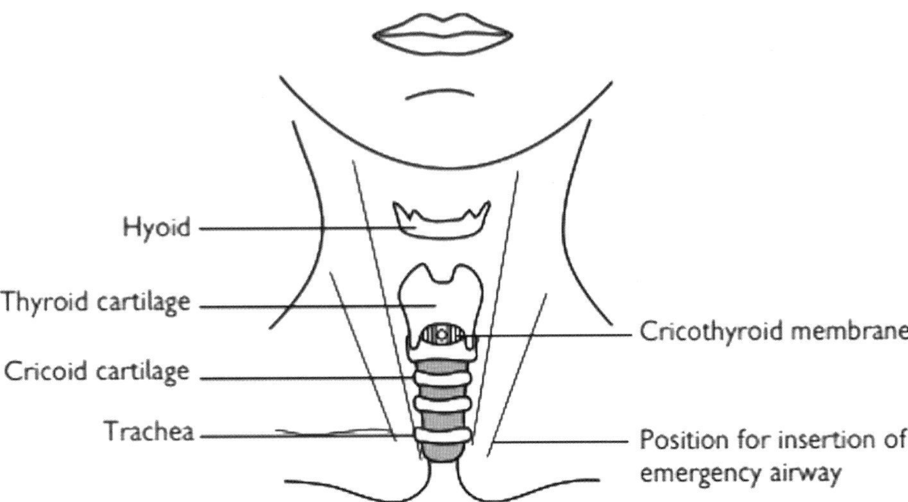

Figure 5.12 Cricothyrotomy Anatomy. Reproduced with permission from: The Oxford American Handbook of Otolaryngology—Blitzer A, Schwartz J, Song P, Young N. Oxford University Press 2008. Figure 8.12, page 187.

Setup

Equipment

- Shoulder roll
- Accordion connector or extension
- Scalpel
- Retractor
- Small cuffless endotracheal tube
- Bag mask resuscitator (e.g., Ambu bag)

For an emergency percutaneous needle cricothyrotomy, also obtain:

- A large-bore IV catheter (size dependent on size of child) attached to a saline-filled syringe
- A 3.0 IV catheter attached to a circuit adapter

Drugs, Dosages, Administration

WARNING!! A standard cricothyrotomy is not appropriate for neonates or infants because even the smallest endotracheal tube is too large to fit through a neonate or infant's cricothyroid membrane. In the case of a neonate or infant, a percutaneous cricothyrotomy may be tried, although this will still be very difficult.

No specialized medications are necessary.

!! **Potential Complications**: Potential complications of an emergency cricothyrotomy include injury to vessels, improper positioning of the airway device, and misidentification of anatomy with a resultant failed airway.

Step-by-Step: Emergency Cricothyrotomy

1. **Position the patient, identify landmarks, and prepare the skin.** Position the patient in extension with a neck or shoulder roll to bring the laryngeal anatomy to prominence and then sterilize the skin. Feel for the center of the thyroid cartilage (because it is larger and more readily palpable), then move your finger downward (caudad) until you feel your finger sink into the cricothyroid membrane.

   >> **Tip on Technique:** The Difficult Airway Society recommends the use of the "laryngeal handshake" to find the cricothyroid membrane, and this technique has been studied in adult patients.[1] This technique involves grasping the entire larynx, close to the chin, with the clinician's nondominant hand (thumb on one side of the larynx, other four fingers on the other side of the larynx) (Figure 5.13). The clinician then slides his or her hand downward, palpating with the index finger for the cricothyroid membrane (Figure 5.14).[1]

2. **Perform the emergency cricothyrotomy.** Make a stab incision with a scalpel of appropriate size through the cricothyroid membrane. Separate the skin with a retractor or hook. Insert an endotracheal tube through the stab wound into the trachea.

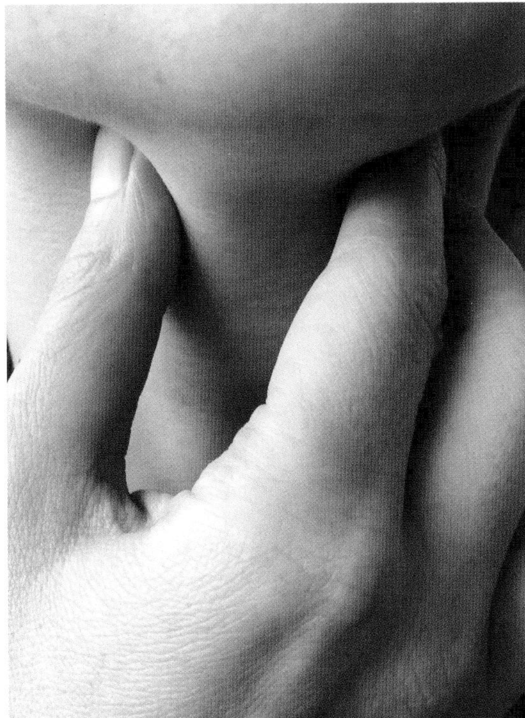

Figure 5.13 Laryngeal handshake: identification of the trachea.

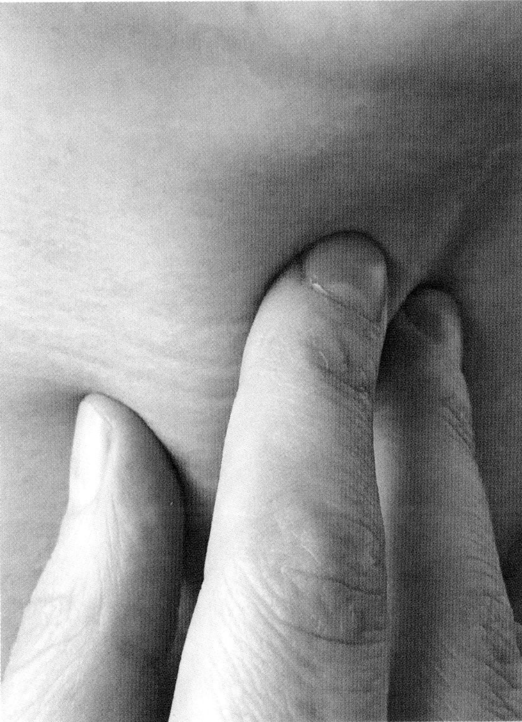

Figure 5.14 Laryngeal handshake: identification of the cricothyroid membrane.

Postoperative Management Considerations: Emergency Cricothyrotomy

Watch the patient carefully because if decannulation occurs, it may be very difficult to re-establish an airway. If long-term ventilatory support is needed, at the team's discretion the cricothyrotomy may be later converted electively to a tracheostomy.[2]

Step-by-Step: Emergency Percutaneous Needle Cricothyrotomy

1. **Position the patient, identify landmarks, and prepare the skin.** Position the patient in extension with a neck or shoulder roll to bring the laryngeal anatomy to prominence and then sterilize the skin. Feel for the center of the thyroid cartilage (because it is larger and more readily palpable), then move your finger downward (caudad) until you feel it sink into the cricothyroid membrane.
2. **Perform emergency percutaneous needle cricothyrotomy.** Puncture the cricothyroid membrane in a caudad direction with an IV catheter attached to a saline-filled syringe, aspirating until air bubbles appear, which indicates an intratracheal position. After confirmatory aspiration of air bubbles, advance the IV catheter into the trachea. Remove the needle and syringe and attach the syringe directly to the IV catheter. Aspirate again to confirm intratracheal location of the catheter. Attach the catheter to a specialized adaptor (called the "3.0 endotracheal tube to IV catheter adaptor") and then to an Ambu bag or other bag valve device.

WARNING!! While performing a needle cricothyrotomy, migration of the IV catheter into the subcutaneous tissue or carotid vessels can easily occur. If this migration is not recognized, and air is introduced into the vasculature, catheter migration will rapidly be a fatal event.

WARNING!! It is very important to allow for adequate exhalation while ventilating through a needle cricothyrotomy; otherwise, auto-PEEP and death will rapidly occur.

WARNING!! A needle cricothyrotomy generally allows for adequate oxygenation and, if the child is still breathing spontaneously, may allow for some ventilation as well until a surgeon can arrive to perform a tracheostomy. The child will have some degree of hypercarbia. Attaching a jet ventilator to this airway in an infant or neonate can cause significant barotrauma or subcutaneous emphysema. Consider gentle hand ventilation, or oxygenate with passive diffusion.

!! **Potential Complications**: Possible complications of a needle cricothyrotomy include injury to blood vessels, improper positioning of the airway device, and misidentification of structures resulting in a failed procedure.

Postoperative Management Considerations: Emergency Percutaneous Needle Cricothyrotomy

Watch the patient carefully because if decannulation occurs, it may be very difficult to re-establish an airway. At the team's discretion, if long-term ventilatory support is needed, the cricothyrotomy may later be converted electively to a tracheostomy.[1]

Foreign Body Aspiration

Introduction

An airway foreign body is a surgical emergency when a patient presents with respiratory compromise. This occurs most commonly in toddlers, owing to their tendency to put nonfood objects into their mouth. Bronchial foreign bodies will be more likely to go into the right mainstem bronchus because of the angle of the bronchus. Removal of the foreign body will be performed by the otolaryngologist, typically under general anesthesia. Occasionally, if complete airway obstruction occurs acutely in the emergency department or operating room, an emergency attempt will first be made to push the foreign body into a bronchus so that one lung can be ventilated, as a temporizing measure until the foreign body can be definitively removed by otolaryngology.

> **WARNING!!** Peanuts are especially difficult to remove because they can crumble or break into smaller pieces. Additionally, unroasted peanuts can cause pneumonitis.

Critical Anatomy

An understanding of basic tracheal and bronchial anatomy is critical when dealing with foreign body aspiration.

Setup

Equipment

- Rigid bronchoscope with ventilating side port
- Array of smaller endotracheal tubes (in the event one-lung ventilation is necessary)

Drugs, Dosages, Administration

As the patient becomes more upset and agitated, increased airway compromise may occur. Intranasal midazolam (0.1–0.2 mg/kg of a 5-mg/mL concentration) or intranasal dexmedetomidine (2 mcg/kg of 100 mcg/mL concentration) can be administered to ensure a smooth inhalation induction in children for whom acquiring an IV preoperatively would precipitate respiratory decompensation.

!! **Potential Complications**: Monitor the patient carefully because the administration of midazolam can result in decreased airway tone and increased respiratory compromise.

Step-by-Step

1. **Conduct a preoperative evaluation and prepare for procedure.** Obtain a past medical history as usual. Review any images that may contribute to localization or identification of the foreign body. Discuss the induction plan with the surgeon. Maintain normothermia by warming the room and placing an underbody warming device.

> **WARNING!!** The clinician must be aware of the fact that placing an IV line preoperatively will upset the patient, and the subsequent agitation could result in real harm due to complete airway obstruction. The clinician must balance the risks versus the benefits of preoperative IV placement.

2. **Position the patient.** Place standard ASA monitors. Ensure working, noninfiltrated IV access. For an inhalation induction, the child can be positioned supine on the operating room table or in the seated position in the anesthesiologist's lap after appropriate monitors are applied. Maintenance of spontaneous ventilation is key. If an IV is already in place, a controlled IV induction with titrated propofol can be performed to maintain spontaneous ventilation.

> **WARNING!!** Frequently, patients with an airway foreign body have copious secretions and a full stomach. A baseline risk for aspiration exists because the airway cannot be secured with an endotracheal tube while bronchoscopy is being performed.

!! **Potential Complications**: Use of nitrous oxide may result in hypoxia in a patient with respiratory compromise. Administer 100% oxygen during induction.

Pearl: Gastric contents can be suctioned after induction and IV placement. Suctioning of gastric contents does not eliminate the aspiration risk but may decrease it.

3. **Induce the patient.** Perform a standard inhalation induction or, if an IV line is already in place, a slowly titrated IV induction. Maintain spontaneous ventilation. Although a risk for aspiration does exist, the clinician will often choose to keep the patient breathing spontaneously during the induction of anesthesia because complete airway obstruction may occur when breathing reflexes are suppressed. Switching to a total IV anesthetic after induction is usually preferred to decrease exposure of OR staff to sevoflurane as well as to maintain a stable and steady state of anesthesia.

> **WARNING!!** If continuing to use an inhalational anesthetic during rigid bronchoscopy, it is difficult to accurately assess the MAC% (minimum alveolar concentration %) of a volatile anesthetic agent in this open system. This could lead to inadequate anesthesia, patient movement, and possible patient injury while the rigid bronchoscope is in place. Consider using an IV anesthetic infusion.

4. **Accomplish foreign body retrieval.** Typically, the otolaryngologist will perform the foreign body retrieval. Assisted ventilation can push the foreign body further down into the bronchial tree, making the foreign body more difficult to access. Occasionally, the foreign body will initially be successfully retrieved from a lower bronchus and then accidentally be dropped and become lodged at a higher point, impairing ventilation to a greater degree. If ventilation is thus significantly impaired, the surgeon must push the object further down the bronchial tree in order to allow ventilation. Once the patient has been adequately ventilated and oxygenated again, then retrieval can proceed.

Caution! If the patient starts to desaturate (either by loss of spontaneous ventilation or inability to ventilate by rigid bronchoscopy) and the surgeon is not imminently about to retrieve the foreign body, have the surgeon remove the rigid bronchoscope and place an endotracheal tube. Take time to oxygenate the patient sufficiently before removing the endotracheal tube and reinserting the rigid bronchoscope. This series of steps may need to be repeated multiple times in a difficult retrieval.

Postoperative Management Considerations

Generally, after a foreign body retrieval, the patient is extubated at the end of the case. If there is significant trauma to the airway or concern for postoperative swelling as seen on bronchoscopy, it is best to place an endotracheal tube at the conclusion of foreign body removal and keep the patient intubated postoperatively.

Gastric Content Aspiration Management

Aspiration of gastric contents may present intraoperatively as frank emesis or may occur silently throughout a case and present only with decreasing SpO_2 intraoperatively. Aspiration can occur at any point during an anesthetic or sedation with an unsecured airway or uncuffed endotracheal tube. Aspiration is more likely in patients who are not appropriately NPO ("nothing by mouth") or who have an anatomic or physiologic abnormality contributing to increased gastric volume, delayed gastric emptying, or poor esophageal sphincter tone. Many of our fragile pediatric patients have a history of "silent aspiration" and are at a much higher aspiration risk during anesthesia. It has recently been suggested that point-of-care ultrasound of gastric volumes can be used to grossly determine gastric volume and to assess perioperative aspiration risk.[3] (see Chapter 3, 'Gastric Ultrasound' in Book 2 in this series, Ultrasound Guided Procedures and Radiologic Imaging for Pediatric Anesthesiologists)

Caution! Even a negative or "empty stomach" point-of-care gastric ultrasound is not a 100% guarantee against aspiration.

Setup

Drugs, Dosages, Administration

In patients with a history of gastroparesis or in patients who are likely to have decreased esophageal sphincter tone (e.g., after a tracheoesophageal repair), consider avoiding oral medications preoperatively.

WARNING!! Bag mask ventilation with higher pressures is used as the initial step to treat laryngospasm but will often inadvertently insufflate the abdomen and therefore increase the likelihood of aspiration of gastric contents. In these cases, place a cuffed endotracheal tube as quickly as is manageable. Additionally, after securing the airway, decompress the stomach with an orogastric tube.

Procedure

If frank emesis is observed, the patient should be immediately positioned laterally, in Trendelenburg position, and with his or her head turned to the side. Suction the airway. Suction through the endotracheal tube if present.

> **Caution!** Radiographic evidence of aspiration pneumonitis takes hours to develop. In children who are otherwise healthy, a chest radiograph, antibiotic prophylaxis, and bronchoalveolar lavage are not typically needed after aspiration.

Note: An FiO_2 of 100% after aspiration is only indicated if the patient's oxygen saturation is decreased from normal.

Postoperative Management Considerations

Not all patients with suspected aspiration need to be admitted postoperatively. Many can be observed in the postoperative care unit and discharged home after a thorough discussion with the parents. Patients with preexisting respiratory conditions and those who are medically fragile are likely to benefit from admission and observation. Use your clinical judgment.

References

1. Drew T, McCaul CL. Laryngeal handshake technique in locating the cricothyroid membrane: a non-randomized comparative study. *Br J Anaesth.* 2018;121(5):1173–1178.
2. Cote CJ, Hartnick CJ. Pediatric transtracheal and cricothyrotomy airway devices for emergency use: which are appropriate for infants and children? *Pediatr Anesth.* 2009;19(Suppl 1):66–76.
3. Van de Putte P, Perlas A. Ultrasound assessment of gastric content and volume. *Br J Anaesth.* 2014;113(1):12–22.

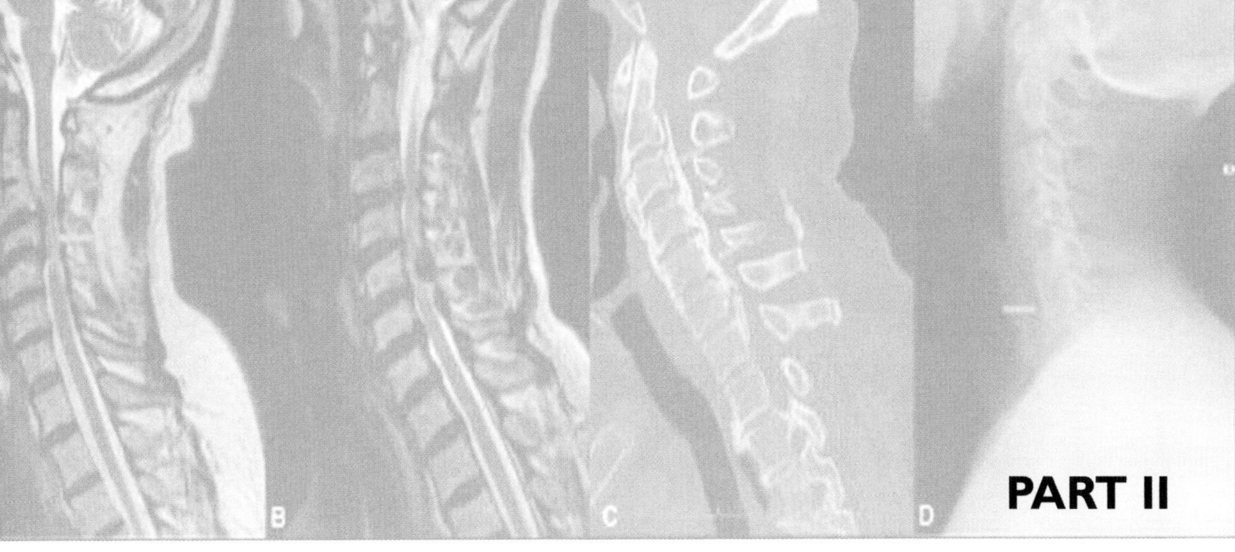

PART II

VASCULAR ACCESS

Chapter 6

Pediatric Fluid Management and Infusion

Elizabeth Dixon and Katiun Attarpour

Introduction

Perioperatively, intravenous (IV) fluids are used for maintenance while a patient is "nothing by mouth" (NPO), to replace insensible losses, and for fluid resuscitation. In cases with significant blood loss, or in patients who come to the operating room anemic and/or coagulopathic, the IV transfusion of blood products may be needed as well. In the pediatric population, cases with significant blood loss represent a small percentage of surgeries. However, when significant blood loss does occur, management of fluids and blood products is critical. Examples of pediatric surgeries with high blood loss in which fluid and/or blood infusion may be necessary include trauma, burns, large tumors, scoliosis repair, craniosynostosis repair, neurosurgery, and cardiac surgery.

Pediatric Fluid Management Principles

Preoperatively, calculate the maximum allowable blood loss (MABL). Items needed to do this are:

- Estimated blood volume for that patient's age (Table 6.1)
- The patient's starting hemoglobin (Hgb)
- The minimum allowable Hgb for that patient, taking into account the patient's underlying medical conditions and pathophysiology, based on your clinical judgment

Overall Fluid Management

Intraoperatively, a patient needs fluid and/or blood for three reasons: maintenance, insensible losses, and surgical blood loss.

Maintenance deficits are calculated based on the 4-2-1 rule. Multiply the first 10 kg of weight by 4, the next 10 kg of weight by 2, and every kg over 20 kg of weight by 1. The result is the patient's hourly maintenance fluid requirement.

$$4\times(\text{first } 10\text{ kg})+2\times(\text{next } 10\text{ kg})+1\times(\text{every kg over } 20\text{ kg})=\text{maintenance deficits}$$

For example, for an 8-kg child, the hourly maintenance fluid rate would be 32 mL of crystalloid.

$$4\times(8\text{ kg})=32$$

For a 20-kg child, the hourly maintenance fluid rate would be 60 mL of crystalloid.

$$4\times(10\text{ kg})+2\times(10\text{ kg})=40+20=60$$

Table 6.1 Estimated Blood Volume by Age

Age	Volume
Premature neonate	100 mL/kg
Neonate	85–90 mL/kg
Infant	80 mL/kg
Child/adult	65–75 mL/kg

Formula to use: Maximum allowable blood loss = estimated blood volume × (starting hemoglobin – minimum allowable hemoglobin)/starting hemoglobin.

For each hour that the patient is NPO, the patient will require this amount of fluid. Generally, half of this deficit is replaced with Lactated Ringer's solution (LR) over the first hour, and the second half is replaced over the next 8 hours. For example, for a 20-kg child, you would replace 30 mL over the first hour and 30 mL extra over the next 8 hours.

Insensible losses are 0 to 10 mL/kg/hr depending on the surgical procedure. For example, a patient with a large abdominal incision and exposed bowel will lose 10 mL/kg/hr. Take caution and use clinical judgment, however, because excessive fluid administration may lead to edema, making the surgery more difficult. Children who are younger, especially those who are preterm, will have a higher amount of insensible fluid loss. Younger patients have higher skin permeability, more body surface area for their weight, and a higher metabolic demand. Insensible fluid loss is also increased by the use of radiant warmers and phototherapy. To preserve body heat and reduce insensible water loss, we suggest using a warming mattress, forced-air warming, and/or a heated humidifier.

Surgical blood loss is particularly hazardous in children, given their low baseline blood volume. Crystalloid can be used initially; however, colloid (e.g., albumin), and blood products must be promptly considered for larger amounts of blood loss, based on clinical judgment and lab measurements. Blood loss and transfusion should additionally be discussed with the surgical team. Normally, mild anemia is tolerated in children when intravascular volume deficits are repleted. In addition to lab values, use clinical indicators including postoperative urinary output, heart rate, respiratory rate, and overall hemodynamic stability to guide transfusion decisions. The development of lactic acidosis is a late sign of inadequate oxygen-carrying capacity.

In general:

- If crystalloid is used to compensate for surgical blood loss, use 3 mL of crystalloid for every 1 mL of blood loss.
- If colloid is used to compensate for surgical blood loss, use 1 mL of colloid for every 1 mL of blood loss.
- If blood products are used to compensate for surgical blood loss, use 1 mL of packed red blood cells (PBRCs) for every 1 mL of blood loss.

Caution! PRBCs may contain large amounts of potassium (5–60 mEq/L, depending on PRBC age). Use caution to avoid hyperkalemia and treat hyperkalemia if it does occur. In children at risk for hyperkalemia (including neonates, large or rapid transfusions, and children with renal insufficiency), the blood bank should take steps to reduce the potassium content of the PBRCs that are provided. This may include washing and/or providing recently donated units. If available, running the PRBCs through a cell saver will reduce potassium even further.[3]

- If greater than 1 blood volume of PRBCs is given, consider giving fresh frozen plasma (FFP) and platelets

Children, especially neonates, have a decreased ability to metabolize citrate. If rapid administration of blood products occurs (>1 mL/kg/min), calcium must also be given. This is especially true for FFP, which is the blood product with the greatest citrate concentration. Transfusion of FFP at rates exceeding 1.0 mL/kg/min can cause severe ionized hypocalcemia leading to myocardial depression and a decreased blood pressure. Therefore, IV calcium chloride (2.5–5 mg/kg) or calcium gluconate (7.5–15 mg/kg) should be administered in a separate IV line when FFP is given, especially when FFP is given rapidly. Check blood calcium levels frequently during blood product administration. Neonates given FFP are at particular risk for hypocalcemia, possibly owing to their lessened ability to mobilize calcium and metabolize citrate. Patients with decreased hepatic function will also have a decreased capability to metabolize citrate.

> **WARNING!!** When giving fluids, it is important to consider the fact that the neonatal kidney is unable to excrete sizeable amounts of extra water or electrolytes, and therefore excessive fluid can easily cause congestive heart failure in a neonate.

A hematocrit of 20% or even slightly less is tolerated in many children; however, this must be determined using your clinical judgment on a case-by-case basis. Patients who do not tolerate a lower Hgb include newborns (especially those born prematurely) and patients in whom an increased oxygen-carrying capacity must be maintained, such as those with respiratory failure or cyanotic congenital heart disease. Keep in mind that neonates and premature infants with a hematocrit less than 30% have a higher incidence of apnea.

Hypoglycemia Management

Children younger than 3 months (especially those younger than 1 month) are at risk for hypoglycemia even with standard NPO times. In these children, a blood sugar is often checked at the beginning of the procedure and treated if hypoglycemic, and 5% dextrose in 0.9% normal saline (NS) (could also be 5% dextrose in LR, or 5% dextrose in 0.45% NS depending on the patient's other metabolic needs) is administered at the current maintenance rate. Giving this solution by "piggyback" infusion can help to decrease the chance of an accidental glucose bolus.

Patients on total parenteral nutrition (TPN) are at particular risk for hypoglycemia, and a dextrose-containing solution should be started at maintenance for these patients during the procedure. Additionally, glucose levels should be checked frequently.

In children with mitochondrial diseases, avoid lactate-containing solutions. These children may also have an increased glucose requirement; monitor carefully.

Types of Infusions

Setting up a Blood Intravenous Administration Set

Introduction

A blood IV administration set includes free-flow IV tubing with two separate spikes that connect into a single filter chamber to allow for the efficient administration of two different fluids (these could be any combination of crystalloids, colloids, blood products, and medications). The filter chamber will contain a 170- to 260-micron filter.

Equipment

- IV fluid appropriate for your patient
- Tubing

Step-by-Step

1. **Before attaching tubing to the patient's IV line, spike the IV bag.** Close both roller clamps: above the filter chamber as well as below the filter chamber. Spike the IV bag with one of the Y-tubing spikes (Figure 6.1).
2. **Prime the tubing.** Unclamp the Y-tubing roller clamp and allow fluid to fill the filter chamber approximately halfway (Figure 6.2). If necessary, squeeze the filter chamber in order to fill. Open the roller clamp below the filter chamber and allow tubing to fill ("prime") to gravity (Figure 6.3).

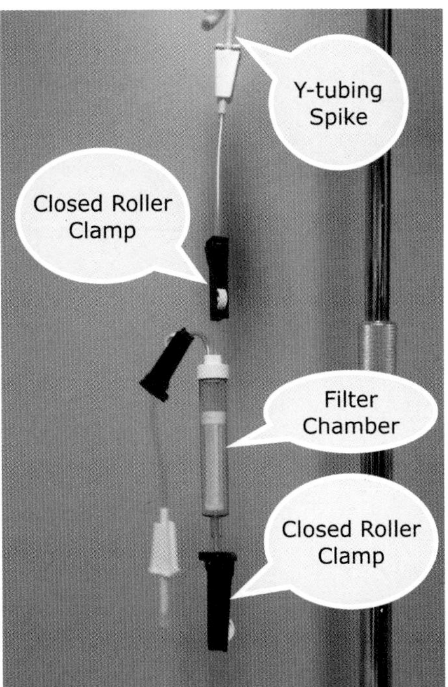

Figure 6.1 Intravenous bag is spiked, and both roller clamps are closed.

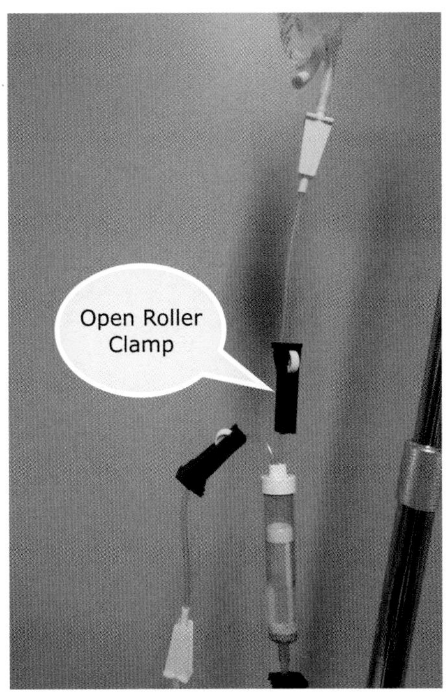

Figure 6.2 Filter chamber is filling with top roller clamp open.

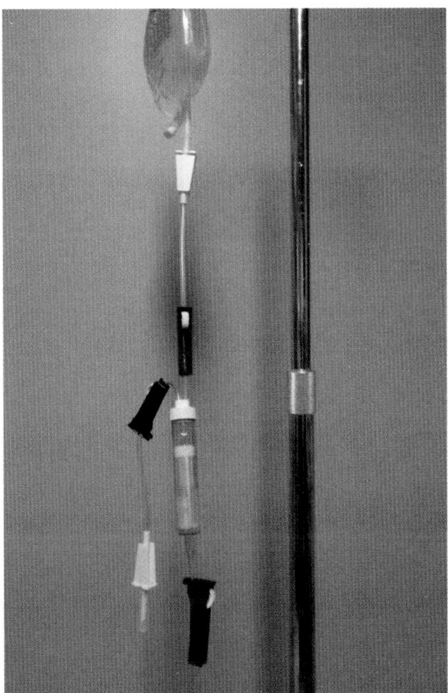

Figure 6.3 Both roller clamps are open with fluid flowing to prime tubing.

> **Caution!** Avoidance of air emboli in infants and small children requires that all air be expelled from IV lines and syringes. To do this, aspirate each injection port to remove air trapped at junctions. Also, before administering a drug intravenously, make sure that no air is trapped in the dead space of the needle or syringe. A volume of air that is clinically inconsequential to an adult may prove disastrous to an infant.

Setting Up a Volume-Control Intravenous Administration Set (Buretrol or Volutrol Tubing)

Introduction

A volume control IV administration set is free-flow IV tubing that uses a 150-mL volumetric cylinder (chamber) to closely control fluid administration.

Clinical Applications

This is most often used for small pediatric patients (<1 year old), when only a small volume of IV fluid is desired.

Equipment

- IV fluid of choice (e.g., crystalloid, colloid)
- Buretrol or Volutrol tubing

>> **Tip on Technique:** To avoid accidental administration of too much fluid, never keep more than 2 hours of maintenance fluid in the chamber.

> **Caution!** Air may be accidentally administered if the Buretrol or Volutrol is allowed to "run dry"—that is, if all of the fluid is already given, air may run into the patient, causing an air embolus.

Step-by-Step

> **WARNING!!** All four of the following steps must be completed, and tubing must be fully primed, with no air bubbles, before attaching the tubing to the patient's IV line.

1. **Spike the IV bag.** Clamp above and below the volumetric chamber (Figure 6.4), and then spike the IV bag.
2. **Fill the volumetric chamber.** Unclamp the clamp above the volumetric chamber (between the IV bag and chamber; Figure 6.5) and allow the chamber to fill to the desired level. Reclamp the clamp above the volumetric chamber.
3. **Prime the tubing.** Unclamp the clamp below the volumetric chamber and allow the tubing to prime to gravity (Figure 6.6).
4. **Raise the volumetric chamber.** Hang the volumetric chamber on the IV pole adjacent to the IV fluid bag to facilitate flow (Figure 6.7).

>> **Tip on Technique:** Always ensure that the flange inside of the volumetric chamber (on the bottom) is open (Figure 6.8). The flange can inadvertently close and inhibit IV flow. Squeezing or lightly tapping the chamber often solves this problem.

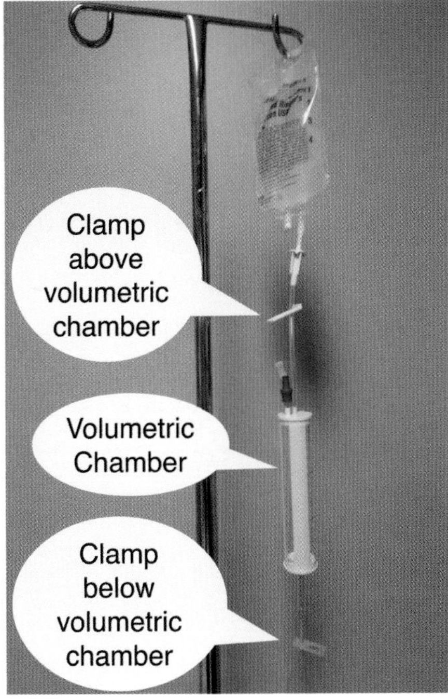

Figure 6.4 Intravenous bag and Buretrol tubing with both clamps clamped.

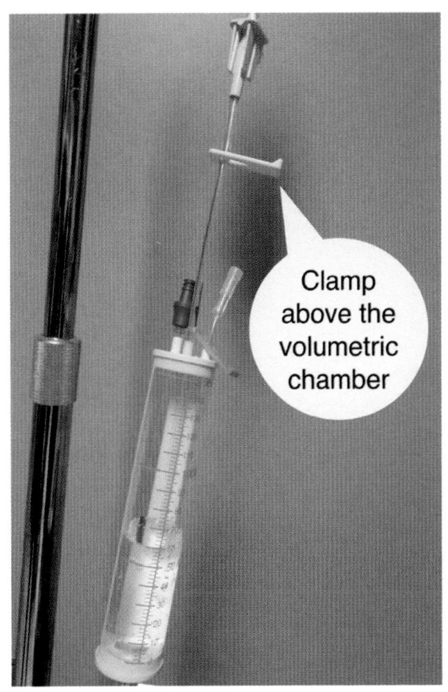

Figure 6.5 Buretrol is filling, and top clamp is unclamped.

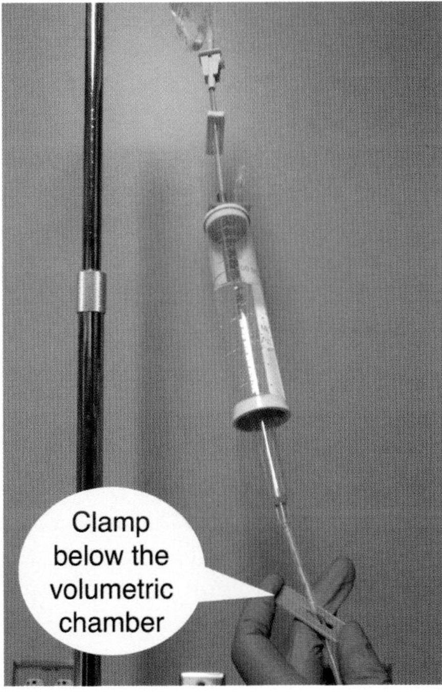

Figure 6.6 Lower Buretrol clamp is being unclamped.

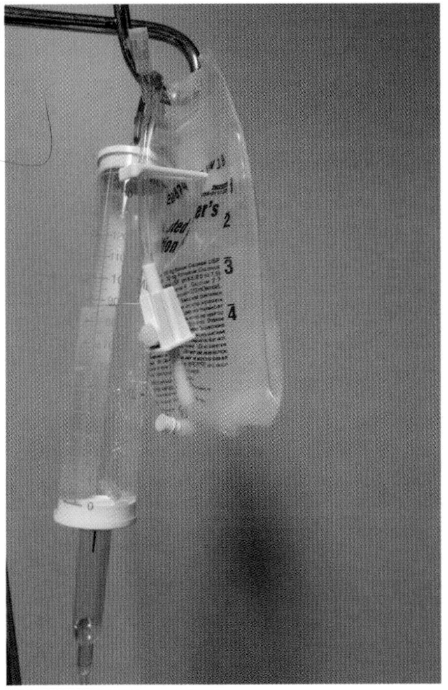

Figure 6.7 Volumetric chamber is hanging on the intravenous pole.

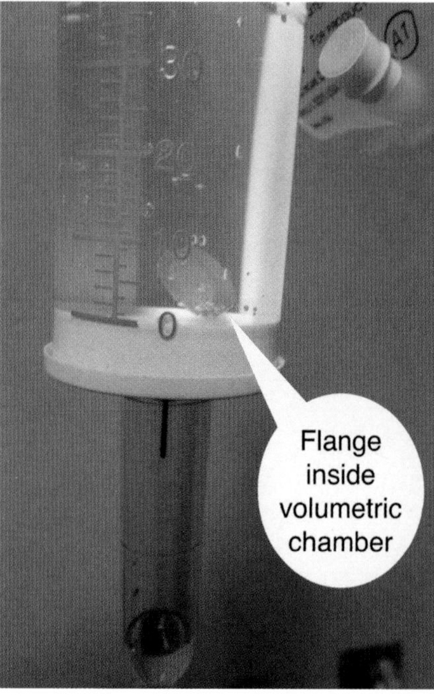

Figure 6.8 Open flange in Buretrol.

Types of Pumps

Smith's Medfusion 4000 Syringe Pump

Introduction

Smith's Medfusion 4000 syringe pump is an infusion pump that uses syringes, from 1 mL up to 60 mL, allowing for precise delivery of medications and fluids while maintaining low fluid volumes.

Clinical Applications

This pump can be used for accurately controlled infusions of IV medications, small volumes of crystalloid and colloid, and blood and blood products.

Equipment

- Smith's Medfusion 4000 syringe pump
- Desired medication or fluid
- Syringe (1–60 mL)
- Compatible tubing. The most commonly used tubing is the standard bore extension set with Luer-Lok. Multiple versions of tubing exist that include a variety of other features, such as a side clamp or stopcock.

WARNING!! If used near a magnetic resonance imaging (MRI) machine, the Smith's Medfusion 4000 syringe pump must be maintained outside of the 150 gauss line and secured to a nonmovable object for MRI (1.5 Tesla) usage.

Pearl: The pump is able to sense an increase in pressure and will sound the alarm if there is a potential occlusion. Reasons for an increase in pressure include viscous medications, a clamped IV line, and positional or kinked IV access. The override occlusion settings can be changed based on provider preference from very sensitive to least sensitive.

Step-by-Step

1. **Turn power on.** Press the power button. Allow the self-test to complete before any further action (Figure 6.9).

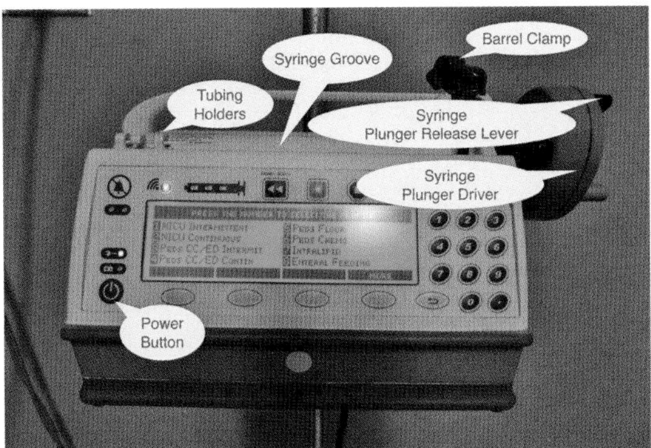

Figure 6.9 Smith's Medfusion 4000 syringe pump.

2. **Load the syringe.** Ensure that the barrel clamp is up and turned away from the syringe groove. The syringe plunger driver should be pulled all the way out by squeezing the syringe plunger release lever. As you place the syringe onto the syringe groove, place the flange of the syringe into the flange clip (Figure 6.10).

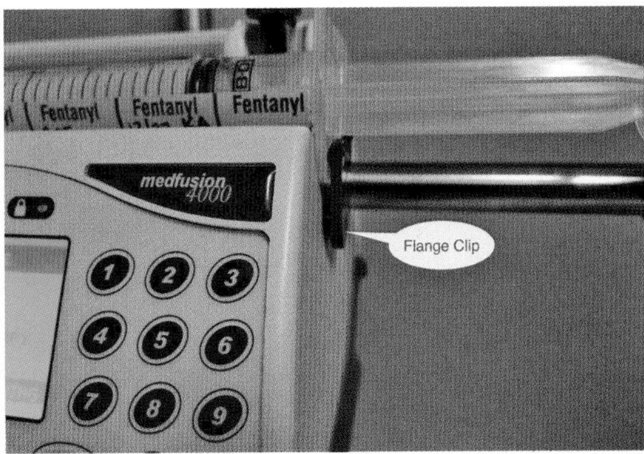

Figure 6.10 Smith's Medfusion 4000 syringe pump. Flange of syringe is placed into flange clip.

Squeeze the syringe plunger release lever and push the drive toward the end of syringe, until the plunger of the syringe is held within the syringe plunger holders. Move the barrel clamp onto the syringe (Figures 6.11–6.13). Thread the tubing through the tubing holders (Figure 6.14).

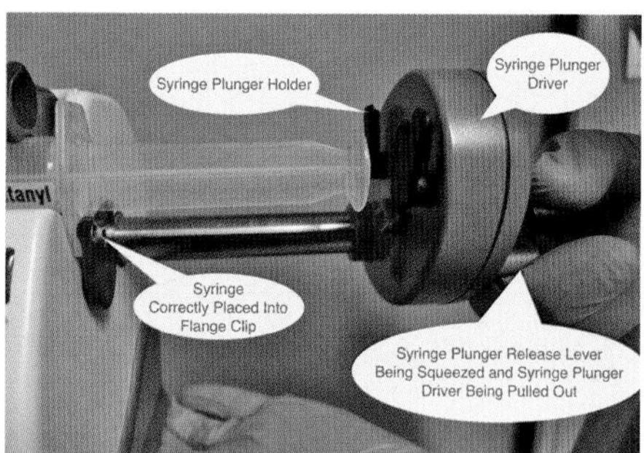

Figure 6.11 Smith's Medfusion 4000 syringe pump. Syringe is placed in flange clip, and syringe plunger driver is pulled out.

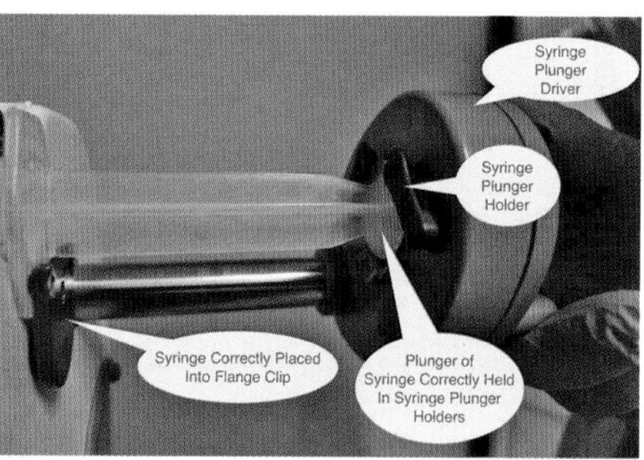

Figure 6.12 Smith's Medfusion 4000 syringe pump: Plunger of syringe is held in syringe plunger holders.

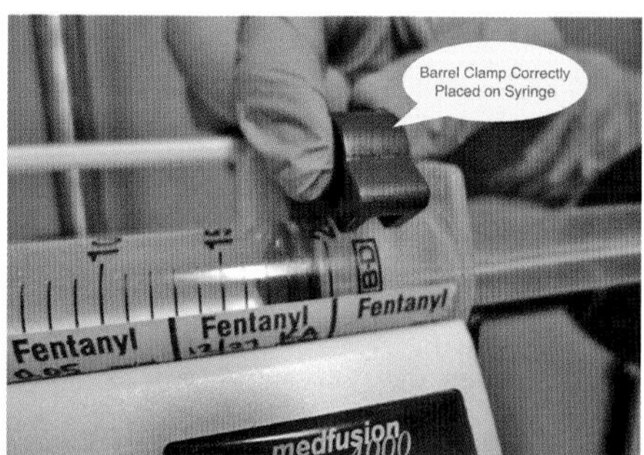

Figure 6.13 Smith's Medfusion 4000 syringe pump. Barrel clamp is on syringe.

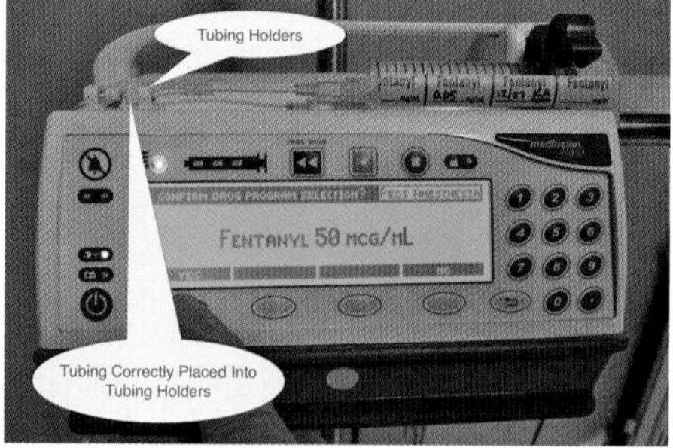

Figure 6.14 Smith's Medfusion 4000 syringe pump. Thread the tubing through the tubing holders.

Select the correct syringe model on the screen (Figure 6.15). Confirm the syringe model, size, and loading (Figure 6.16).

Pearl: Most commonly, an alarm indicating improper syringe placement results from the improper placement of (1) the flange clip, (2) the plunger driver, or (3) the barrel clamp. When the pump sounds the alarm, it will display a picture with instructions (Figure 6.17).

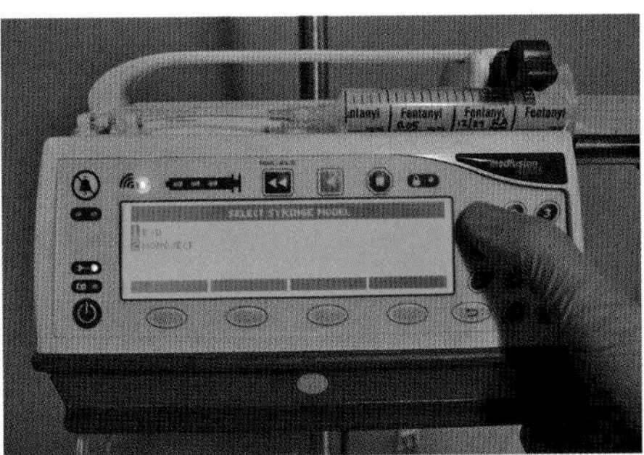

Figure 6.15 Smith's Medfusion 4000 syringe pump. Select the correct syringe model on the screen.

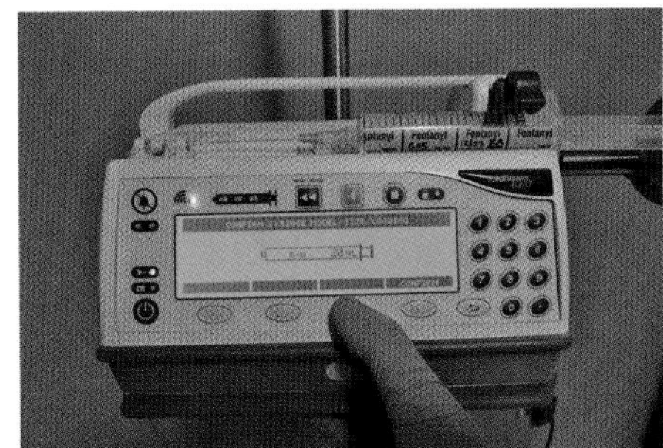

Figure 6.16 Smith's Medfusion 4000 syringe pump. Confirm the syringe model, size, and loading.

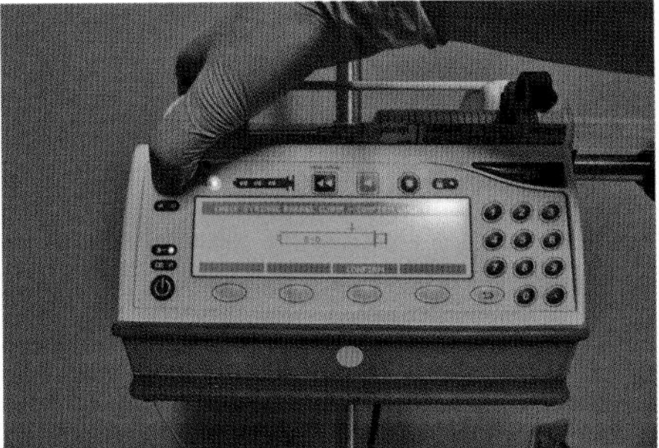

Figure 6.17 Smith's Medfusion 4000 syringe pump. Troubleshooting the alarm.

3. **Program an infusion for delivery.** There will be a series of screen confirmations. Use the number keys to do the following: Select Profile. Select Category. Select Drug. Program Infusion Parameters (this may include entering the patient's weight and the desired dose).

> **Caution!** Always ensure that the drug concentration in the profile matches the drug concentration of the medication you will be delivering.

Prime the pump and administration set (skip this step if the administration set was already primed).

> **Caution!** DO NOT prime any syringe while tubing is connected to the patient.

Confirm all settings and press start.

>> **Tip on Technique:** Always use the smallest syringe size possible for the medication you are administering. The minimum recommended infusion rate is dependent on the syringe model and size and whether FlowSentry (rapid occlusion detection) is enabled. For example, for a 50-mL syringe with FlowSentry enabled, the minimum recommended infusion rate is 0.6 mL/hr. See the manufacturer's literature for further recommendations.

4. **Program a bolus dose.** After the infusion is programmed, program a bolus dose, if needed, using the "options" soft key OR the "prime/bolus" key. Confirm selections and press start to deliver the bolus. The infusion will resume administration after the bolus is delivered.

   Note: For both loading and bolus dose delivery, if the pressure in the line is too high, an occlusion alarm may occur. After sounding the alarm, the pump will continue delivering the loading/bolus dose at 70% of the initial rate.

5. **Program standby mode, if desired.** To delay the programmed infusion to start later, choose the "options" soft key and press the number key for "standby"; if the infusion has already been started, you will need to press the pause button. Enter the amount of time for the infusion to be held (up to 24 hours) and press enter. The pump will display a countdown of the standby time remaining. The pump will sound the alarm when the standby time is complete. The clinician can begin the infusion at any time while in standby by pressing the "start" button.

Baxter SIGMA Spectrum Infusion Pump

Introduction

This pump uses the Dose Error Reduction System (DERS), which is an extensive library of drugs, including dosage and infusion rate information to prevent drug infusion errors. This preprogrammed drug library should be used whenever possible. The pump also includes a BASIC mode, which should only be used when a drug is not present in the library.

Clinical Applications

This pump can be used for administration of IV fluids as well as continuous and intermittent medication infusions.

Equipment

- Baxter SIGMA Spectrum infusion pump
- IV fluid of choice
- Compatible Baxter IV tubing

WARNING!! The SIGMA Spectrum infusion pump is not MRI compatible.

Step-by-Step

1. **Prime the tubing.** Clamp the tubing using either the roller clamp or slide clamp. Spike the IV infusion bag and fill the drip chamber about halfway. Open the clamp and allow the tubing to prime to gravity, ensuring that no air is in the tubing. Clamp tubing using the slide clamp, about 6 to 8 inches below the upper fill chamber (Figure 6.18).

2. **Load the tubing into the pump.** Insert the slide clamp into the keyhole on the top of the pump (Figure 6.19). This will open the door of the pump and turn the pump on. Load the tubing from the top to the bottom, pressing on loading points 1 through 4 until the screen displays three green bars and checkmarks. This indicates that the tubing is properly loaded (Figure 6.20). Close the door and remove the slide clamp from the top of the pump (Figure 6.21). Open the roller clamp, if closed.

Caution!	After priming the tubing and loading it into the pump, open the roller clamp and slide the clamp out BEFORE connecting the infusion to the patient. Opening these clamps may result in a bolus of up to 0.2 mL. Similarly, closing the door of the pump while the tubing is connected to the patient may also result in a bolus of drug.

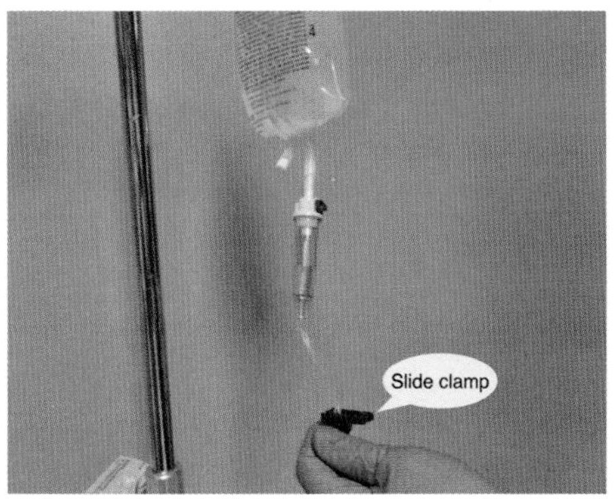

Figure 6.18 Baxter SIGMA infusion pump. Intravenous tubing clamped with tubing primed.

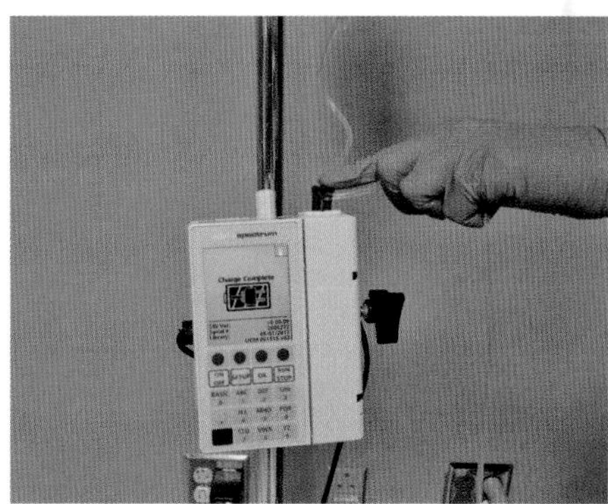

Figure 6.19 Baxter SIGMA infusion pump. The slide clamp is inserted into the keyhole.

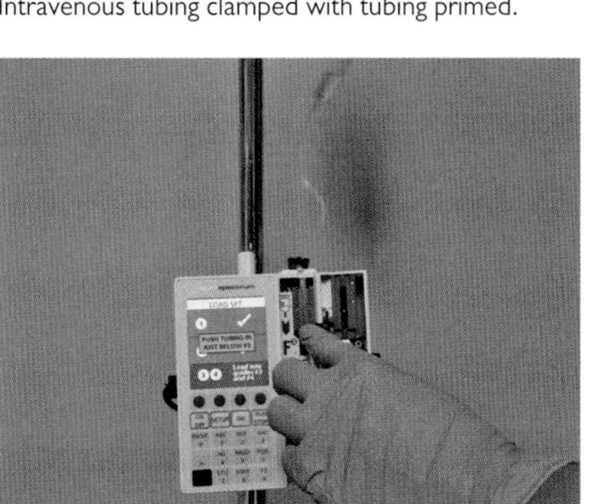

Figure 6.20 Baxter SIGMA infusion pump. Loading the tubing into the pump.

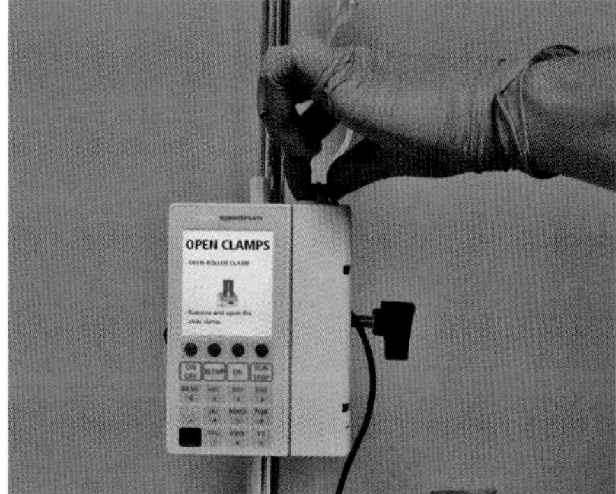

Figure 6.21 Baxter SIGMA infusion pump. Pump door is closed, and the slide clamp is removed from the pump.

3. **Program the pump.** After turning the pump on, a "New Patient?" prompt will appear. Select "Yes" to clear previous programming. The pump will display a series of prompts to program a specific infusion. These prompts will include information regarding the care area, drug, concentration, and volume to be infused. BASIC mode may also be used ONLY if the intended infusion is not listed in the drug library.
4. **Select desired mode.** Press "Run/Stop" to start the infusion. Press "Hold" to place the pump in standby mode.

> **Caution!** The infusion rate for "minidrip" infusion sets (60 drips/mL) should not exceed 200 mL/hr. The infusion rate for sets with back check valves should not exceed 500 mL/hr.

Cardinal AlarisPC Infusion Pump

Introduction

The Cardinal AlarisPC Pump module allows for continuous or intermittent delivery of fluid, blood, blood products, and medications. The PC unit is the main interface of the Alaris system for point-of-care programming and monitoring. Clinicians can attach up to four IV infusion modules onto a single PC unit, allowing for efficient use of space and organization of infusions.

Clinical Applications

The Cardinal AlarisPC Pump module is used for infusions of medications and IV fluids.

Equipment

- The Alaris Pump Module (Figure 6.22)
- IV fluid of choice
- Alaris compatible tubing

> **Caution!** The Alaris Pump Module allows for a maximum of four infusion/monitoring modules. Any modules in excess of four will not be recognized.

> **WARNING!!** The Alaris infusion pump is not MRI compatible and is not compatible with Stereotaxis Technology.

Step-by-Step

1. **Attach module.** Position the free module at a 45-degree angle to the PC unit (or another module), aligning the IUI connectors. Continue to rotate the free module down against the PC unit (or another module) until the release latch clicks in place (Figure 6.23).

   >> **Tip on Technique:** Modules can be attached either to the side of the PC unit or to the side of another module. The process for attachment and detachment is the same, whether it is the PC unit or module.

   Pearl: Modules are always displayed from left to right. If a module is added to the left of other modules, the modules will be reidentified. Module identification does not interfere with active infusion or monitoring of an activated module.

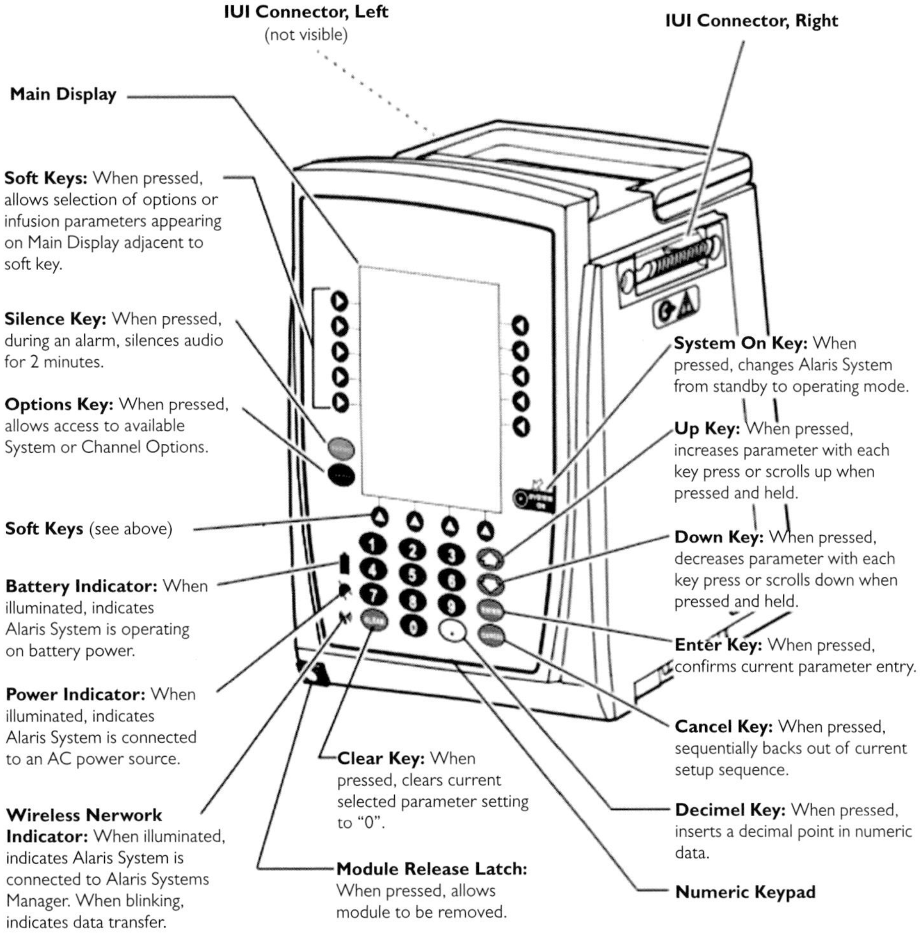

IUI Connector, Left (not visible)

IUI Connector, Right

Main Display

Soft Keys: When pressed, allows selection of options or infusion parameters appearing on Main Display adjacent to soft key.

Silence Key: When pressed, during an alarm, silences audio for 2 minutes.

Options Key: When pressed, allows access to available System or Channel Options.

Soft Keys (see above)

Battery Indicator: When illuminated, indicates Alaris System is operating on battery power.

Power Indicator: When illuminated, indicates Alaris System is connected to an AC power source.

Wireless Nerwork Indicator: When illuminated, indicates Alaris System is connected to Alaris Systems Manager. When blinking, indicates data transfer.

Clear Key: When pressed, clears current selected parameter setting to "0".

Module Release Latch: When pressed, allows module to be removed.

System On Key: When pressed, changes Alaris System from standby to operating mode.

Up Key: When pressed, increases parameter with each key press or scrolls up when pressed and held.

Down Key: When pressed, decreases parameter with each key press or scrolls down when pressed and held.

Enter Key: When pressed, confirms current parameter entry.

Cancel Key: When pressed, sequentially backs out of current setup sequence.

Decimel Key: When pressed, inserts a decimal point in numeric data.

Numeric Keypad

Figure 6.22 Alaris Pump Module, Model 8015.

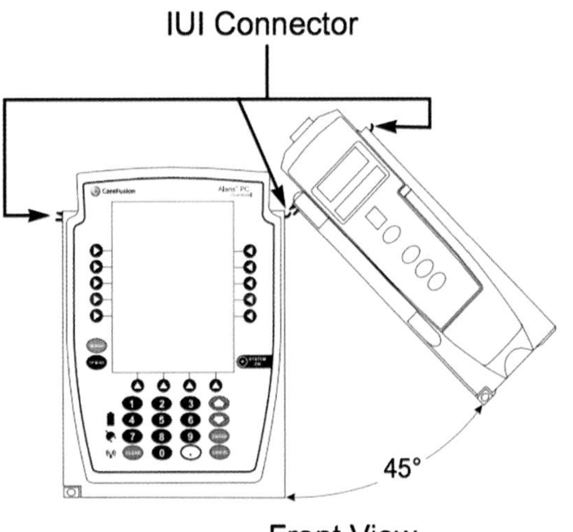

Figure 6.23 Alaris Pump Module, Model 8015. Free module is at a 45-degree angle to the PC unit.

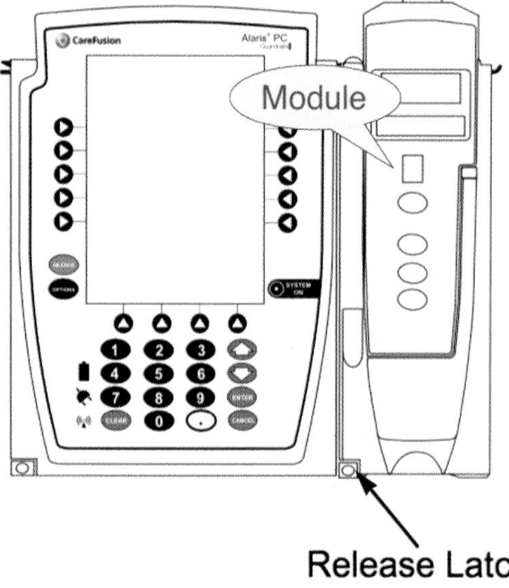

Figure 6.24 Alaris Pump Module, Model 8015. Front view is shown of the PC unit and module connected, with an *arrow* pointing to the release latch.

2. **Power on the system, select a new patient, and program the module.** Push the "System On" key which begins a system self-test. At the end of the self-test, a "New Patient?" screen appears. Selecting the "Yes" soft key clears all previous parameters from memory. Program the module with your desired infusion.

   Note: For System Options please see: http://www.carefusion.com/Documents/guides/user-guides/IF_Alaris-System-8015-v9-19_UG_EN.pdf.

3. **Detach module (if desired).** The module must be powered off before detaching. Push the module release latch (Figure 6.24) and then rotate the module up and away from the PC unit (or attached module) to disengage their IUI connectors. The Alaris System will now recognize the new configuration and display module position(s) (A, B, or C, from left to right) on the main display.

References

1. Miller RD, ed. *Miller's Anesthesia.* 7th ed. Philadelphia, PA: Elsevier; 2009.
2. Alaris PC Unit User Manual. Available at http://www.carefusion.com/Documents/guides/user-guides/IF_Alaris-System-8015-v9-19_UG_EN.pdf.
3. Westphal-Varghese B, Erren M, Westphal M, et al. Processing of stored packed red blood cells using autotransfusion devices decreases potassium and microaggregates: a prospective, randomized, single-blinded in vitro study. *Transfus Med.* 2007;17(2):89–95.

Chapter 7
Peripheral Intravenous Line Access

Tristan Levey, Andrew Wuenstel, and Amanda Foley

Introduction

To start a peripheral intravenous (IV) line, identify the site, place the tourniquet proximal to the IV site, clean the skin, stabilize the vein, and insert the catheter. When a "flash" of blood return is seen, advance the needle slightly, thread the catheter, connect the catheter to tubing, and secure with a sterile dressing.

Clinical Applications

Peripheral IV access is used to administer IV fluids or medications.

Contraindications

A peripheral IV should be avoided at any site with infection, compression, or proximal obstruction.

Critical Anatomy

Common IV access sites in children are the metacarpal, saphenous, cephalic, median, and scalp veins. These veins vary in size, depth, and difficulty.

A. **Metacarpal/dorsal hand veins** are on the dorsal aspect of the hand and typically arise from adjacent digital veins and form a network that usually provides several targets for access, although there is significant variation. These veins form the cephalic vein (radial side) and basilic vein (ulnar side) as they converge (Figure 7.1).

>> **Tip on Technique:** Hand veins are superficial and move easily, making anchoring difficult. During IV insertion, the skin should be held taut but without compressing the vein.

>> **Tip on Technique:** Before removing the needle from the catheter, use your finger to compress the vein just proximal to the catheter tip to prevent bleeding while you hook up the IV tubing.

Pearl: For 'blind' placement of an IV into a metacarpal vein that cannot be visualized, it is helpful to remember that a metacarpal vein is often located between the fourth and fifth metacarpal bones on the dorsum of the hand.

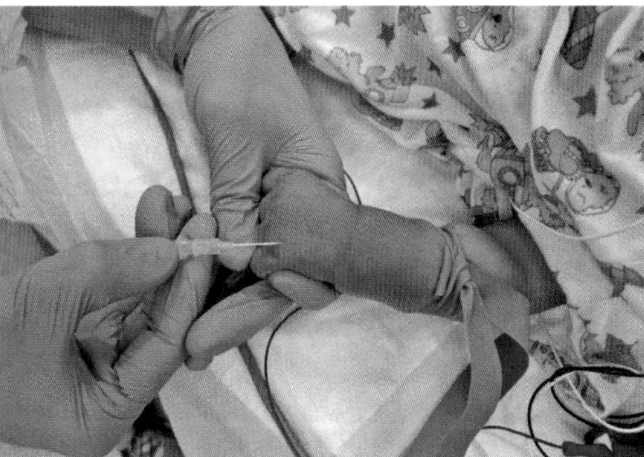

Figure 7.1 Needle approaching a metacarpal hand vein.

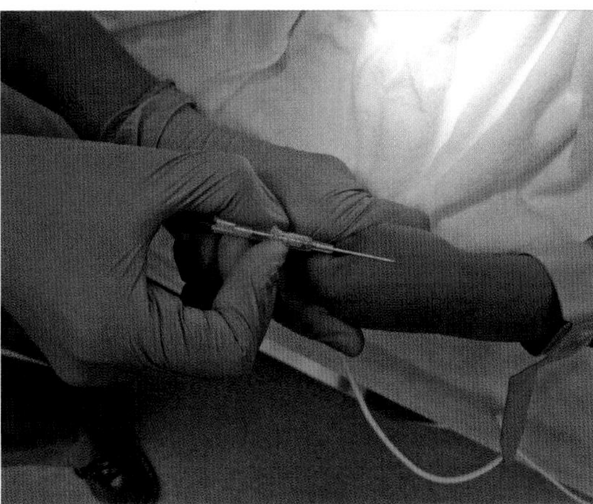

Figure 7.2 Needle approaching the cephalic vein.

B. **The cephalic vein** arises from the lateral (radial) side of the dorsal venous network before curving around the wrist to run along the anterolateral forearm, where it is frequently easily accessed. It continues on this course up the arm, but more proximally it is less superficial (Figure 7.2).

Pearl: The cephalic vein is commonly known as the "intern's vein" because it is both large and superficial, making it an easy target for access.

C. **The median cubital vein** runs from the cephalic vein medially toward the basilic vein diagonally across the antecubital fossa and is reliably present if not always visible.

>> Tip on Technique: Although easy to access, an IV in the antecubital fossa is susceptible to disruptions in flow if the patient's forearm is flexed. An arm board may help to preserve an antecubital IV in a patient who cannot reliably keep the forearm extended.

Note: In about 20% of patients, the median cubital vein divides at the antecubital fossa into basilic (medial) and cephalic (lateral) components. It is the basilic (medial) vein that runs superficial to the median nerve and brachial artery and vein in this variant of the population.

WARNING!!	The medial nerve, brachial artery, and brachial vein are under the median vein and can be accidentally punctured if the needle goes too deep. These deeper structures are separated by the bicipital aponeurosis fascial plane from the superficial veins.

D. **The greater saphenous vein** is formed on the foot from the dorsal vein of the great toe and the dorsal venous arch of the foot. It ascends anteriorly to the medial malleolus and superiorly up the medial calf (Figure 7.3).

Pearl: The saphenous vein is frequently accessed blindly given that it is the largest superficial vein of the lower extremity with relatively little variation in its course.

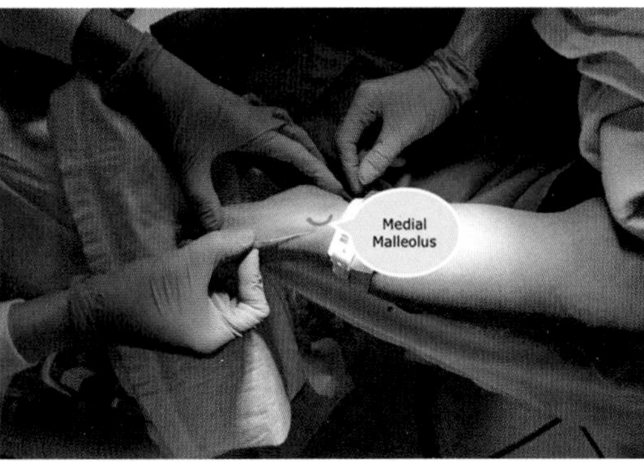

Figure 7.3 Needle approaching the saphenous vein.

E. **The superficial veins of the scalp** can be used as a last resort to obtain superficial IV access in an infant or small child. The scalp veins are popular because there is minimal subcutaneous tissue to traverse and the scalp has very little motion after the IV is placed. Many clinicians target the superficial temporal veins, which originate in the preauricular space and divide into the frontal and parietal branches as they spread anteriorly or superiorly, respectively, over the scalp. There is significant variation in the venous network of the scalp, but veins usually run adjacent to their corresponding artery. The tourniquet used to promote venous engorgement when placing the line is created by placing a rubber band around the infant's head like a headband.

>> **Tip on Technique:** When placing a scalp catheter, the clinician should sit or stand at the head of the bed.

>> **Tip on Technique:** The clinician may choose to place the patient in a slight head-down position for gravity to promote venous engorgement. If the potential IV site is hairy, shave the site before placing the IV to make it easier to secure with tape.

Setup

Equipment

- Tourniquet
- Alcohol or chlorhexidine swabs (avoid chlorhexidine in newborns)
- Peripheral IV catheter (14–24 gauge, depending on ease of insertion and requirements)
- Gauze
- IV tubing
- Tape to secure catheter

>> **Tip on Technique:** Have all equipment you may need available and nearby when you perform the procedure (see step 1).

Drugs, Dosages, Administration

If the IV line is being placed in an awake patient, sedation, local anesthetic, or a distraction device may be needed. Commonly used drugs include topical EMLA cream (Eutectic Mixture of Local Anesthetics, containing lidocaine 2.5% and prilocaine 2.5%) or subcutaneous lidocaine. Devices for distraction include J-Tip and Buzzy.

>> **Tip on Technique:** If using EMLA cream, apply at least 20 to 30 minutes in advance of placing the IV catheter to allow time for the local anesthetic to work.

WARNING!!	Prilocaine, one of the components of EMLA cream, can cause methemoglobinemia in some patients in large doses.
WARNING!!	If using local anesthetics, carefully calculate the maximum dose (including that which will be given intravenously during surgery and by the surgeon) to prevent local anesthetic systemic toxicity (LAST). See Chapter 15: Local Anesthetic Systemic Toxicity Treatment

Step-by-Step

1. **Prepare for the procedure.** Have all equipment you may need available, including multiple catheters and sizes.

   >> **Tip on Technique:** Applying a warm compress to the IV site can increase vasodilation and make IV placement easier.

   >> **Tip on Technique:** Before starting, loosen the catheter from the needle by advancing the catheter slightly off of the needle and then returning the catheter to its original position. This helps the catheter to advance easily during IV placement.

2. **Position the patient, identify landmarks, and prepare the skin.** Position the patient so that the vein being accessed is parallel to the trajectory of the dominant arm of the person performing the procedure.

   >> **Tip on Technique:** Lowering the IV site to below the level of the heart will increase venous engorgement, increasing the likelihood of success.

   Choose the IV insertion site and position the patient. The tourniquet is placed proximally to the desired IV site, and the skin is disinfected. For an awake patient, administer subcutaneous local anesthetic at the IV site (if EMLA was not already used) and/or use a distraction method.

   >> **Tip on Technique:** Place the tourniquet proximally on the upper extremity to allow for multiple site attempts. Avoid bony areas because it will be difficult to compress the vein adequately.

3. **Insert the needle into the peripheral vein.** Anchor the vein with the thumb of your nondominant hand. The angle of approach should be less than 30 degrees. The more parallel the approach to the vein, the less risk for going "through and through," or puncturing the back wall of the vein. Insert the IV catheter and advance until you see a "flash" of blood in the catheter, indicating vascular puncture. In larger peripheral IVs, the practitioner usually sees blood continually flow back into the catheter, which helps confirm that the catheter is still in the vein. After obtaining blood return, decrease the angle of your needle, parallel to the vein. A common mistake is to try to thread the catheter immediately after blood return is obtained. After blood return is obtained, the needle and catheter must first be advanced

together, before threading the catheter, because a short distance exists between the tip of the needle and the start of the catheter (~1 mm for a 24-gauge IV, ~5 mm for a 14-gauge IV).

> **Caution!** Try to avoid placing a peripheral IV line over a joint or crease (e.g., wrist, metacarpophalangeal joint) because it will be more easily displaced.

>> **Tip on Technique:** Preferentially start at a branch point, if visualized, because the vein is more stable at this point, which will help to prevent "rolling."

>> **Tip on Technique:** If the vein is long enough, begin more distally. If the first attempt is unsuccessful, cannulation of the same vein can then be attempted more proximally. However, if you attempt to place an IV line and fail, you may create a hole in the vessel. A failed attempt may also cause the vessel to spasm and therefore make a more proximal location on the same vessel more difficult to cannulate.

4. **Thread the catheter and remove the tourniquet.** Thread the catheter off of the needle into the vein and then remove the tourniquet.

> **WARNING!!** Always remove the tourniquet after the IV line is placed. Keep track of all sharps used during insertion to avoid accidental needle sticks to patients or medical staff.

5. **Test and secure tubing.** Tighten the connection between the IV catheter and tubing while trying not to move or rotate the catheter. Ensure adequate flow of IV fluids and the absence of infiltration. Place a sterile dressing so that the IV site and surrounding skin are visible through the bandage. Ensure that that patient is positioned for the surgery or procedure so that flow through the peripheral IV is not impeded.

>> **Tip on Technique:** Loop the IV tubing without kinking and tape it in place. This loop will help prevent the peripheral IV from being pulled out if the tubing is pulled on. Occasionally, if the tip of the catheter is against a vein, valves in the vein may prevent flow in the IV line. In that case, you may need to retract the skin or catheter a few millimeters to achieve return of flow.

> **WARNING!!** Ensure the catheter is secured TIGHTLY to the tubing. Remember to remove all of the sharps from the area.

Postoperative Management Considerations

Patients should be monitored closely. Complications of peripheral IV line placement include infiltration and hematoma. Later complications also include infection, thrombophlebitis, and inadvertent administration of medications into the surrounding tissues if the IV is infiltrated. Infiltration is more common in the pediatric population, affecting up to 11% of hospitalized children. Premature infants are especially susceptible.

Further Reading

Bergvall E, Sawyer T. Scalp vein catheterization technique: catheterization of scalp veins, complications. *Emedicinemedscapecom*. 2017. Available at: http://emedicine.medscape.com/article/1348863-technique#c2.

Moore K, Dalley A, Agur A. *Clinically Oriented Anatomy*. 1st ed. London: Lippincott Williams & Wilkins; 2010.

Reynolds P, MacLaren R, Mueller S, et al. Management of extravasation injuries: a focused evaluation of noncytotoxic medications. *Pharmacotherapy*. 2014;34(6):617–632.

Riker M, Kennedy C, Winfrey B, et al. Validation and refinement of the difficult intravenous access score: a clinical prediction rule for identifying children with difficult intravenous access. *Acad Emerg Med*. 2011;18(11):1129–1134.

Chapter 8
Pediatric Intraosseous Placement

Samuel C. Seiden

Introduction

Intraosseous access permits rapid delivery of most fluids and medications when venous access is not possible. Intraosseous access is achieved by introducing a hollow needle into the bone marrow, either by punching or drilling through the bone cortex, so that the tip of the needle is located within the marrow space. The bone marrow is highly vascularized, and fluids and medications that are delivered into the bone marrow will quickly be absorbed into the systemic circulation.

There are several options for devices for obtaining intraosseous access. For the manual technique, products such as the Cook (Bloomington, IN) or Jamshidi™ (Carefusion, San Diego, CA) intraosseous infusion needle are popular. When using a manual device, the intraosseous space is entered using a continuous, rotational force at the desired site. Other options include an intraosseous drill, such as the EZ-IO® (Vidacare, Shavano Park, TX), or an intraosseous automatic injection device, such as the NIO™ (PerSys Medical, Houston, TX) or BIG (Bone Injection Gun, WaisMed Company, Houston, TX).

Although manual devices (Figure 8.1) are lightweight and easy to carry, the drill or automatic injection device (Figure 8.2) may help to regulate the amount of pressure that is used to access the bone marrow cavity and may also indicate when the intramedullary space is entered. Using a drill may lessen the probability that the practitioner will "skive" or "slip" off of the bone when attempting to enter the intramedullary space. Use of a drill or automatic injection device might also decrease the time required to obtain access or increase the probability of success on the first attempt; in one small study of 107 paramedics using adult mannequin models, "success rates for first intraosseous injection attempt were higher for the BIG (91.59%) than EZ-IO® (82.66%) or Jamshidi (47.66%)." Mean procedure time was 2.0 ± 0.7 for the BIG device vs

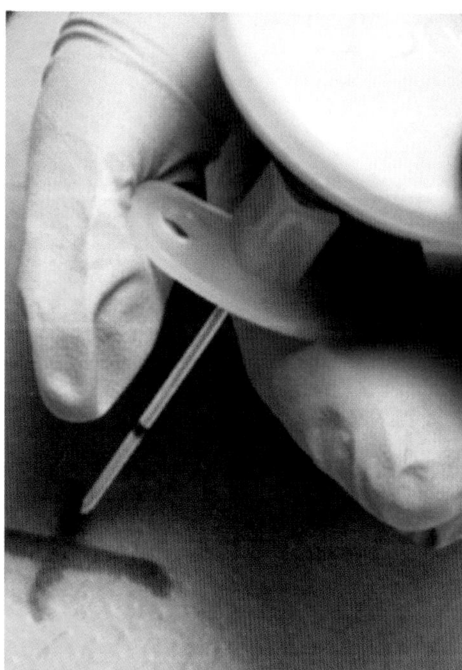

Figure 8.1 Intraosseous insertion site with manual device about to enter the skin.

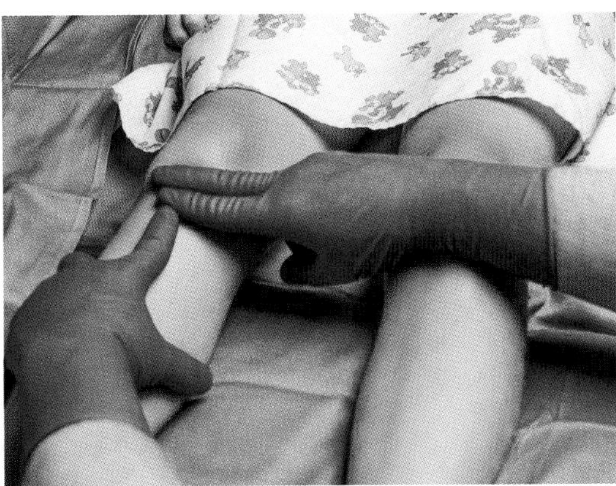

Figure 8.2 Proximal Tibia Intraosseous Site: Landmark identified two fingerbreadths below the base of the patella and one fingerbreadth medial in a child on the flat surface of the bone.

3.1 ± 0.9 minutes for the EZ-IO® device vs 4.2 ± 1.0 minutes for the Jamshidi device."[1] Many intraosseous needles are approved for specific indications in a given country. Medications that have been reported as safe and effective when administered by the intraosseous route include vasoactive drugs, neuromuscular blocking agents, antibiotics, propofol and other hypnotics, blood, albumin, and crystalloid. Hypertonic or alkaline solutions should be avoided or diluted.[2]

Clinical Applications

Because the intraosseous space does not collapse, it can be used as a rapid source of vascular access in patients who are volume depleted or in whom vascular access cannot be obtained by peripheral or central routes. The most recent American Heart Association/American Academy of Pediatrics guidelines for Pediatric Advanced Life Support state that in an emergency situation, "intraosseous (IO) access can be quickly established with minimal complications by providers with varied levels of training. Limit the time spent attempting to establish peripheral venous access in a critically ill or injured child."[3] This guideline also states that, in an emergency, "IO access is a rapid, safe, effective, and acceptable route for vascular access in children."[3]

Note: Analysis of blood samples drawn from an intraosseous site may damage a blood gas machine or laboratory equipment or yield inaccurate results. Veldhoen et al.[4] concluded that using a single-use, cartridge-based analyser could prevent bone marrow from damaging laboratory equipment. This study also compared intraosseous with intravenous blood samples in hemodynamically stable patients, using the i-STAT point-of-care device, and found that the values obtained were clinically acceptable for pH, base excess, sodium, ionized calcium, and glucose and that "the intraclass correlation coefficient was excellent (>0.8) for comparison of intraosseous and intravenous base excess, and moderate (around 0.6) for bicarbonate, sodium and glucose."[4] Another study that compared intraosseous and arterial samples found that similar values for hemoglobin, hematocrit, pH, glucose, and lactate were obtained; potassium levels, base excess, and bicarbonate were higher in the IO sample; and sodium and ionized calcium values were slightly lower.[5]

Contraindications

Absolute contraindications to intraosseous access include a fracture at or proximal to the desired site of cannulation, infection, and underlying bone disease or infection at the site. Intraosseous vascular access is also contraindicated in the presence of bone diseases (e.g., osteogenesis imperfecta, osteoporosis, and other diseases that place the patient at an increased risk of fracture), a history of trauma or fracture at the chosen site, and prosthetics, such as a rod or a nail, in the extremity being used (look for scars). A site should not be reused for at least 1 to 2 days after removal of a prior intraosseous needle.

!! **Potential Complications:** Severe complications include loss of bone or limb; neonates in particular are at increased risk.[6] Other complications include fracture of the bone from intraosseous placement and/or prolonged bone healing,[7] osteomyelitis (risk decreased when intraosseous line is removed within a few hours of insertion), impact on future bone growth (although this was not seen in one small study[8]), compartment syndrome, and loss of the bone or limb.

Critical Anatomy

The most commonly used insertion sites are the proximal tibia, distal tibia, proximal humerus and for infants/children only, the distal femur. Of these sites, the proximal humerus may be the preferred site in teenagers and adults because it the least painful, is closest to the central circulation, and has a high flow rate.

Note: Each device may be approved only for certain insertion sites, which may also be specific to the country in which it is used. For example, the US Food and Drug Administration has approved the EZ-IO® for use in the proximal tibia, distal tibia, proximal humerus, and distal femur for infants and children

Proximal tibia. This site drains to the popliteal vein. The intraosseous needle should be inserted two fingerbreadths below the base of the patella and one fingerbreadth medial on the flat surface of the bone. Pinch the sides of the tibial bone between your fingers to isolate the proximal tibia. In children younger than 2 years, the tibial tuberosity may not be fully developed. If the tibial tuberosity is not identifiable, the lower aspect of the patella should be palpated, and the insertion site will be two fingerbreadths (approximately 3 cm) below the patella and one fingerbreadth medial. If the tibial tuberosity is palpable, the insertion site will be one fingerbreadth medial to the tibial tuberosity (Figures 8.2 and 8.3).

Distal tibia. This site drains to the great saphenous vein. Place one finger directly over the medial malleolus. Move two fingerbreadths or approximately 3 cm proximally and palpate the anterior and posterior tibial borders to confirm the flat center aspect of the bone. Orient the intraosseous needle perpendicular to the flat aspect of the bone before insertion (Figure 8.4).

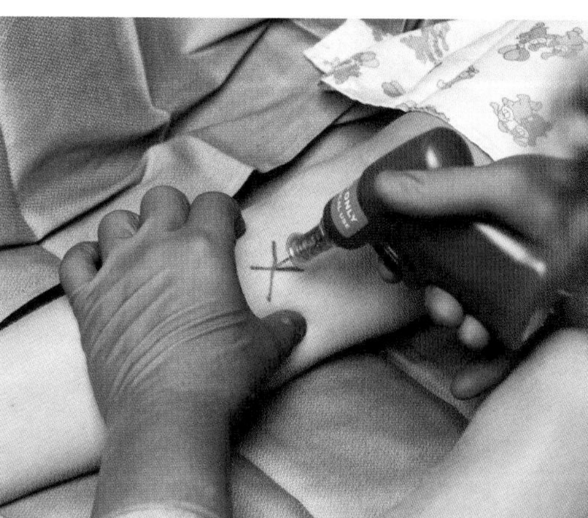

Figure 8.3 Proximal Tibia Intraosseous Insertion: Pinch the sides of the proximal tibia between your fingers to isolate the bone. Insert the needle perpendicular to the flat surface of bone.

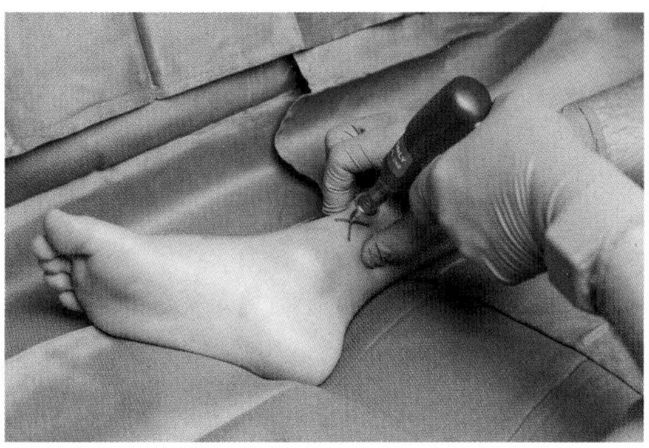

Figure 8.4 Distal Tibia Intraosseous Insertion: Place one finger directly over the medial malleolus and move 2 fingerbreadths or approximately 3 cm proximal and palpate anterior and posterior tibia borders to confirm the flat center aspect of the bone. Insert the needle perpendicular to the flat surface of the bone.

Proximal humerus. This site drains to the axillary vein. It should be used only when the relevant anatomy can be clearly identified and is generally only used in older teenagers and adults (i.e., after bone growth is complete). The humerus should be internally rotated before insertion in order to best facilitate entrance to the intramedullary space and to rotate the brachial plexus away from the insertion site. This can be accomplished by placing the patient's palm flat over the umbilicus, although this may be impractical in a draped patient whose arms are at his or her sides. Alternatively, the arm should be rotated prone so that the thumb points in the posterior direction. The practitioner should use his or her thumb to palpate the humerus until a notch or groove is felt; this is the greater tubercle or surgical neck of the humerus, where the bone juts out just slightly. The intraosseous insertion site is approximately 1 cm higher (proximal) at the most prominent point. The patient should avoid lifting his or her arm after the line has been inserted because this may cause impingement from the acromion process and potential displacement of the intraosseous line (Figures 8.5 and 8.6).

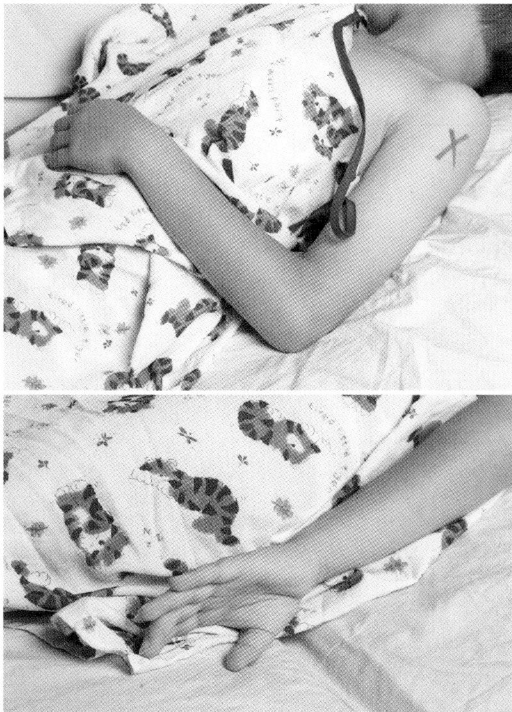

Figures 8.5 and 8.6 Proximal Humerus Intraosseous Insertion: The arm is placed in one of two positions for intraosseous insertion into the humerus. Option 1 (Figure 8.5): The humerus is internally rotated by placing the palm flat over the umbilicus. Option 2 (Figure 8.6): The arm is rotated prone so that the thumb faces posteriorly.

Distal femur (infant/child). The stretched out leg should be secured so that it cannot bend during placement and until the IO catheter is removed. Insertion site is just proximal to patella (maximum 1 cm) and 1–2 cm medial to midline.

Setup

Equipment

- Sterile prep
- Intraosseous needle: Depending on the age, insertion site, and amount of adipose tissue present, the correct size of needle should be selected to ensure that a sufficient amount of needle reaches the medullary space while maintaining sufficient needle length above the skin to adequately secure the needle (Figure 8.7).
- Sterile dressing
- Sterile gloves

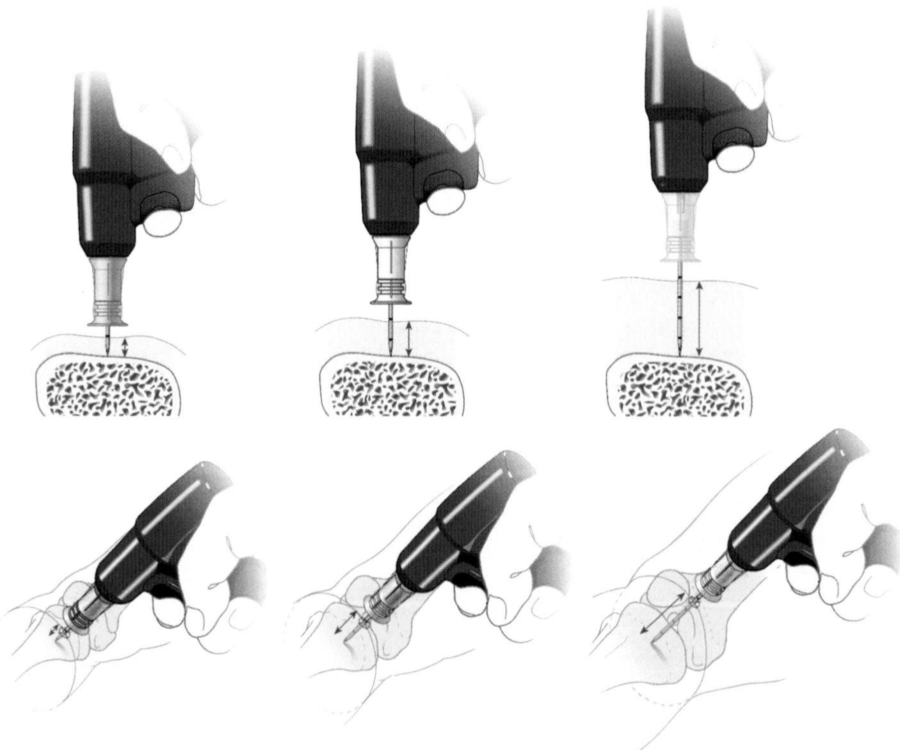

Figure 8.7 When inserting an intraosseous needle, allow sufficient needle length so that when the needle touches bone at least one black line or approximately 1 cm of needle remains outside of the skin. The reason for this is to ensure that, when the needle is inserted into the bone, it will reach the medullary space. Age, insertion site, and adipose tissue affect the needle choice as does the brand of intraosseous needle being inserted. Picture used with permission.

- Fenestrated drape
- Local anesthetic (if indicated)—1% lidocaine
- 5-mL syringe
- 50-mL syringe
- Fluids with tubing
- Pressure bag
- Blood sample tubes (crossmatch, electrolytes)

Step-by-Step

1. **Prepare for the procedure.** If the patient is conscious, after disinfecting the skin, lidocaine can be administered at the skin and infiltrated down to the periosteum. Also, lidocaine can be given through the intraosseous line before the infusion begins to decrease pain during injection. In awake patients injection into the intraosseous space is quite painful, whereas placement of the IO needle itself causes less discomfort.
2. **Position the patient, identify landmarks, and prepare the skin.** Place the patient in a comfortable position with full access to the desired intraosseous site. Disinfect the skin and apply a sterile drape over the insertion area.
3. **Insert the intraosseous needle from the skin to the bone.** The insertion site should be held with the nondominant hand. Press the needle set through the skin, perpendicular to the surface, until the tip touches the bone. At least 5 mm of the intraosseous needle (one black line) must be visible above the skin at the point where the tip of the needle touches the bone. If less than 5 mm of needle is visualized above the skin, a longer needle should be considered because the needle might otherwise be too short to enter the medullary space.
4. **Insert the intraosseous needle into the bone**.

   For manual intraosseous devices (e.g., Jamshidi, Cook): Simultaneously apply steady manual pressure and perform a twisting motion to "screw" the needle into the bone.

   For an automatic intraosseous device (e.g., the EZ-IO®): Squeeze the driver trigger, and apply a minimal amount of gentle, steady pressure. Immediately release the driver trigger when a sudden "give" or "pop" is felt; this indicates entry into the medullary cavity. It is important to remember to "**stop when you feel the pop**." It is especially important to remember to use minimal pressure for pediatric patients. Pediatric patients have softer and smaller bones, leading to a higher risk for needle displacement if excessive force is used.

Caution! Make sure that your hand is not behind the insertion site. If the needle passes completely through the bone with your hand behind the insertion site, a needlestick injury might occur.

5. **Remove the stylet and connect the infusion set.** After the needle is correctly positioned, remove the stylet and connect the infusion set. While infusing, watch for signs of infiltration. Place a sterile dressing. Stabilize with either a specialized IO stabilization device or with sterile gauze (so the catheter does not move from side to side). The location of the catheter in the correct location should be confirmed with the following methods: (1) stability of the catheter; (2) ability to aspirate; (3) physiological or pharmacologic changes with medication administration; and (4) adequate flow rate. To maintain flow, a pressure bag can be placed over the intravenous fluid bag and inflated to approximately one third of mean arterial pressure.

Pearl: After 5 years of age, a significant portion of the red marrow has been converted to less vascular, yellow marrow, which has a much higher fat component. This makes access more difficult, decreases the maximum infusion rate, and may increase the risk for fat emboli.

6. **Confirm intraosseous placement with color Doppler ultrasound, if feasible.** Color Doppler ultrasound can be used to visualize flow in the intraosseous space (with a correctly placed intraosseous line) as well as extraosseous flow (with an incorrectly placed intraosseous line).[9] Use a linear probe in the transverse (preferred) or sagittal plain to visualize the bone that has been accessed. With color Doppler, flow toward the probe will appear red, and flow away from the probe will appear blue. Power Doppler will detect lower velocity flow, but does not give information as to the direction of flow. [9]

Postoperative Management Considerations

Do not leave an intraosseous catheter inserted for more than 24 hours. Obtain IV or central venous access as soon as possible and remove the intraosseous line once this access is obtained. Monitor the insertion site frequently for signs of extravasation or osteomyelitis. A post insertion x-ray is recommended in children to assess for possible fracture. For removal: Attach a luer-lock syringe to the hub. Keep the hub and syringe in alignment. Take care to avoid bending the needle. As you remove the needle, rotate it clockwise while pulling it straight out. After removal, apply a sterile dressing.

References

1. Kurowski A, Timler D, Evrin T, et al. Comparison of 3 different intraosseous access devices for adult during resuscitation: randomized crossover manikin study. *Am J Emerg Med.* 2014;32(12):1490–1493.
2. Fiser DH. Intraosseous infusion. *N Engl J Med.* 1990;322(22):1579–1581.
3. Kleinman ME, Chameides L, Schexnayder SM, et al. Part 14: pediatric advanced life support: 2010 American Heart Association Guidelines for Cardiopulmonary Resuscitation and Emergency Cardiovascular Care. *Circulation.* 2010;122(18 Suppl 3):S876–908.
4. Veldhoen ES, de Vooght KM, Slieker MG, et al. Analysis of blood gas, electrolytes and glucose from intraosseous samples using an i-STAT((R)) point-of-care analyser. *Resuscitation.* 2014;85(3):359–363.
5. Jousi M, Saikko S, Nurmi J. Intraosseous blood samples for point-of-care analysis: agreement between intraosseous and arterial analyses. *Scand J Trauma Resusc Emerg Med.* 2017;25(1):92.
6. Suominen PK, Nurmi E, Lauerma K. Intraosseous access in neonates and infants: risk of severe complications—a case report. *Acta Anaesthesiol Scand.* 2015;59(10):1389–1393.
7. Ginsberg-Peltz J. Time to bone healing after intraosseous placement in children is ill defined. *Pediatr Emerg Care* 2016;32(11):799–800.
8. Fiser RT, Walker WM, Seibert JJ, et al. Tibial length following intraosseous infusion: a prospective, radiographic analysis. *Pediatr Emerg Care.* 1997;13(3):186–188.
9. Tsung JW, Blaivas M, Stone MB. Feasibility of point-of-care colour Doppler ultrasound confirmation of intraosseous needle placement during resuscitation. *Resuscitation.* 2009;80(6):665–668.

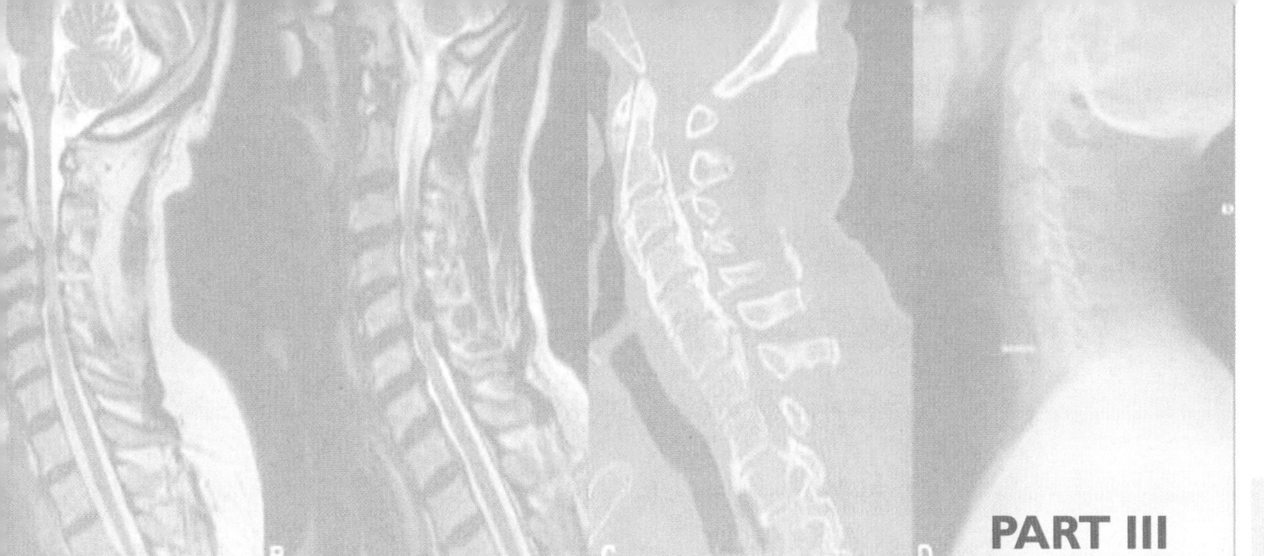

REGIONAL ANESTHESIA

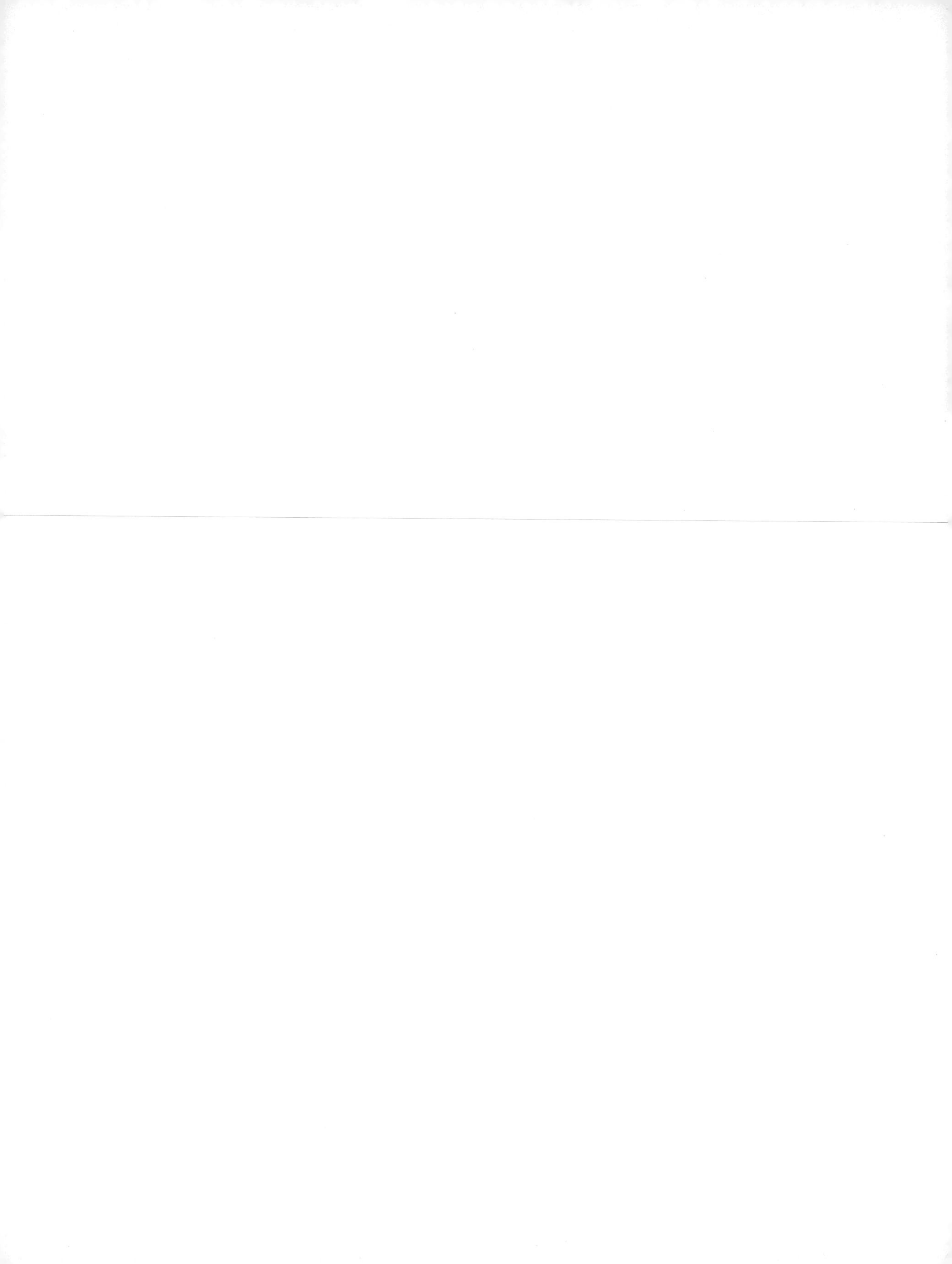

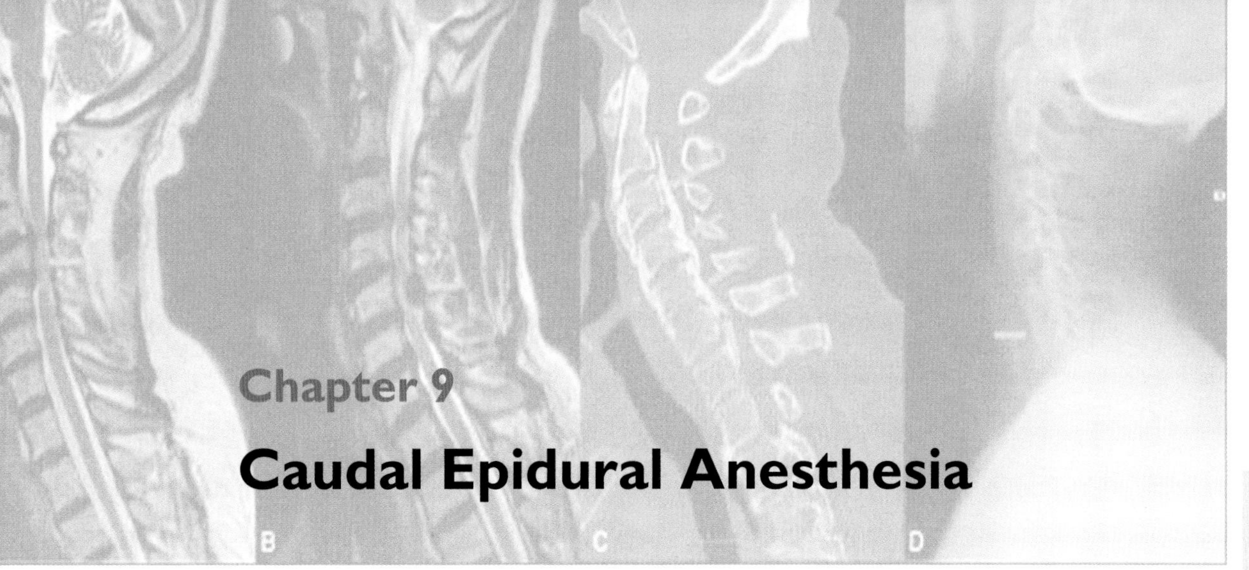

Chapter 9
Caudal Epidural Anesthesia

Jared R. E. Hylton and Jorge A. Pineda

Caudal Epidural Anesthesia Fundamentals

Introduction

Caudal epidural anesthesia (CEA) in pediatric patients was first described in 1933 as a replacement for general anesthesia in 83 children undergoing transurethral surgery,[1] and since that time it has been shown to be useful in a variety of surgeries. The popularity of this block stems from its efficacy, simplicity, speed, and relative safety. The caudal approach to the epidural space can be used for the administration of local anesthetic and adjunct medications for either surgical anesthesia or postoperative analgesia. This technique is most commonly applied to surgical procedures occurring below the umbilicus and is frequently used as a single injection technique to be performed after induction of general anesthesia and before surgical incision for augmentation of general anesthesia and postoperative pain control. For longer procedures, a catheter can be placed to facilitate repeat dosing at the conclusion of surgery. Alternatively, more cephalad dermatomes can be anesthetized with an epidural catheter threaded to the desired level. The benefits of caudal epidural anesthesia extend beyond postoperative analgesia and include decreased intraoperative anesthetic requirements and a reduction in the neuroendocrine stress response to surgery.[2,3]

As with any procedure, caudal epidural anesthesia has risks. The most common risk is a failed or incomplete block. The rate of complete or partial failure in the setting of a large teaching hospital is 3 to 11%, with rates increasing especially in children older than 7 years.[8] Other risks and potential complications include local anesthetic systemic toxicity, dural puncture, intraosseous injection, penetration of the sacrum, bleeding, and infection.

Recently published data from the Pediatric Regional Anesthesia Network (PRAN) collaborative group showed that the incidence of a positive test dose for caudal block placement was 0.1% in 18,650 patients.[7] Similar to intravenous (IV) injection, intraosseous injection leads to rapid systemic uptake with the potential risk for local anesthetic toxicity and cardiovascular collapse.

Unlike epidural anesthesia in adults, caudal epidural anesthesia, as well as high spinal and epidural anesthesia, is generally not associated with hypotension in patients younger than 6 to 8 years,[9] thought to be secondary to the relatively low basal sympathetic tone at this age.

Clinical Applications

Traditionally, caudal epidural anesthesia has most frequently been used as a single-shot technique for urologic or lower abdominal surgical procedures such as inguinal hernia repair, orchiopexy, and hypospadias repair. This technique can also be applied to gastrointestinal tract surgery involving the lower abdomen as well as lower extremity orthopedic surgery.

In certain cases, depending on the level of surgeon and anesthesiologist comfort, neuraxial anesthesia can be used as the sole anesthetic, with the infant given a pacifier for soothing. Additional evidence is needed to determine whether the use of neuraxial anesthesia as the primary anesthetic in neonates without preoperative or intraoperative sedative medications will reduce the risk for post-operative apnea.[4]

Contraindications

The contraindications for caudal epidural anesthesia are similar to those for spinal or lumbar and thoracic epidural anesthesia. Absolute contraindications include (1) parent refusal; (2) coagulation disorders; (3) current use of anticoagulation medication; (4) active infection at the site of injection, such as diaper rash, active cellulitis, pilonidal cyst, meningitis, or osteomyelitis of the sacrum; (5) trauma at the site of injection; (6) congenital malformation of the spinal cord (spina bifida) or vertebral bodies; and (7) a tethered spinal cord.

Be familiar with current American Society of Regional Anesthesia and Pain Medicine (ASRA) guidelines regarding anticoagulation and bleeding disorders in the setting of neuraxial anesthesia before performing any neuraxial anesthetic. These guidelines are available at http://www.asra.com.

Exercise caution with patients who present with a sacral dimple because it may be associated with spina bifida occulta, and caudal epidural anesthesia is contraindicated. Also, severe scoliosis may distort normal sacral anatomy and increase difficulty. We advise caution in using bupivacaine in pediatric patients with underlying cardiac dysfunction because this local anesthetic is known to have relatively higher potential for cardiac toxicity. Systemic infection or sepsis may also be considered a relative contraindication to caudal epidural anesthesia.

Critical Anatomy

The caudal space is an extension of the epidural space found between the termination of the dural sac and the termination of the sacral canal.[10] The sacral canal contains the terminus of the dural sac and filum terminale, sacral and coccygeal components of cauda equina, epidural fat, and the valveless sacral epidural vein plexus that generally ends at S4 but may extend through the canal.[11]

The sacral hiatus (Figure 9.1) is a U-shaped or V-shaped structure formed from the lack of dorsal fusion of the fifth and fourth sacral vertebral arches. It is limited laterally by the sacral cornua and is covered by the sacrococcygeal ligament, which is the sacral continuation of the ligament flava. The cornua of the sacral hiatus (sacral cornu) are most easily palpated as two bony ridges approximately 0.5 to 1.0 cm apart. Alternatively, the operator may first palpate the L4–L5 intervertebral space in the midline and then palpate in the caudal direction until the sacral hiatus is appreciated. The correct location is often located at the level of the beginning of the crease of the buttocks. One way of locating the hiatus is to picture the hiatus along with the bilateral posterior superior iliac spines forming an equilateral triangle.

Infant and neonatal spinal cord anatomy differs in distinct ways from the anatomy of older children and adults. The conus medullaris (termination of the spinal cord) in neonates and infants is at L3 and does not reach the adult level at L1 until approximately 1 year of age. Similarly, the termination of the dural sac is at approximately S4 at birth and then shifts to S2 by 1 year of age as the infant grows. In neonates the sacrum is narrower and flatter relative to that in adults, making the approach to the subarachnoid space more direct and thus making

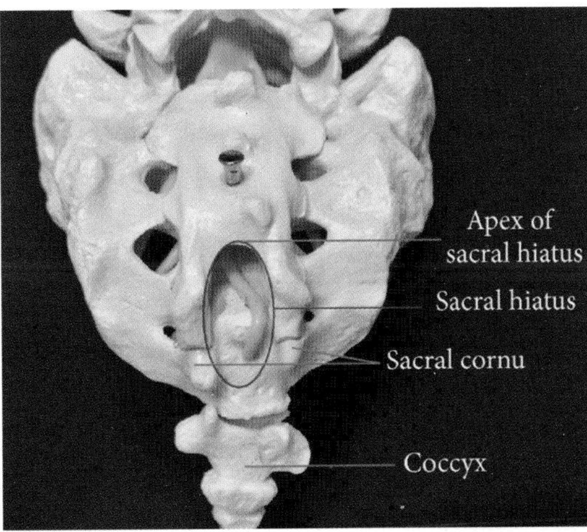

Figure 9.1 Posterior view of sacrum and sacral hiatus. (Image from Kao SC, Lin CS. Caudal epidural block: an updated review of anatomy and techniques. *Biomed Res Int.* 2017;2017:921714. Permissions confirmed as open access.)

dural puncture more likely. At birth, the sacrum is only partially ossified, and neonates may be at greater risk for complications because the largely cartilaginous sacrum may make the recognition of intraosseous injection more difficult.

Setup

Equipment

For a single-shot caudal epidural anesthesia technique, the minimum equipment required includes:

- Sterile gloves
- Disinfecting solution (alcohol or iodine based)
- 22- or 20-gauge angiocatheter needle and catheter system
- Sterile towels
- Local anesthetic solution
- Test dose solution
- Towel roll or pillow for positioning under patient knees

For all caudal epidural anesthesia procedures, the patient should be connected to standard American Society of Anesthesiology (ASA) monitors, the patient should have IV access, and airway management and resuscitation equipment and medications should be available.

Needle choice is largely based on anesthesiologist preference and experience. Some prefer to use a 22-gauge spinal needle or "B bevel" needle, claiming that this needle provides superior tactile feedback for passage through the sacrococcygeal ligament. We prefer to use a 22-gauge nonsafety angiocath needle because we feel there is no disadvantage in tactile feedback. In addition, we are concerned about a theoretically increased risk for dural puncture when advancing a sharp spinal needle into the caudal space after passage through the sacrococcygeal ligament. We feel there is less risk for dural puncture with advancing a plastic catheter off of the needle of the angiocatheter system into the epidural space versus advancing a spinal needle.

Before starting the case, gather all necessary equipment for a caudal epidural anesthetic. Based on the patient's body weight and desired level of sensory block, calculate an appropriate dose of local anesthetic and adjuvant (if desired).

Drugs, Dosages, Administration

This section will cover single-injection dosing of CEA medications. For dosing of continuous caudal epidural catheters, please see Chapter 11, Epidural Anesthesia.

Local Anesthetics

Given the goal of prolonged postoperative analgesia, a long-acting local anesthetic is typically used, commonly ropivacaine, bupivacaine, or levobupivacaine (not currently available in the United States), although none of these has superior efficacy.[12] Any neuraxial medication must be preservative free, with that particular formulation approved for neuraxial use. In general, if a motor block is desired, a more concentrated form of bupivacaine is used, while ropivacaine is preferred if the goal is to minimize motor block. Ropivacaine has a more favorable safety profile with regard to cardiac toxicity.

Two important considerations dictate the volume and concentration of local anesthetic used for caudal epidural anesthesia. First, the level of sensory blockade desired is dictated by the volume of local anesthetic used (Table 9.1).

Second, the higher concentration of local anesthetic can be used to produce a denser sensory block and facilitate a lighter plane of general anesthesia, taking care to avoid toxic doses of local anesthetic.

Table 9.1 Local Anesthetic Dosage for Single-Shot Caudal Epidural Anesthesia

Desired Caudal Dermatomal Coverage	Example Procedure	Dosage (mL/kg) (not to exceed 20 mL total[14])	Local Anesthetic
Sacral, low lumbar	Urogenital procedure	0.5–0.75 (for 0.1 or 0.125% concentration only)	0.1–0.2% ropivacaine or 0.125–0.25% bupivacaine
Lumbar, low thoracic	Inguinal hernia repair, lower extremity procedures	1.0	0.1–0.2% ropivacaine or 0.125% bupivacaine
Lumbar, low-mid thoracic	Abdominal incision	1.0–1.25	0.1% ropivacaine or 0.125% bupivacaine

WARNING!! It is important to calculate the allowable total local anesthetic dose by weight and to stay below this maximum dose in order to decrease the risk for local anesthetic systemic toxicity (LAST). This calculation should include all local anesthetics, including those given by the surgeon, IV local anesthetic given by the anesthesiologist, and EMLA or subcutaneous lidocaine given before starting an IV.

Test Dose

We recommend using a 1-mL test dose of local anesthetic with 1:200,000 epinephrine to monitor both heart rate and blood pressure changes in order to assist in the detection of an accidental intravascular catheter. It is important to note that an epidural test dose is not a perfectly sensitive or specific marker of intravascular or intraosseous placement.

Adjuvants

Adjuvant medications used in addition to local anesthetics can prolong the duration of postoperative analgesia (Table 9.2). It is important to note that all adjuvant medications administered by the neuraxial route must be preservative free and approved for neuraxial use (may be manufacturer dependent, even for the same drug).

Landmark-Based, Single-Shot Caudal Epidural Anesthesia

Introduction

Readers should refer to the earlier Caudal Epidural Anesthesia Fundamentals section at the beginning of this chapter for background information, clinical applications, contraindications, critical anatomy, equipment, and drugs, dosages, and administration information for this procedure.

Step-by-Step

1. **Place the patient in the lateral decubitus position.** After placement of standard ASA monitors, induction of general anesthesia and appropriate airway management, place

Table 9.2 Adjuvant Medications for Single-Shot Caudal Epidural Anesthesia*

Medication†	Dose	Maximum Dose	Side Effects/Caution
Epinephrine	5 MICROgrams/mL (1:200,000)	Unknown	Used only in small amounts (15 MICROgrams) as part of the local anesthetic solution for a test dose. In excessive doses, may cause myocardial infarction and cardiac arrest
Clonidine	1 MICROgram/kg	2 MICROgrams/kg	Sedation, hypotension, and bradycardia at high doses. Avoid in young infants.
Dexmedetomidine	1 MICROgram/kg	Unknown	Possible bradycardia at higher doses.
Morphine	75–100 MICROgrams/kg	100 MICROgrams/kg	Respiratory depression (can be delayed 6–12 hours), pruritis, urinary retention, nausea.
Dexamethasone	0.1 mg/kg	Unknown	No major side effects reported

* Based on reported trials.

† Must be preservative free and approved for neuraxial use.

the patient in the lateral decubitus position (Figure 9.2) to prepare for caudal epidural anesthesia. The goal is to minimize any rotational misalignment of the spinal column to maintain the sacrum as flat as possible relative to the anesthesiologist in order to optimize the midline approach of needle advancement. This can be accomplished with a towel roll placed between the knees, knees flexed to the chest, and mild flexion of the spinal column.

Caution! While positioning and preparing for caudal epidural anesthesia, exposed infants and neonates in particular, but also young children, can experience significant heat loss, potentially leading to deleterious side effects associated with hypothermia. We recommend taking measures to prevent heat loss such as warming the operating room, using an underbody forced-air warming device, or placing warm blankets over the patient's upper body and head.

>> **Tip on Technique:** Although clinician preferences may vary, we recommend placing the patient into right lateral decubitus position so that the anesthesia machine monitors can be easily viewed while performing the procedure.

>> **Tip on Technique:** It is helpful to obtain a stool to sit facing the patient's back at approximately eye level to optimize ergonomics. Positioning the patient to minimize the medial-to-lateral spinal curvature will help the clinician visualize the path of the spinal column and will assist the clinician in advancing the needle in a midline fashion. A pillow

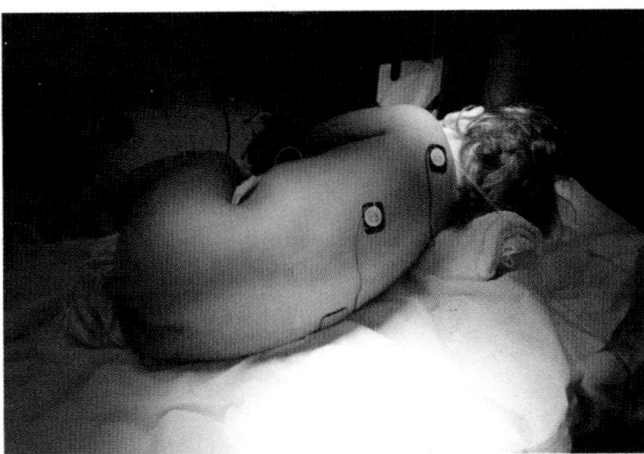

Figure 9.2 A child in lateral decubitus position.

or towel roll placed between the patient's legs can help rotate the patient's pelvis into a neutral position, thus minimizing any rotational distortion of the spinal column.

!! **Potential Complications:** Carefully watch the airway at all times while moving and positioning the patient in order to prevent inadvertent airway dislodgment.

2. **Identify landmarks and sterilize the skin.** After positioning the patient, it is often useful to palpate and identify the anatomical landmarks previously discussed. If uncertainty in identifying the sacral cornu and hiatus is encountered, reposition the patient to optimize anatomical variables; the decision whether to use ultrasound should be undertaken before skin preparation and draping. After identifying the sacral hiatus, prepare the skin over the hiatus with a chlorhexidine- or iodine-based antiseptic solution.

WARNING!! Alcohol-based skin preparation solutions are a potential fire hazard in the operating room, especially when electrocautery is used for the surgical procedure. When using alcohol-based skin prep, do not allow excess preparation solution to pool around or under the patient. Ensure that the alcohol-based skin preparation solution is completely dry and that any excess is wiped away with towels before preparing the patient for surgery.

>> **Tip on Technique:** We recommend cleaning the skin with antiseptic solution in a circular pattern to create a zone of prepped skin with an approximate radius of 4 cm from the center of the hiatus. Be careful to not wipe superiorly from the gluteal crease toward the hiatus to avoid fecal contamination.

3. **Advance the needle.** After the patient is prepped and draped in the typical sterile fashion, using sterile technique the you should again locate the sacral cornu and hiatus. We recommend using the second and fourth digits to palpate the cornu while simultaneously locating the hiatus with the third digit. After the apex of the hiatus is located, finger positioning should be maintained over the aforementioned anatomical landmarks, and needle puncture should occur just rostral to the your third digit with the needle advanced in the midline. You should visualize

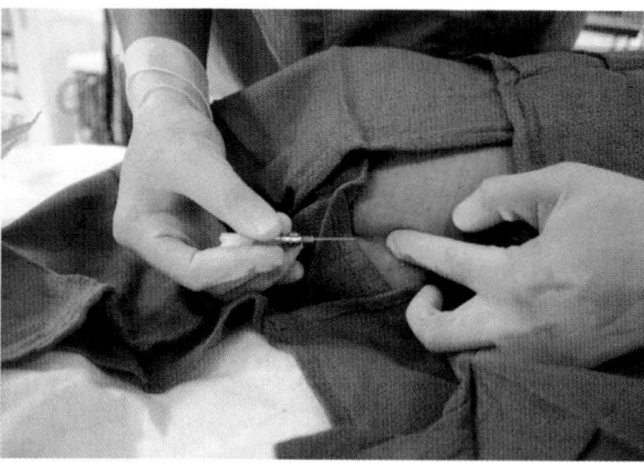

Figure 9.3 Hand positioning for palpation of landmarks and needle advancement. Note that in this image, the anesthesiologist's second digit of the left hand is directly over the apex of the hiatus, while the right hand is preparing to insert the needle just rostral to the second digit in a midline fashion, advancing the needle inferior to superior.

advancement of the needle directly at the center of the sacral hiatus in a midline fashion (Figure 9.3).

Caution! Care must be taken not to advance the needle too far into the epidural space after advancement through the sacrococcygeal ligament in order to avoid inadvertent dural puncture.

>> **Tip on Technique:** With regard to the angle of the needle during advancement, we recommend initially inserting the needle at an angle of 60 to 90 degrees relative to the skin. As the needle is advanced directly into the sacral hiatus, resistance will be encountered that signifies that the needle has entered the sacrococcygeal ligament. After entering the sacrococcygeal ligament, the needle angle should be flattened to an angle of less than 30 degrees relative to the skin, and then the needle should be slowly advanced in a midline fashion until a loss of resistance is appreciated. Some authors describe a tactile sensation, described as a "pop," as the needle advances through the sacrococcygeal ligament into the caudal epidural space. In clinical practice, the passage of the needle through the ligament into the epidural space can be more subtle than this classic description. Needle advancement should cease when a loss of resistance is appreciated.

!! **Potential Complications:** During advancement of the needle during the initial steep angle, care should be taken not to force the needle against high resistance. High resistance to needle advancement likely means that an osseous structure has been encountered, such as the sacrum or floor of the hiatus. The needle should be withdrawn and the angle of advancement flattened to avoid further advancement into bony structures.

4. **Advance the catheter (if using an angiocatheter).** After you have appreciated a loss of resistance, the needle is likely within the caudal epidural space. You should then stabilize the needle and catheter system with your dominant hand, and then slide the catheter over and off the needle with your nondominant hand. Within the epidural space, the catheter should be easy and smooth to advance. After the angiocatheter is in place, retract/remove the needle (Figure 9.4).

>> **Tip on Technique:** If resistance is encountered to catheter advancement, the needle/catheter unit may still be within the sacrococcygeal ligament or may be within

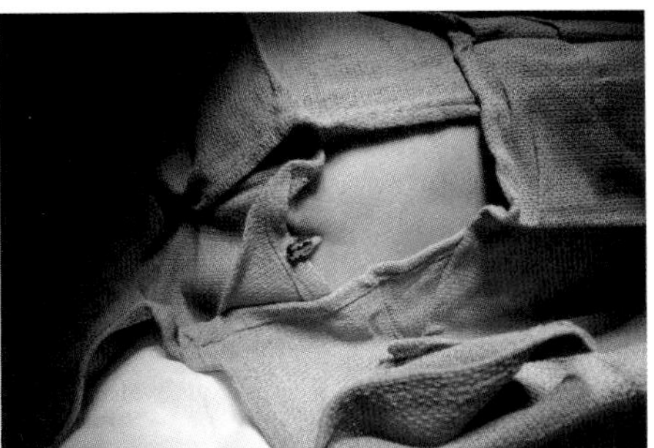

Figure 9.4 Completion of angiocatheter advancement into the caudal epidural space.

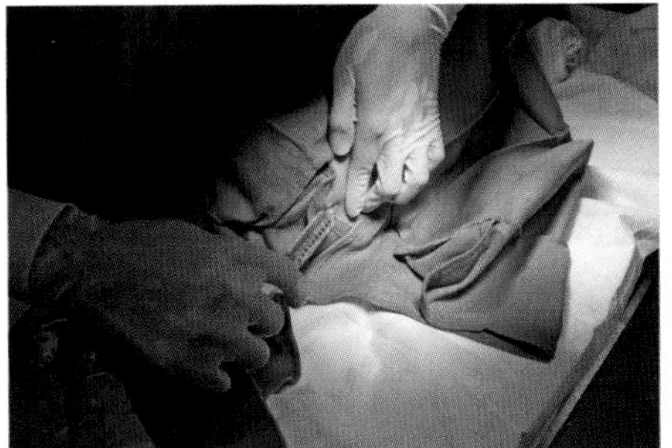

Figure 9.5 Medication is injected while simultaneously palpating the caudal catheter insertion site to help rule out subcutaneous injection.

subcutaneous soft tissue. Check to make sure that the needle has been advanced midline. The catheter can be pulled back onto the needle, and the entire unit can be advanced slightly in an attempt to reach the epidural space. Care must be taken not to advance the needle too far within the epidural space in order to avoid dural puncture.

Note: After removing the needle, the catheter should remain firmly anchored in place by the sacrococcygeal ligament. If the catheter deviates off to one side or appears "floppy," it is likely that the catheter is simply within subcutaneous tissue and not truly within the epidural space.

5. **Inject the local anesthetic.** While maintaining sterile conditions, attach your medication syringe directly to the caudal catheter. Aspirate gently, ensuring no return of blood or cerebrospinal fluid (CSF). We recommend first administering a 1-mL test dose of local anesthetic mixed with preservative-free 1:200,000 epinephrine to assist with intravascular detection. If no blood pressure or heart rate changes are detected after 1 minute, the remainder of the appropriate local anesthetic dose may be injected through the caudal catheter. Inject the medication incrementally over a full minute, intermittently aspirating from the syringe to ensure no return of CSF or blood (Figure 9.5).

>> Tip on Technique: While injecting medication with the dominant hand, it is useful to place the nondominant hand over the catheter insertion site to stabilize the catheter. Palpation over the catheter site during injection can assist in detection of a subcutaneously placed catheter because the clinician will feel a tactile sensation of swelling and firming of the patient's subcutaneous tissue if the catheter is not in the epidural space. If this is encountered, the caudal catheter should be removed and replaced.

!! Potential Complications: During medication injection, potential complications include intravascular or intraosseous injection, local anesthetic toxicity, or subcutaneous injection.

>> Tip on Technique: For longer procedures, some anesthesiologists prefer to dose the caudal both before and after the surgery to optimize both the intraoperative and postoperative benefits of caudal epidural anesthesia. If desired, a short length of IV extension tubing, such as a "J-loop" or microbore tubing, can be flushed with the local anesthetic solution and attached to the caudal catheter. After pre-incision injection of an appropriate dose of local anesthetic, this catheter and tubing unit can be secured with tape and sterile dressing and left for the duration of the surgery in order to facilitate repeat dosing at the end of surgery. Ensure that the catheter and tubing are appropriately padded to reduce the risk for skin breakdown or ulceration. After the surgical procedure, ensure catheter removal and site coverage with a sterile dressing.

Postoperative Management Considerations

You should ensure that motor function has returned before the patient is discharged.

Caudal Epidural Anesthesia with Continuous Catheter Placement

Introduction

Readers should refer to the earlier Caudal Epidural Anesthesia Fundamentals section at the beginning of this chapter for background information, clinical applications, contraindications, critical anatomy, equipment, and drugs, dosages, and administration information for this procedure.

Step-by-Step

1. **Place the patient in the lateral decubitus position.** After induction of general anesthesia and appropriate airway management, place the patient in the lateral decubitus position (Figure 9.2) to prepare for caudal epidural anesthesia. The goal is to minimize any rotational misalignment of the spinal column to maintain the sacrum as flat as possible relative to the anesthesiologist and optimize the midline approach of needle advancement. This can be accomplished with a towel roll placed between the knees, knees flexed to the chest, and mild flexion of the spinal column.

Caution! While positioning and preparing for caudal epidural anesthesia, exposed infants and neonates in particular, but also young children, can experience significant heat loss, potentially leading to deleterious side effects associated with hypothermia. We recommend taking measures to prevent heat loss such as warming the operating room, using an underbody forced-air warming device, or placing warm blankets over the patient's upper body and head.

>> **Tip on Technique:** Although clinician preferences may vary, we recommend placing the patient in the right lateral decubitus position so that the clinician can continuously view the monitors on the anesthesia machine while performing the technique.

>> **Tip on Technique:** It is helpful to obtain a stool to sit facing the patient's back at approximately eye level to optimize ergonomics. Positioning the patient to minimize the medial-to-lateral spinal curvature will help you visualize the path of the spinal column and will assist the clinician in advancing the needle in a midline fashion. A pillow or towel roll placed between the patient's legs can help rotate the patient's pelvis into a neutral position, thus minimizing any rotational distortion of the spinal column.

!! **Potential Complications:** Carefully watch the airway at all times while moving and positioning the patient in order to prevent inadvertent airway dislodgment.

2. **Identify landmarks and sterilize the skin.** Palpate and identify the anatomical landmarks. If uncertainty in identifying the sacral cornu and hiatus is encountered, reposition the patient to optimize anatomical variables; the decision whether to use ultrasound should be undertaken before skin preparation and draping. After identifying the sacral hiatus, prepare the skin over the hiatus with chlorhexidine- or iodine-based antiseptic solution.

WARNING!! Alcohol-based skin preparation solutions are a potential fire hazard in the operating room, especially when electrocautery is used for the surgical procedure. When using alcohol-based skin prep, do not allow excess preparation solution to pool around or under the patient. Ensure that the alcohol-based skin preparation solution is completely dry and that any excess is wiped away with towels before preparing the patient for surgery.

>> **Tip on Technique:** We recommend cleaning the skin with antiseptic solution in a circular pattern to create a zone of prepped skin with an approximate radius of 4 cm from the center of the hiatus. Be careful not to wipe superiorly from the gluteal crease toward the hiatus due to the risk of fecal contamination.

3. **Prepare the caudal epidural kit.** After appropriately positioning the patient and palpation and confirmation of landmarks, prepare the caudal epidural kit. These kits will vary by institution. The basic components should include a caudal epidural needle, epidural catheter, antiseptic solution, epidural catheter filter, sterile drape, sterile towel, and sterile dressing. Note that an 18-gauge needle is needed for caudal epidural catheter placement.

Caution! Catheter placement likely carries with it a higher risk for infectious complications. It is prudent for the anesthesiologist to perform a complete sterile scrub and don sterile gown and gloves as well as to drape out the entire procedural area with sterile drapes before performing the epidural catheter placement.

4. **Measure the caudal epidural catheter.** After the patient is prepped and draped in the typical sterile fashion, proceed with estimating the length of epidural catheter that will be threaded cephalad into the caudal space. This can be accomplished by identifying the dermatomal level at which sensory blockade is desired and, while maintaining sterile conditions, holding up the catheter to the patient with the tip at the desired dermatome.
5. **Insert and advance the needle.** After the patient is prepped and draped in the typical sterile fashion, using sterile technique you should again locate the sacral cornu and hiatus. We recommend using the second and fourth digits to palpate the cornu while simultaneously locating the hiatus with the third digit. When the apex of the hiatus is located, needle puncture should occur just rostral to the third digit with the needle advanced in the midline (Figure 9.3).

Caution! To avoid inadvertent dural puncture, care must be taken not to advance the needle too far into the epidural space.

>> **Tip on Technique:** We recommend initially inserting the needle at an angle of 60 to 90 degrees relative to the skin. As the needle is advanced directly into the sacral hiatus, resistance will be encountered that signifies that the needle has entered the sacrococcygeal ligament. After entering the sacrococcygeal ligament, the needle angle should be flattened to an angle of less than 30 degrees relative to skin and the needle should be slowly advanced in a midline fashion until a loss of resistance is appreciated. Some authors describe a tactile sensation, described as a "pop," as the needle advances through the sacrococcygeal ligament into the caudal epidural space. In clinical practice, the passage of the needle through the ligament into the epidural space can be more subtle than this classic description. Needle advancement should cease when a loss of resistance is appreciated.

!! **Potential Complications:** During advancement of the needle, care should be taken to avoid forcing the needle against high resistance. High resistance to needle advancement is likely from encountering an osseous structure, such as the sacrum or floor of the sacral hiatus. The needle should be withdrawn and the angle of advancement flattened to avoid further advancement into bony structures.

4. **Advance the epidural catheter.** After you appreciate a loss of resistance, the needle is likely within the caudal epidural space. You should then stabilize the needle with your dominant hand, and then slide the catheter into the needle with your nondominant hand in a cephalad direction. If the catheter is in the epidural space, the catheter should be easy and smooth to advance. After the catheter is in place, retract/remove the needle from the unit. Next, withdraw the stylette from the catheter (if a stylette is present), remove the needle from the patient, and attach the filter to the catheter (Figure 9.6).

   Note: Typical caudal epidural catheter kits come with a styletted epidural catheter to help prevent coiling and assist with advancement of the catheter.

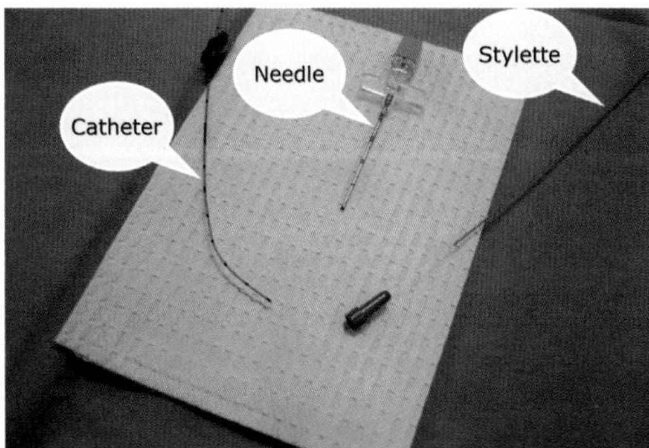

Figure 9.6 Caudal epidural catheter needle and catheter with stylette. Note the end of the stylette with a blue plastic cap as well as the black demarcation lines on the epidural catheter, which are used to note a specific depth by centimeter.

>> **Tip on Technique:** If resistance to catheter advancement is encountered, this may be because the needle/catheter unit is still within either the sacrococcygeal ligament or subcutaneous soft tissue.

8. **Confirm caudal epidural catheter placement, if desired.** After the caudal epidural catheter is advanced to the predetermined depth and before dressing, an epidurogram can be obtained using fluoroscopy. Between 0.5 and 2 mL (MAX) of iopamidol nonionic contrast can be injected through the catheter to confirm placement (Figure 9.7).

>> **Tip on Technique:** Noting how the contrast spreads within the epidural space can provide an understanding of the approximate volume of local anesthetic solution needed to cover the desired dermatomal levels.

9. **Inject the local anesthetic.** While maintaining sterile conditions, attach the medication syringe directly to the caudal catheter. Aspirate gently to ensure no return of blood or CSF. We recommend then first administering a 1-mL test dose of local anesthetic mixed with preservative-free 1:200,000 epinephrine to assist with detection of an intravascular catheter. If blood pressure or heart rate changes are detected after 1 minute, the remainder of the appropriate local anesthetic dose may be injected through the caudal catheter. Inject the medication in an incremental fashion, intermittently aspirating from the syringe to ensure no return of CSF or blood.

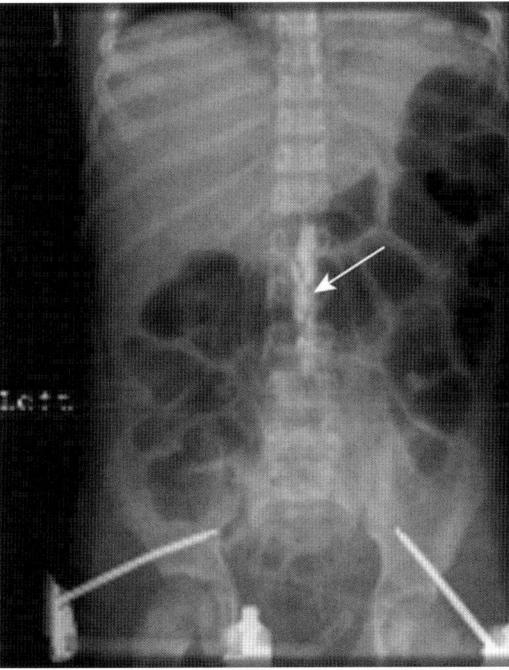

Figure 9.7 Epidurogram. After injection of contrast into the epidural space, an epidurogram shows a characteristic midline "bubbly" appearance (*arrow*). (Used with permission from Cote CJ, et al. *A Practice of Anesthesia for Infants and Children*. 5th ed. Figure 41-7. Copyright 2013, Elsevier Saunders, Page 850.)

>> **Tip on Technique:** While injecting the medication with the dominant hand, it is useful to hold the catheter with the nondominant hand at the insertion site to stabilize the catheter. Palpation over the catheter site during injection can also assist in detection of a subcutaneously placed catheter because the anesthesiologist will feel a tactile sensation of swelling and firming of the patient's subcutaneous tissue if the catheter is not in the epidural space. If swelling is encountered, the caudal catheter should be removed and replaced.

!! **Potential Complications:** During medication injection, potential complications include intravascular or intraosseous injection, local anesthetic toxicity, or subcutaneous injection.

10. **Dress the caudal catheter.** Given the approximation of the caudal catheter insertion point to the anus, contamination with fecal material and subsequent infectious complications is of special concern. With this in mind, it bears special mention to meticulously dress the caudal catheter to ensure stability and prevent soiling from fecal material.

    >> **Tip on Technique:** Our preferred method of securing the caudal catheter involves using benzoin skin adhesive and Steri-Strips over the catheter before application of a sterile transparent dressing. This technique can aid in stabilization of the catheter to help prevent inadvertent dislodgment of the catheter. After application of the transparent dressing, application of an appropriately sized sterile 1000 drape (3M, Maplewood, MN) or similar product at the caudad end of the transparent dressing can assist in containment of fecal material away from catheter insertion site. A drape placed in this fashion has been nicknamed the "mud flap."

Postoperative Management Considerations

The pediatric anesthesiologist should appropriately dose and write orders for the initial local anesthetic solution to be administered in the postoperative period through the caudal epidural catheter. The patient should be monitored and seen daily by an acute pain team, which should consist of a pediatric anesthesiologist specially trained in acute pain and regional anesthesia. This acute pain team should be available 24 hours a day to address any issues related to the catheter. Daily monitoring of the patient should be tailored to adjust local anesthetic dosing to optimize pain management as well as evaluate for complications related to catheter placement.

Special Considerations for Ultrasound-Guided Caudal Epidural Anesthesia

Ultrasound-Guided Anatomy

The sacral hiatus is easiest to see in the transverse view over the midline with an out-of-plane approach (Figure 9.8). With this view, the sacral cornua appear as two inverted U-shaped hyperechoic structures (Figure 9.8). The base of the sacral bone and sacrococcygeal ligament appear as two parallel bandlike structures situated between the cornua (Figure 9.8). Alternatively, the sacral hiatus can be viewed in the longitudinal plane at the midline (Figure 9.9).

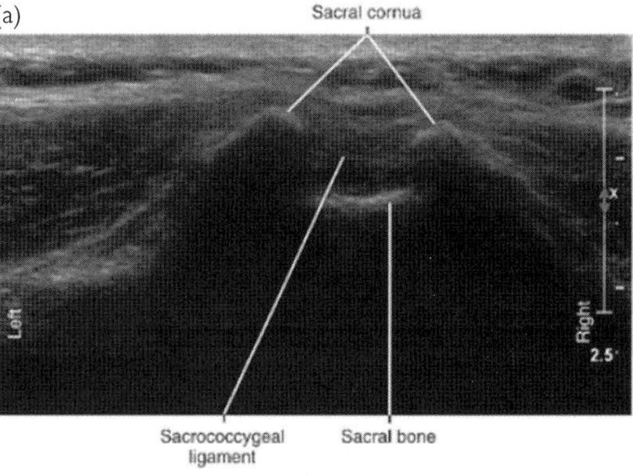

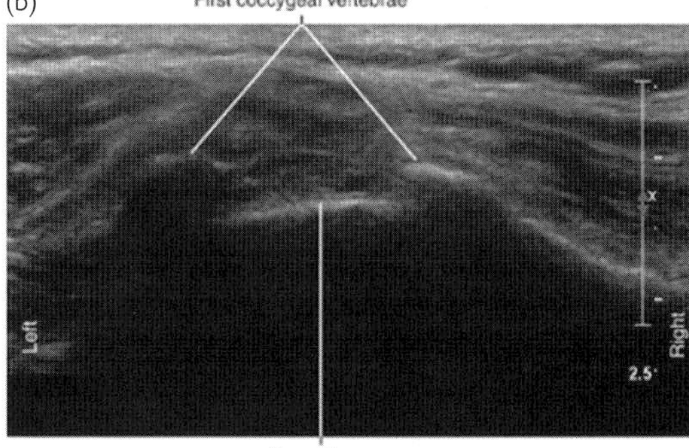

Figure 9.8 Transverse view of sacral cornua. (Used with permission from Gray AT. *Atlas of Ultrasound-Guided Regional Anesthesia*. 2nd ed. Figure 56-2. Copyright 2013 Saunders Elsevier, Page 262.)

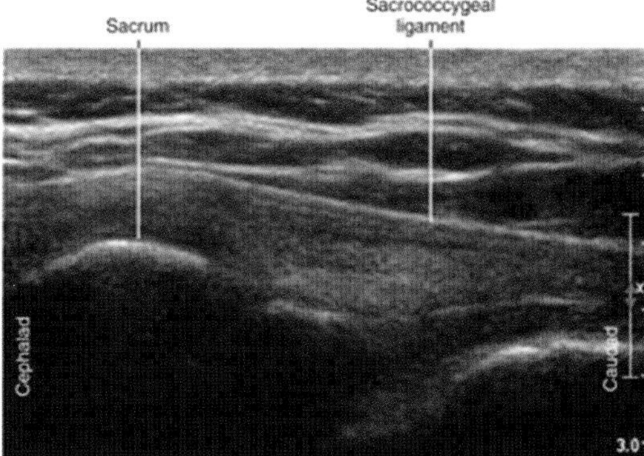

Figure 9.9 Longitudinal view of sacrum, highlighting view of sacrococcygeal ligament. (Used with permission from Gray AT. *Atlas of Ultrasound-Guided Regional Anesthesia*. 2nd ed. Figure 56-1. Copyright 2013 Saunders Elsevier, Page 261.)

Procedural Concerns

Some experts raise concerns about performing an ultrasound-guided neuraxial block under direct guidance for two reasons: (1) potential neurotoxicity of the ultrasound gel and (2) increased difficulty maintaining sterility. For these reasons, the following sequence of steps has been proposed for ultrasound-guided caudal epidural anesthesia:[13]

1. Palpate the location.
2. Confirm with ultrasound and then wipe off ultrasound gel. Place the sterile probe cover over the ultrasound probe.
3. Prep and drape the caudal epidural site in your typical sterile fashion, including sterile gloves, gown, and mask.
4. Insert needle per your usual technique into the caudal epidural space.
5. Confirm needle placement with ultrasound using sterile ultrasound gel. After the needle position is confirmed, inject under visualization, taking care to avoid contaminating the needle placement site with ultrasound gel.
6. During injection of the local anesthetic solution, ultrasound imaging should show the hypoechoic local anesthetic solution filling the space between the sacrum and sacrococcygeal ligament, in essence pushing the ligament away from the sacrum.

Further Reading

1. Campbell M. Caudal anesthesia in children. *J Urol.* 1933;30:245–249.
2. Nakamura T, Takasaki M. Metabolic and endocrine responses to surgery during caudal analgesia in children. *Can J Anaesth.* 1991;38:969–973.
3. Teyin E, Derbent A, Balcioglu T, et al. The efficacy of caudal morphine or bupivacaine combined with general anesthesia on postoperative pain and neuroendocrine stress response in children. *Pediatr Anesth.* 2006;16:290–296.
4. Jones LJ, Craven PD, Lakkundi A, et al. Regional (spinal, epidural, caudal) versus general anesthesia in preterm infants undergoing inguinal herniorrhaphy in early infancy. *Cochrane Database Syst Rev.* 2015;(6):CD003669.
5. Peterson KL, DeCampli WM, Pike NA, et al. A report of two hundred twenty cases of regional anesthesia in pediatric cardiac surgery. *Anesth Analg.* 2000;90(5):1014–1019.
6. Nguyen KN, Byrd HS, Tan JM. Caudal analgesia and cardiothoracic surgery: a look at postoperative pain scores in a pediatric population. *Paediatr Anaesth.* 2016;26(11):1060–1063.
7. Suresh S, Long J, Birmingham PK, et al. Are caudal blocks for pain control safe in children? An analysis of 18650 caudal blocks from the Pediatric Regional Anesthesia Network (PRAN) database. *Anesth Analg.* 2015;120(1):151–156.
8. Veyckemans F, Van Obbergh LJ, Gouverneur JM. Lessons from 1100 pediatric caudal blocks in a teaching hospital. *Reg Anesth.* 1992;17:119–125.
9. Johr M, Berger TM. Caudal blocks. *Paediatr Anaesth.* 2012;22(1):44–50.
10. Standring S. *Gray's Anatomy: The Anatomical Basis of Clinical Practice.* 40th ed. London: Churchill Livingstone Elsevier, 2008:749–761.
11. Lees D, Frawley G, Taghavi K, et al. A review of the surface and internal anatomy of the caudal canal in children. *Paediatr Anaesth.* 2014;24(8):799–805.
12. Dobereiner EF, Cox RG, Ewen A, et al. Evidence-based clinical update: Which local anesthetic drug for pediatric caudal block provides optimal efficacy with the fewest side effects? *Can J Anaesth.* 2010;57(12):1102–1110.
13. Taenzer AH. Personal communication with editor. January 2019.
14. Lee B, Koo BN, Choi YS, et al. Effect of caudal block using different volumes of local anaesthetic on optic nerve sheath diameter in children: a prospective, randomized trial. *Br J Anaesth.* 2017;118(5):781–787.

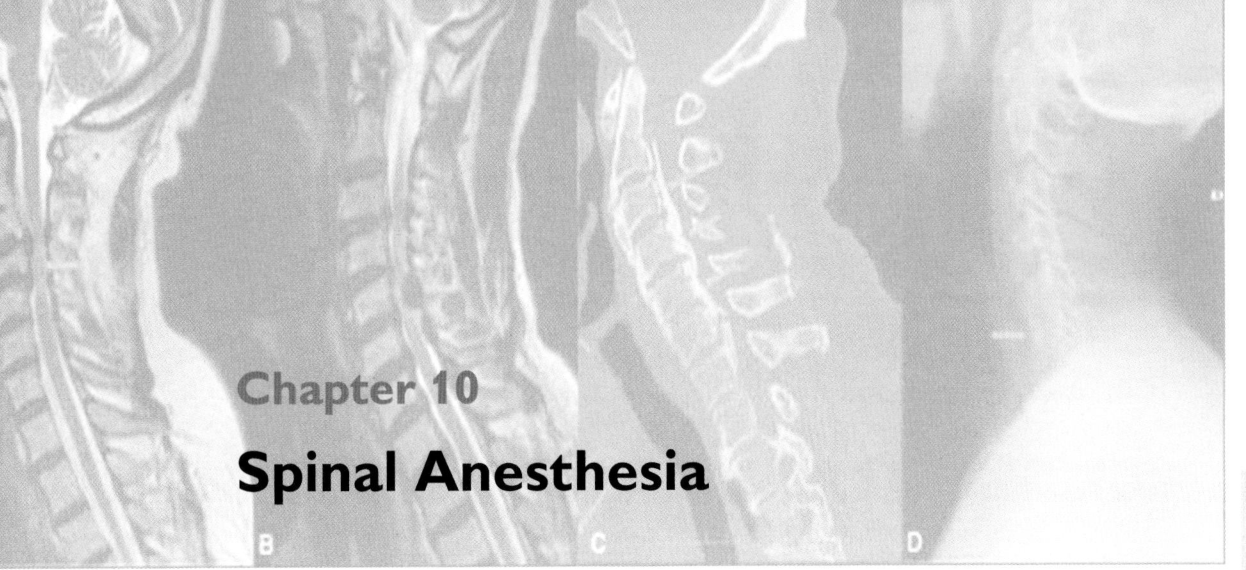

Chapter 10

Spinal Anesthesia

Alina Lazar

Introduction

Spinal anesthesia is the injection of local anesthetics and additives into the subarachnoid space, providing analgesia by creating a sensory block and providing suitable surgical conditions by creating a motor block. After positioning the patient and sterilizing the skin, the puncture site is infiltrated with 1% lidocaine, and the spinal needle is inserted in the midline at the L3–4 or L4–5 interspace. When cerebrovascular fluid appears at the tip of the needle, the desired medications are injected, and the needle is removed.[1]

Clinical Applications

In the pediatric population, spinal "intrathecal" anesthesia can be used as an alternative to general anesthesia for lower extremity and abdominal surgery in high-risk patients (e.g., premature or former premature infants, teenagers with malignant hyperthermia susceptibility or chronic respiratory disease).[2] Preservative-free morphine injected into the intrathecal space can also be used for postoperative pain control, for example, after scoliosis repair.

Contraindications

Contraindications for performing a spinal anesthetic include lack of parental consent, low conus medullaris position of the spinal cord, coagulopathy, infection at the puncture site, bacteremia/sepsis, increased intracranial pressure, uncontrolled seizures, hemodynamic instability, and anatomic deformities. Spinal block is controversial in children with neuromuscular diseases (particularly central core disease) or in the presence of a ventriculoperitoneal shunt (risk for shunt infection and dural leak).[3]

All anesthesiologists should be familiar with current American Society of Regional Anesthesia and Pain Medicine (ASRA) guidelines regarding anticoagulation and bleeding disorders in the setting of neuraxial anesthesia before performing any neuraxial anesthetic. These are available at http://www.asra.com.

WARNING!! Spinal anesthesia is absolutely contraindicated in infants with spinal cord abnormalities, including a low conus medullaris position of the spinal cord, occult spinal dysraphism, spinal cord tethering, or a thickened filum terminale. Ultrasound may help identify these anomalies, which are more common in infants with urogenital anomalies. The presence of a hairy nevus or sacral dimple above the gluteal cleft could indicate occult spinal dysraphism.[4]

Critical Anatomy

The conus medullaris ends at the L3 level in neonates and reaches adult levels by the second year of life. During flexion of the spine, the intercristal (Tuffier) line bisects the L5 vertebra. The ligamentum flavum is very soft in children, and a "pop" may not be perceived when the dura is penetrated. The distance from skin to subarachnoid space (in millimeters) can be estimated by the formula: weight (kg) × 2 + 7.[5] Therefore, the estimated distance from the skin to the subarachnoid space in a 10-kg child is 27 mm, or 2.7 cm.

Setup

Equipment

- A 22- or 25-gauge styletted "pencil point" (Quincke) needle (see Table 10.1 for recommended needle lengths)

Table 10.1 Spinal Needle Length Based on Patient Age

Age (years)	Needle Length (inches)
<2	1.5
2–12	2.5
>12	3.5

- Airway management equipment in age-appropriate sizes
- Induction agents
- Resuscitation agents
- Standard American Society of Anesthesiologists (ASA) monitors

WARNING!! Nonstyletted (intravenous [IV] catheter and hypodermic) needles should NOT be used because they carry the risk for the creation of lumbar epidermoid tumors from the inadvertent deposition of skin tags.

Pearl: In infants, the use of a 'Slip Tip' tuberculin syringe may offer greater precision in drug delivery compared with a Luer-Lock syringe.

Drugs, Dosages, Administration

The dose and duration of action of commonly used local anesthetics and additives are shown in Tables 10.2 and 10.3, respectively. Epinephrine and clonidine prolong the duration of a spinal block by at least 30% in children, significantly longer than in adults. Spinal opioids, alone or in addition to local anesthetics, also prolong analgesia.[2]

Pearl: Because of a proportionally higher cerebrospinal fluid (CSF) volume, the amount of drug required for spinal anesthesia is greater per kilogram in children than in adults. Fast drug reabsorption and rapid CSF turnover also shorten the duration of spinal anesthesia in children.

Table 10.2 Local Anesthetic Doses and Duration of Action for Spinal Anesthesia

Type of Local Anesthetic	Doses Based on Weight			Duration Range (mean), in minutes
	<5 kg	5–15 kg	>15 kg	
Bupivacaine 0.5% isobaric or 0.75% hyperbaric	0.5–1* mg/kg	0.4 mg/kg	0.3 mg/kg	30–180 (80)
Tetracaine 0.5% hyperbaric†	0.5–1* mg/kg	0.4 mg/kg	0.3 mg/kg	35–240 (90)
Ropivacaine 0.5% isobaric	0.5–1* mg/kg	0.5 mg/kg	0.5 mg/kg	34–210 (96)

*Larger doses are used to achieve higher (mid-upper thoracic) sensory block and longer duration of anesthesia.
† Hyperbaric tetracaine is prepared by mixing equal volumes of tetracaine 1% and dextrose 10%.

Table 10.3 Additives Used for Spinal Anesthesia

Type	Dose (MICROgrams/kg)
Epinephrine	2–3
Morphine	4–15
Fentanyl	0.2–2
Clonidine	1–2

WARNING!! It is important to calculate the allowable total local anesthetic dose by weight and to stay below this maximum dose in order to decrease the risk for local anesthetic systemic toxicity (LAST). This calculation should include all local anesthetics, including that given by the surgeon, IV local anesthetic given by the anesthesiologist, and EMLA or subcutaneous lidocaine given before starting an IV. See Chapter 15, Local Anesthetic Systemic Toxicity Treatment.

Caution! Infants and young children (especially former premature infants) who receive a spinal anesthetic are at an especially high risk for developing postoperative apnea, even if they have not received additional sedative or anesthetic medications.[1] Careful monitoring is essential.

!! **Potential Complications:** If large doses of local anesthetics are administered or if the child is placed in the Trendelenburg position (or if the legs are raised, e.g., for a diaper change) too quickly after a block, high or total spinal anesthesia may result. In awake infants, this manifests as oxygen desaturation and apnea. Under anesthesia, the presence of a high or total spinal may become apparent when spontaneous respirations do not occur during attempted emergence. Biphasic respiratory depression can also be caused by intrathecal opioids. The first phase is soon after injection, similar to that caused by IV opioids. The second phase typically occurs 6 to 12 (although up to 24) hours later and is due to the rostral migration of morphine in the CSF and subsequent action on the brainstem's respiration centers. Continuous pulse oximetry and ready access to naloxone are essential for the first 24 hours after the administration of intrathecal opioids.

!! **Potential Complications:** Clonidine may cause transient hypotension and apnea. Opioids may lead to itching.

>> **Tip on Technique:** Elevating the head of the infant off of the table 45 degrees when the infant is in the lateral decubitus position increases CSF pressure and may increase the success rate for a spinal anesthetic.

Before starting the case, gather all the necessary equipment. Based on the patient's body weight and desired level of sensory block, calculate an appropriate dose of local anesthetic and adjuvant (if desired).

>> **Tip on Technique:** It may be useful to gather all supplies on a mobile flat surface, such as a Mayo stand.

>> **Tip on Technique:** The dose of local anesthetic (with additives, if used) should be calculated and prepared in a syringe before dural puncture. Add a volume of local anesthetic equal to the volume of the spinal needle dead space (usually 0.1 mL) to the calculated volume of local anesthetic.

Step-by-Step

1. **Prepare before the procedure.** If the patient will be awake during the procedure, apply a small amount of EMLA (eutectic mixture of local anesthetics) or lidocaine 4% (LMX-4) to the lumbar area and cover with an occlusive dressing for 1 hour (for EMLA) or 30 minutes (for lidocaine), before the spinal block to reduce patient discomfort during insertion of the spinal needle (Figure 10.1). Older patients may also benefit from an anxiolytic before the procedure. For all procedures, the patient should be connected to standard ASA monitors, the patient should have IV access, and airway management and resuscitation equipment and medications should be immediately available. If the patient will be under general anesthesia for the procedure, induce the patient, secure IV access, and manage the airway per your institution's standards.

   !! **Potential Complications:** Patient age <32 weeks, anemia, concomitant administration of acetaminophen, and large doses of EMLA increase the risk for methemoglobinemia after EMLA administration.

   Note: Because hemodynamic stability is maintained after spinal anesthesia in infants, a preprocedure IV fluid bolus is typically NOT administered.

2. **Position the patient.** Place the patient in one of two positions: sitting (if the patient will be awake or lightly sedated during the procedure) or the lateral decubitus position (if the patient will be under general anesthesia or heavily sedated). In either position, an assistant should maintain the patient's back firmly in a flexed position.

   Sitting position. Position the patient with maximal hip flexion to widen the interspinous space. This position also increases CSF pressure by creating a hydrostatic column, aiding the clinician in recognizing when the dural puncture has occurred. We advise placing a

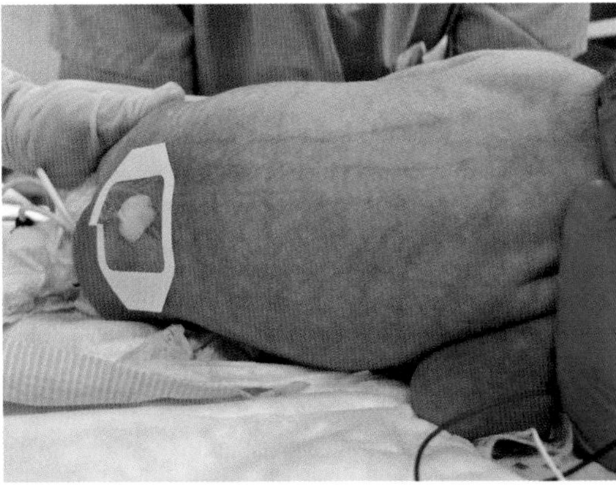

Figure 10.1 Topical EMLA anesthesia application before the spinal block.

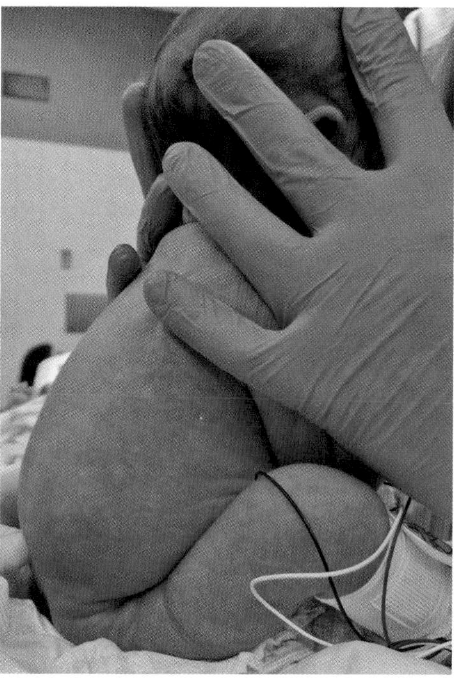

Figure 10.2 Sitting position with hips maximally flexed and head supported.

folded towel under the infant to create more room to attach the syringe to the spinal needle (Figure 10.2).[6]

>> **Tip on Technique:** If the patient will be awake for the procedure, consider placing the blood pressure cuff on the lower extremity so that compression from the blood pressure cuff does not disturb the patient during surgery.

Lateral decubitus position: For larger, more vigorous infants, placement in the lateral decubitus position may also help to stabilize the patient and prevent rotation of the spine (Figure 10.3).

>> **Tip on Technique:** If the block is being performed by a right-handed clinician, placing the patient in the left lateral decubitus position facilitates palpation of the landmarks with the left hand, while the syringe/needle is in the right hand for the procedure.

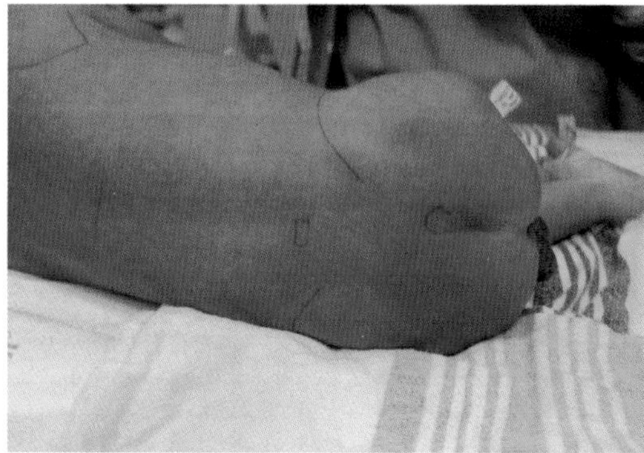

Figure 10.3 Lateral decubitus position with landmarks identified.

3. **Identify anatomical landmarks and prepare the skin.** Ultrasonography may be used to delineate anatomy. Cleanse the skin with betadine or chlorhexidine, and use sterile technique (including sterile gloves) throughout the procedure.

WARNING!!	Both chlorhexidine and povidone-iodine (Betadine) are neurotoxic and should be completely dry before inserting a spinal needle to prevent tracking of these fluids into the subarachnoid space. Avoid chlorhexidine in infants younger than 6 months.
WARNING!!	Alcohol-based skin preparation solutions are a potential fire hazards in the operating room, especially when electrocautery is used for the surgical procedure. When using an alcohol-based skin prep, do not allow excess preparation solution to pool around or under the patient. Ensure that the alcohol-based skin preparation solution is completely dry and that any excess is wiped away with towels before preparing the patient for surgery.

4. **If the patient is awake, comfort and/or sedate the patient.** Comfort awake infants with a pacifier dipped in sucrose "sweeties" (Figure 10.4). Administer sedation judiciously according to your clinical judgment. If topical anesthesia was not applied preoperatively, inject a small amount (<0.25 mL) of 1% lidocaine with a 25- to 30-gauge needle into the skin and subcutaneous tissue at the puncture site in awake or sedated children (Figure 10.5).

   Note: Some pediatric surgeons will perform hernia repair or urogenital procedures in awake infants under spinal anesthesia alone without general anesthesia. Previously, for those procedures, when possible, spinal anesthesia without sedation was recommended for preterm or former preterm infants to prevent apnea.[7] Newer studies, however, suggest that the risk for apnea may be the same in infants who receive a spinal anesthetic alone or with sedation.[1]

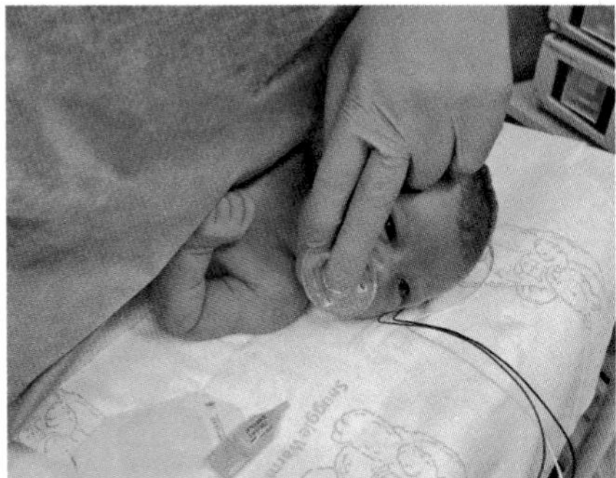

Figure 10.4 Infant being soothed with a pacifier dipped in sucrose.

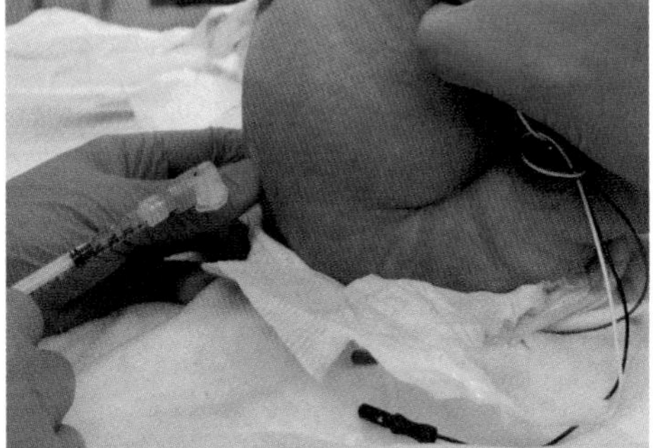

Figure 10.5 Skin infiltration with local anesthetic using a tuberculin syringe.

5. **Insert the spinal needle and inject medication into the subarachnoid space.** Insert the spinal needle into the midline of the back over the spinous process at the L3–4 or L4–5 interspace, perpendicular to the skin or angled up slightly, with the bevel facing cranially (Figure 10.6). In infants, remove the stylet promptly (0.5 cm), and advance the needle slowly to prevent passing the needle beyond the subarachnoid space and entering the venous plexus. Resistance to needle advancement may increase slightly as the needle enters the ligaments. If CSF is not obtained after the first pass, withdraw the needle slowly, adjust the position of the needle relative to the patient's sagittal plane, and attempt advancement again. When CSF is seen exiting the needle, slowly inject the drug (over at least 10 seconds), remove the needle, and immediately place the patient into a supine position.

> **WARNING!!** Raising the infant's legs (to place the electrocautery pad or for other reasons) can cause an excessively high blockade level. Placing a small shoulder roll can help to reduce rostral spread of local anesthetic.

> **Caution!** AVOID injecting the drug rapidly or using the barbotage method (repeated injection of anesthetic and withdrawal of CSF). Rapid injection or barbotage may cause a high or total spinal block.

Note: Flow is slower through smaller needles. Especially when a very small (e.g., 25-gauge) needle is used, a delay may occur between entrance of the needle tip into the subarachnoid space and the appearance of CSF at the needle hub. Advance the needle incrementally and very slowly.

6. **Evaluate block level.** Assess the level of the spinal block; in awake patients, profound muscle weakness in the lower extremities and a lack of response to a firm skin pinch in the dermatomal area that will be operated on should be observed to confirm block level.

Note: Supplemental local anesthesia may be given by the surgeon if needed during the latter part of surgery when the spinal block regresses. Be cognizant of the total dose of local anesthetic to avoid local anesthetic systemic toxicity.

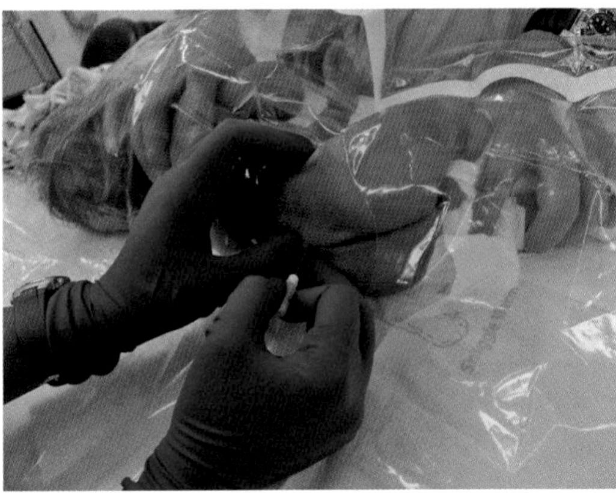

Figure 10.6 Insertion of the spinal needle.

7. **Sedate the patient for the surgical procedure, if needed.** Because deafferentation from a spinal block produces sedation, during surgery infants require nothing more than soothing music, a warm blanket, a pacifier or finger to suck on, and occasionally drops of an oral sucrose solution. Older children may be sedated or encouraged to listen to music or to watch videos, and often require general anesthesia in addition to the spinal anesthetic.

   >> **Tip on Technique:** For surgeries in infants with spinal anesthesia only, use soft restraints to prevent an infant's arm from reaching onto the sterile field and to prevent the infant's legs from moving as the motor block regresses.

Postoperative Management Considerations

Postoperative complications from a spinal block are infrequent. They include postdural puncture headache, transient radicular symptoms, back pain, and arachnoiditis.

Caution! In infants (especially if premature), intraoperative hypoxemia, apnea, and bradycardia may occur even in the absence of a high block or sedation administration.[8] Postoperative monitoring should be continued for at least 12 hours after surgery. Patients who receive subarachnoid morphine or clonidine should be monitored for apnea for 24 hours postoperatively.

Further Reading

Gupta A, Saha U. Spinal anesthesia in children: a review. *J Anaesthesiol Clin Pharmacol.* 2014;30(1):10–18.

References

1. Davidson AJ, Morton NS, Arnup SJ, et al; General Anesthesia Compared to Spinal Anesthesia (GAS) Consortium. Apnea after awake regional and general anesthesia in infants: the General Anesthesia Compared to Spinal Anesthesia Study—comparing apnea and neurodevelopmental outcomes, a randomized controlled trial. *Anesthesiology.* 2015;123:38–54.
2. Williams RK, Adams DC, Aladjem EV, et al. The safety and efficacy of spinal anesthesia for surgery in infants: the Vermont Infant Spinal Registry. *Anesth Analg.* 2006;102:67–71.
3. Lopez T, Sanchez FJ, Garzon JC, Muriel C. Spinal anesthesia in pediatric patients. *Minerva Anestesiol.* 2012;78:78–87.
4. Lederhaas G. Spinal anaesthesia in paediatrics. *Best Pract Res Clin Anaesthesiol.* 2003;17:365–376.
5. Arthurs OJ, Murray M, Zubier M, et al. Ultrasonographic determination of neonatal spinal canal depth. *Arch Dis Child Fetal Neonatal Ed.* 2008;93:F451–F454.
6. Shenkman Z, Hoppenstein D, Litmanowitz I, et al. Spinal anesthesia in 62 premature, former-premature or young infants—technical aspects and pitfalls. *Can J Anaesth.* 2002;49:262–269.
7. Welborn LG, Rice LJ, Hannallah RS, et al. Postoperative apnea in former preterm infants: prospective comparison of spinal and general anesthesia. *Anesthesiology.* 1990;72:838–842.
8. Davidson A, Frawley GP, Sheppard S, et al. Risk factors for apnea after infant inguinal hernia repair. *Paediatr Anaesth.* 2009;19:402–403.

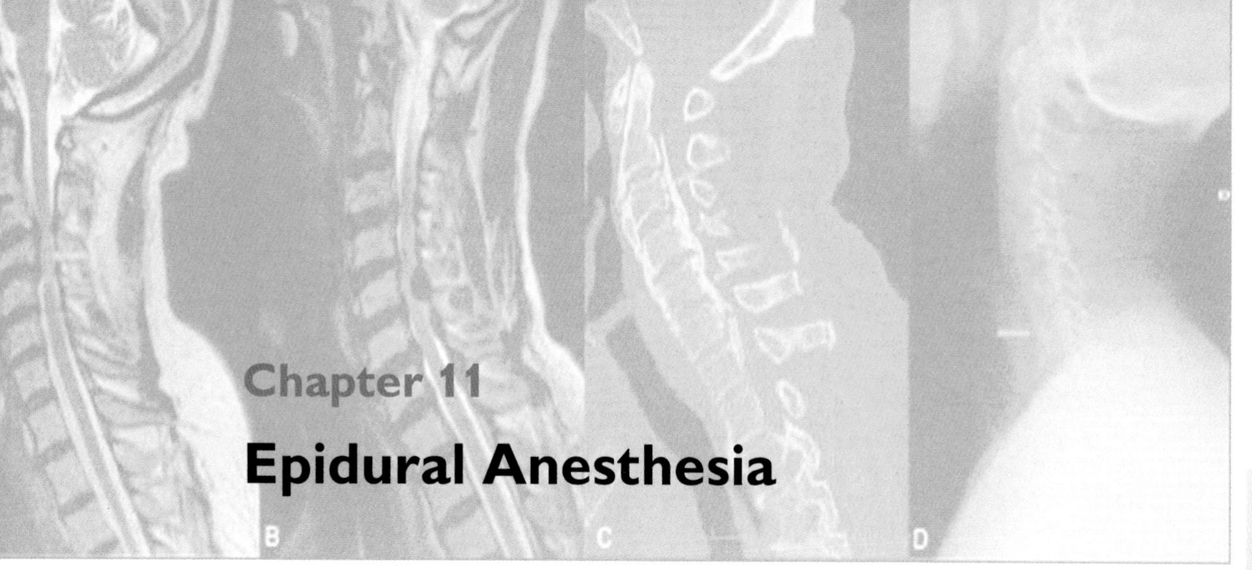

Chapter 11

Epidural Anesthesia

Alina Lazar

Introduction

During epidural anesthesia, local anesthetics and adjuvants are administered into the epidural space by a single-shot, intermittent, or continuous technique.

Clinical Applications

Epidural analgesia is used for open thoracic surgery, major intra-abdominal surgery with extensive surgical dissection, major lower extremity surgery, and long-term pain management.

Contraindications

Epidural anesthesia is contraindicated in children with uncorrected coagulopathy (platelet count <100,000/mm^3 or prothrombin time [PT]/partial thromboplastin time [PTT] >1.5 times control), hemophilia, von Willebrand disease or other coagulopathies, liver disease causing coagulopathy, skin infection at the insertion site, bacteremia/sepsis, or lack of parental consent. The presence of a ventriculoperitoneal shunt is a relative contraindication.

All anesthesiologists should be familiar with current American Society of Regional Anesthesia and Pain Medicine (ASRA) guidelines regarding anticoagulation and bleeding disorders in the setting of neuraxial anesthesia before performing epidural anesthesia. These are available at http://www.asra.com.

Critical Anatomy

In infants, the tip of the conus medullaris and dural sac are located lower in the spinal column than in adults. Additionally, because the epidural space contains less fat and fibrous tissue than in adults, in infants it is easier to insert an epidural catheter at a lower level and then to thread it up to a higher level. In infants younger than 6 months, the vertebral column remains cartilaginous, and epidural catheters can be visualized with ultrasonography. In infants, for the initial placement of the needle, there is a more subtle "give" as the ligamentum flavum is pierced than in adult patients. As a general rule, the depth of the epidural space is 1 mm/kg of body weight (e.g., the depth of the epidural space in a 10-kg child would be 10 mm). However, because wide variation exists in the depth of the epidural space, a test for loss of resistance is performed as soon as the epidural needle has entered the supraspinous ligament.

Setup

Equipment

- Tuohy needles of a suitable size: 3.5 inch, 18 gauge (for adult-sized patients); 3 inch, 18 gauge (for children); and 3 inch, 19 gauge (for infants <5 kg). The short (3-inch) needles are marked at 0.5-cm intervals.

  Note: Smaller gauge and shorter needles are used when appropriate because they are easier to handle, and the smaller bevel is a better fit for the narrow epidural space.

- Catheters: 20 gauge (adult size) and 21 gauge (for small infants)

  Note: The coil-reinforced catheters can be visualized easily by radiographic examination even in the absence of a stylet.

> **Caution!** Pediatric epidural catheters may not have the same depth markings as adult catheters.

Drugs, Dosages, Administration

Loading volumes of 0.25% bupivacaine or 0.2% ropivacaine are 0.3 mL/kg for thoracic epidurals and 0.5 mL/kg for lumbar epidurals. A dose of half of the initial bolus can be given 90 minutes after the initial dose. The first step in planning an epidural infusion is to determine the maximal amount of acceptable local anesthetic that may be infused per hour (Table 11.1). Infusions that combined local anesthetic (see Table 11.1) and opioid and/or clonidine (Table 11.2) are administered at 0.1 to 0.3 mL/kg/hr. Patient-controlled epidural anesthesia (PCEA) can be used in children as young as 5 years. A common PCEA bupivacaine regimen for a child is a basal rate of 0.2 mg/kg/hr, bolus of 0.1 mg/kg/hr, lockout interval of 15 minutes, and maximum hourly rate of 0.4 mg/kg/hr.[1]

> **WARNING!!** It is important to calculate the allowable total local anesthetic dose by weight and to stay below this maximum dose in order to decrease the risk for local anesthetic systemic toxicity (LAST). This calculation should include all local anesthetics, including that given by the surgeon, IV local anesthetic given by the anesthesiologist, and EMLA or subcutaneous lidocaine given before starting an IV. Coordinate this with operating room staff. See Chapter 15, Local Anesthetic Systemic Toxicity Treatment

!! **Potential Complications:** Potential complications include local anesthetic systemic toxicity, pruritus, nausea and vomiting, urinary retention, respiratory depression, and sedation.

> **Caution!** In neonates and infants, cardiac dysrhythmias and apnea may be the presenting symptoms of local anesthetic systemic toxicity.

Table 11.1 Maximum Rates of Commonly Used Local Anesthetics Epidural Infusions in Pediatric Patients

Drug (common concentrations)	Rate (mg/kg/hr) *		
	0–2 Months	**3–6 Months**	**>6 Months**
Bupivacaine (0.05%, 0.1%)	0.25	0.3	0.4
Ropivacaine (0.1%)	0.3	0.4	0.4

* Infusion rates should not exceed 15 mL/hr. In neonates, limit infusion duration to 48 hours (concern for cumulative toxicity).

Table 11.2 Recommended Rates of Adjuvants for Continuous Epidural

Drug	Dose* (mcg/kg/hr)	Typical Concentration (mcg/mL)		
		Neonates (0–2 months)	**Infants**	**Children**
Fentanyl	0.1–0.5	1-2	2 (2-5)	5 (2-5)
Hydromorphone	1	NR	NR	10-20
Morphine	2.5	NR	NR	25-50
Clonidine†	0.1	NR	0.4	0.4-1 (lumbar epidural tip) 0.4-0.6 (thoracic epidural tip)

*Larger doses of opioids are indicated for opioid-tolerant patients.
† When clonidine is added to an epidural solution, the epidural opioid dose should be reduced by 50%.
NR = not recommended.

Pearl: In the absence of hypovolemia, epidural anesthesia in children younger than 8 years is associated with remarkable cardiovascular stability. If hypotension in a child with an epidural occurs in the absence of surgical bleeding, suspect subarachnoid or subdural catheter placement.

Before starting the case, gather all necessary equipment for an epidural anesthetic. Based on the patient's body weight and desired level of sensory block, calculate an appropriate dose of local anesthetic and adjuvant (if desired).

Caution! Double-check your patient's allergies before preparing medications and antiseptic solutions.

>> Tip on Technique: It may be useful to gather all supplies on a mobile flat surface.

Step-by-Step

1. **Conduct a preoperative evaluation; prepare.** Epidural anesthesia is commonly administered in children under general anesthesia. Cooperative children and teenagers may tolerate the procedure awake with minimal/light sedation (fentanyl and midazolam). For all procedures, the patient should be connected to standard American Society of Anesthesiologists (ASA) monitors, the patient should have intravenous (IV) access, and airway management and resuscitation equipment and medications should be immediately available.
2. **Position the patient, identify landmarks, and prepare the skin.** If the child is under general anesthesia, he or she should be placed in the lateral decubitus position with the knees drawn up to the chest. In children under minimal/light sedation, the sitting position may be used, in which case an assistant maintains the curvature of the back.

Caution! Attempting epidural anesthesia in an awake, uncooperative, or a heavily sedated patient may increase risk if the patient moves during the procedure.

Use a sterile technique, including sterile gloves, throughout. Identify the anatomic landmarks, prepare the skin with a sterile disinfecting solution, and apply a sterile drape over the insertion area. In awake/lightly sedated patients, infiltrate the skin with 1% lidocaine (Figure 11.1).

Pearl: In both children and adults, the intercristal line (a horizontal line reaching across the highest portions of both of the iliac crests) bisects the L5 vertebra.

WARNING!! Alcohol-based skin preparation solutions are a potential fire hazard in the operating room, especially when electrocautery is used for the surgical procedure. When using alcohol-based skin prep, do not allow excess preparation solution to pool around or under the patient. Ensure that the alcohol-based skin preparation solution is completely dry and that any excess is wiped away with towels before preparing the patient for surgery.

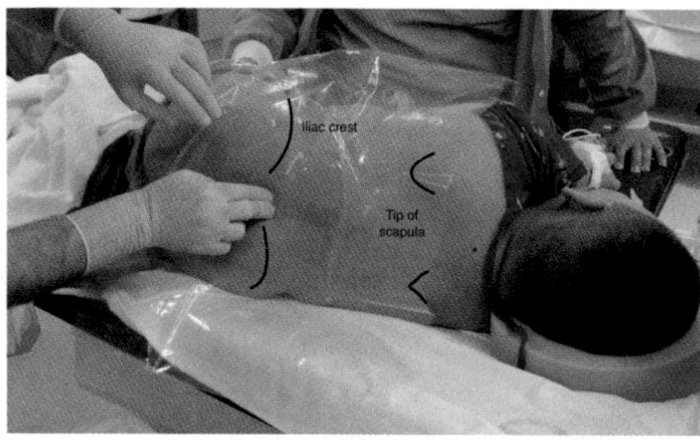

Figure 11.1 Patient in lateral decubitus position with anatomic landmarks demonstrated.

3. **Insert the needle into the epidural space.** For the lumbar approach, in younger children insert the needle at the L4–5 or L5–S1 spinal interspace, and in older children insert the needle at the L3–4 interspace (Figure 11.2). In children, the epidural needle is typically inserted midline. The needle insertion angle is 75 degrees pointing cephalad for lumbar vertebral levels, and slightly steeper (although not as steep as in adults) for thoracic vertebral levels. For older children, some anesthesiologists prefer the paramedian approach, in which the needle is inserted slightly lateral to the midline, advanced to a lamina, and "walked off" the superior edge of the lamina until the ligamentum flavum is reached. Advance the needle with the stylet in place until the interspinous ligament is reached.

Caution! In children, the resistance to advancement through the ligamentum flavum may not be perceived as different from the resistance through the interspinous and supraspinous ligaments.

Advance the saline-filled needle is using either the incremental two-handed technique (checking for loss of resistance after each minimal advancement; Figure 11.3), or with continuous thumb pressure on the syringe plunger as the epidural needle is advanced (i.e., Bromage grip).

Caution! Direct thoracic insertion of a needle in anesthetized children is high risk and should only be performed by anesthesiologists highly experienced in this technique.

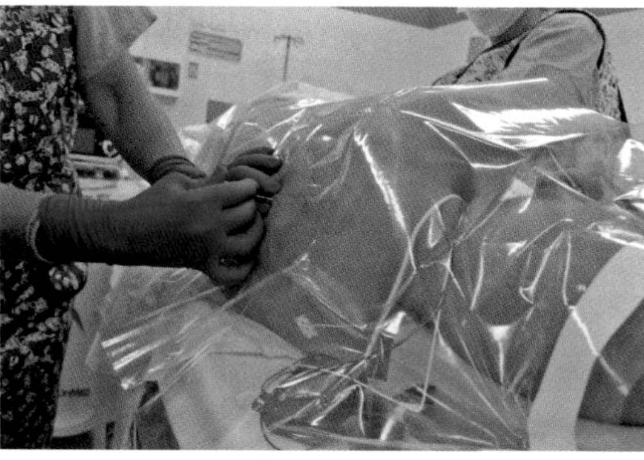

Figure 11.2 Epidural needle insertion.

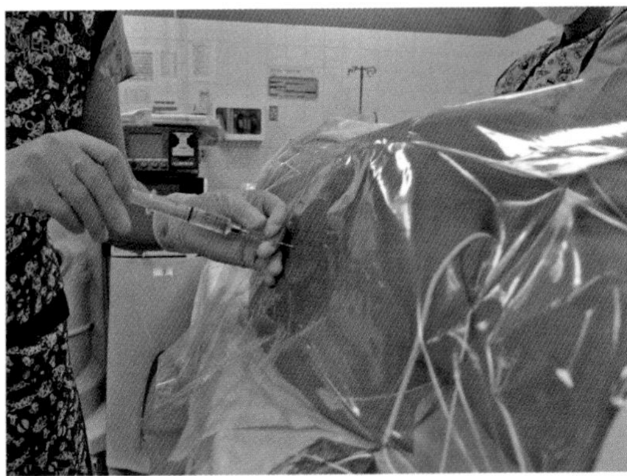

Figure 11.3 Loss of resistance to saline.

Caution! Because of an increased risk for venous air embolism, neurologic injury, and patchy block, the loss of resistance to air technique is generally not used in children.[2]

>> **Tip on Technique:** Making a small skin nick with a 22-gauge needle at the epidural site before inserting the epidural needle decreases the pressure required to advance the needle through the skin and decreases the likelihood of having the needle advance too far and accidentally puncture the dura.

!! **Potential Complications:** Given the small distance from the skin to the epidural space, there is a 10% risk for dural puncture in children.[3] Postdural puncture headache (PDPH), however, is rare in the pediatric population. This may be because children have a lower cerebrospinal fluid (CSF) pressure (because of their shorter stature). Additionally, young patients' inability to articulate symptoms may explain the low incidence of PDPH. The management of PDPH in children includes bed rest, hydration, analgesics, antiemetics, caffeine, and—rarely—an epidural blood patch. Epidural hematoma and neurologic injury are rare in children; however, direct trauma to the spinal cord has been reported in both awake and anesthetized patients undergoing neuraxial anesthesia.

4. **Insert the epidural catheter and administer the test dose.** Epidural catheter advancement in children is associated with greater resistance than in adults. Advance the catheter until 1.5 to 2 cm are in the epidural space. For example, if the epidural space is reached with the needle 2 cm into the skin, threading the catheter so that 4 cm are in the patient (4 cm mark at entrance to skin) will achieve the desired goal of 2 cm of catheter in the epidural space. Remove the epidural needle while being careful to avoid pulling out the epidural catheter (going slowly and pushing the catheter in slightly with each pulling out motion of the needle can assist with avoiding catheter dislodgment). Next, hold the catheter tip below the level of the insertion point (Figure 11.4) and examine the catheter for the presence of blood or CSF (if either is seen, the catheter must be removed). Tightly attach the injection port to the end of the epidural catheter (will vary by manufacturer) and aspirate from this port, again looking for blood or CSF. After aspiration, inject a test dose (0.1 mL/kg of 1–1.5%

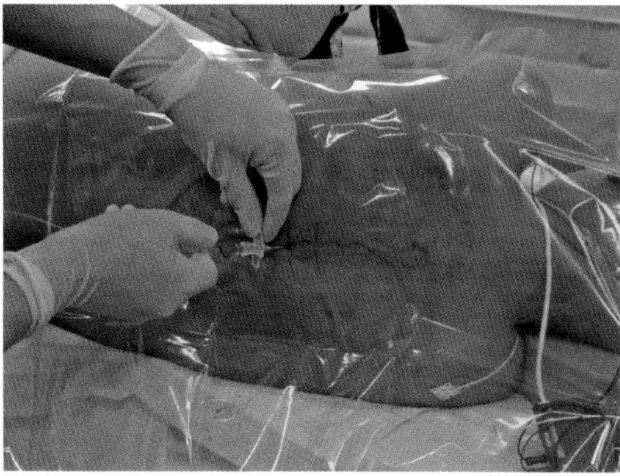

Figure 11.4 Epidural catheter insertion.

lidocaine containing epinephrine 1:200,000, maximum 3 mL) through the epidural catheter. If the catheter is malpositioned, intravascular injection is signaled by an increase in the heart rate, hypertension, or changes in T-wave appearance on the electrocardiogram.

>> **Tip on Technique:** Some anesthesiologists will deliberately choose a needle insertion point a few levels below the desired dermatome and thread the catheter 3 to 5 cm into the epidural space, up to the desired level. This technique allows more of the catheter to be in situ, which may reduce the risk for dislodgment.

> **Caution!** A negative test dose reduces but does not eliminate the possibility of intravascular injection.[4] Of note, T-wave changes, which may indicate intravascular local anesthetic injection, are unreliable during total IV anesthesia.[5]

>> **Tip on Technique:** Advancement of an epidural catheter to a thoracic level through a needle inserted into the epidural space at the lumbar level is less successful than through a needle inserted caudally.[6] However, if a lumbar position is chosen, advancement to thoracic levels is more successful from a high lumbar level than from a lower lumbar level. Success with threading a catheter to the thoracic level can be impeded by the fact that many catheters coil within the epidural space close to the insertion point. When the catheter is far from the desired location, larger volumes of local anesthetics or the addition of opioid can improve the block quality.

5. **Verify the catheter tip position.** Ordinarily, verifying the position of a catheter inserted in the proximity of the surgical dermatome is not needed. However, catheters threaded from a more distant vertebral level do not always arrive at their desired level, and their placement must be verified. The tip of a radiopaque catheter can be easily visualized radiographically. Injection of contrast through the catheter may help identify subdural or intravascular placement and predict analgesic coverage.[7] With ultrasound-guided placement, catheter tip advancement is visualized in real time[8] but requires the help of an experienced assistant. Take care to ensure that ultrasound gel is kept far from the epidural insertion site because the potential for neurotoxicity of the ultrasound gel is unknown.

Caution! Catheters may migrate cephalad after the patient's position is changed from prone or lateral to supine.[9] Compared with firm inelastic epidural catheters, more stretchy and elastic epidural catheters may be predisposed to inward migration postoperatively in active patients owing to a gripping motion of the catheter by the ligamentum flavum.[10]

Pearl: Compared with adults, children require a significantly higher volume of local anesthetic per kilogram of body weight to achieve the same dermatomal spread. Therefore, the catheter tip must be positioned at the level of the surgical incision.

6. **Secure the epidural catheter.** Secure the epidural catheter with a liquid topical adhesive, clear occlusive dressing, and tape (Figure 11.5).

Note: Epidural catheters migrate in approximately 40% of cases. A catheter that migrates may perforate dura or a blood vessel, advance to a high thoracic or cervical area, or be dislodged.

Note: Leakage of infusion fluid around the catheter insertion site is a common problem in small infants because the epidural space may be shallow (e.g., <1 cm deep), and the tissues through which the catheter passes are not dense.

>> Tip on Technique: Application of a liquid topical adhesive, such as Dermabond, over the insertion site decreases problems with catheter leakage or migration. Other products for catheter fixation can result in problems; for example Mastisol may cause skin tears upon removal of dressings, and Steri-Strips may create kinks in the catheter. Commercial fixation devices, such as the SIMS Portex Lockit device, and catheter tunneling may also be used.

!! Potential Complications: Potential clinical manifestations of a migrated epidural catheter are a high neuraxial block, Horner syndrome, bradycardia, local anesthetic toxicity, or loss of effective analgesia.

Postoperative Management Considerations

If the epidural catheter remains in place after surgery, it should be carefully managed by the anesthesiologist or acute pain service to ensure correct dose-infusion rates, lack of migration, and

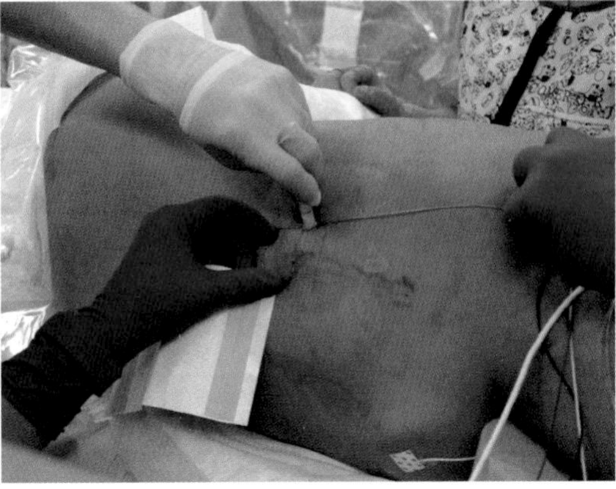

Figure 11.5 Securing the epidural catheter.

success in controlling postoperative pain. Any concern for postoperative coagulopathy (e.g., from intraoperative blood loss, medications given, liver dysfunction) should be addressed before catheter removal.

References

1. Saudan S, Habre W, Ceroni D, et al. Safety and efficacy of patient controlled epidural analgesia following pediatric spinal surgery. *Paediatr Anaesth.* 2008;18(2):132–139.
2. Brown TC, Eyres RL, McDougall RJ. Local and regional anaesthesia in children. *Br J Anaesth.* 1999;83(1):65–77.
3. Dalens B, Tanguy A, Haberer JP. Lumbar epidural anesthesia for operative and postoperative pain relief in infants and young children. *Anesth Analg.* 1986;65(10):1069–1073.
4. Sethna NF, McGowan FX Jr. Do results from studies of a simulated epidural test dose improve our ability to detect unintentional epidural vascular puncture in children? *Paediatr Anaesth.* 2005;15(9):711–715.
5. Polaner DM, Zuk J, Luong K, Pan Z. Positive intravascular test dose criteria in children during total intravenous anesthesia with propofol and remifentanil are different than during inhaled anesthesia. *Anesth Analg.* 2010;110(1):41–45.
6. Shenkman Z, Hoppenstein D, Erez I, et al. Continuous lumbar/thoracic epidural analgesia in low-weight paediatric surgical patients: practical aspects and pitfalls. *Pediatr Surg Int.* 2009;25(7):623–634.
7. Taenzer AH, Clark CT, Kovarik WD. Experience with 724 epidurograms for epidural catheter placement in pediatric anesthesia. *Reg Anesth Pain Med.* 2010;35(5):432–435.
8. Willschke H, Bosenberg A, Marhofer P, et al. Epidural catheter placement in neonates: sonoanatomy and feasibility of ultrasonographic guidance in term and preterm neonates. *Reg Anesth Pain Med.* 2007;32(1):34–40.
9. Simpao AF, Gurnaney HG, Schwartz AJ, et al. Cephalad migration of pediatric caudal epidural catheters associated with change from prone to supine position. *Anesthesiology.* 2012;117(6):1353.
10. Thompson ME, Aasheim H. Migrating thoracic epidural catheter in an infant. *Paediatr Anaesth.* 2012;22(3):285–287.

Chapter 12

Pediatric Complex Regional Pain Syndrome: Stellate Ganglion and Lumbar Sympathetic Blocks

Sarah Choxi

Introduction

Complex regional pain syndrome (CRPS) is a chronic, localized pain condition following an injury, typically affecting a distal extremity. Signs and symptoms manifest as abnormal sensory, motor, vasomotor, and sudomotor changes that exceed the expected clinical course of the inciting event in both magnitude and duration, resulting in significant functional impairment.

CRPS broadly refers to CRPS types I and II. The majority of CRPS diagnoses that involve children are in late childhood or early adolescence, with a mean age of onset between 12 and 13 years, noting a higher frequency among females.[5] CRPS type I is the more common diagnosis, and the lower extremity is more commonly involved than the upper extremity. Early recognition of the signs and symptoms, followed by rapid implementation of a multidisciplinary treatment approach— including physical therapy (PT), psychotherapy, pharmacotherapy, and sympathetic nerve blocks, is a major factor in improving outcome and preventing treatment-resistant CRPS and chronic pain.[1,2,3] Sympathetic nerve blocks are typically performed by anesthesiologists who have additional fellowship training in these procedures during a chronic pain fellowship.

Clinical Applications

Intense PT is critical in treating childhood CRPS; however, PT is often limited by severe pain. Therefore, a method for pain relief should be coordinated with the physical therapist to relieve the patient's pain throughout the sessions. Although the pathophysiology of CRPS is unclear, multiple mechanisms are implicated, including peripheral and central sensitization as well as sympathetically mediated pain. Peripheral nerve blockade can treat the somatic component of CRPS pain, while sympathetic blockade may alleviate pain that is sympathetically mediated.

Stellate ganglion blocks are useful for sympathetically mediated upper extremity pain, and lumbar sympathetic blocks are helpful for treatment of lower extremity sympathetically mediated pain. Single-shot sympathetic blocks should be coordinated with PT sessions to improve participation and pain relief. Both peripheral nerve and sympathetic blocks can reduce pain and facilitate PT. Nerve blocks also often result in resolution of physical changes associated with CRPS and a decreased need for pharmacological drugs, including opioids.[6-8]

Pearl: Diagnosis of pediatric CRPS is based on clinical criteria identified through a thorough history and physical examination. Orthopedic, infectious, vascular, and rheumatologic disorders should be ruled out first.[9]

Pearl: The Budapest criteria have been validated with a sensitivity of nearly 100% and a specificity of 70 to 80% in the adult population; however, these criteria have not been formally validated in the pediatric population.

Budapest Criteria for the Clinical Diagnosis of CRPS

1. Continuing pain that is disproportionate to any inciting event[1]
2. At least one *symptom* in three of the four following categories reported by the patient:
   Sensory: Hyperesthesia or allodynia
   Vasomotor: Temperature asymmetry, skin color changes
   Sudomotor: Edema or sweating changes
   Motor: Decreased range of motion, motor dysfunction or trophic changes
3. At least one *sign* at time of evaluation in two or more of the following categories:
   Sensory: Hyperalgesia or allodynia
   Vasomotor: Temperature asymmetry (<1° C) or skin color changes

Sudomotor: Edema or sweating changes

Motor: Decreased range of motion or trophic changes

4. There is no other diagnosis that better explains the signs and symptoms

Pearl: Treatment is focused on return to function using PT, occupational therapy, and cognitive behavioral therapy.[9]

Contraindications

If any of the following are present, the procedures below should NOT be performed: patient or guardian refusal, local infection or neoplasm, or bleeding diathesis.

Critical Anatomy

The **stellate ganglion block** is for sympathetically mediated pain of the head, neck, and upper extremity. The stellate ganglion is formed by fusion of the inferior cervical and first thoracic sympathetic ganglia. The stellate ganglion is typically identified lateral to the lateral border of the longus colli muscle and anterior to the first rib and the transverse process of the seventh cervical vertebra.

The stellate ganglion block is commonly performed at the anterior tubercle of the transverse process of C6 (Chassaignac tubercle) to reduce the likelihood of a pneumothorax (Figure 12.1). The anterior tubercle of the transverse process of C6 is readily palpable in most patients.

The **lumbar sympathetic block** is for sympathetically mediated pain of the lower extremities. The lumbar sympathetic chain consists of four to five paired ganglia spanning over the anterolateral surface of the second through fourth lumbar vertebrae (Figure 12.2).

Stellate Ganglion Block

Setup

Equipment

- C-arm for fluoroscopy
- 25-gauge 1.5-inch needle
- 25-gauge 3.5-inch spinal needle

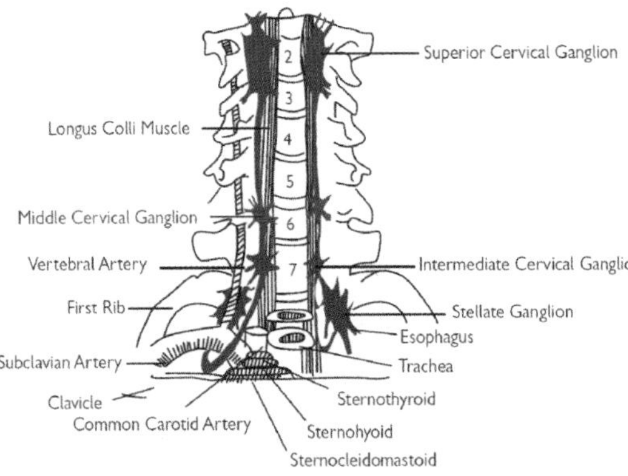

Figure 12.1 Cervical sympathetic chain and surrounding anatomy. (Reproduced with permission from Diwan S, Baqai A. The stellate ganglion block. In: Gupta A, ed. *Interventional Pain Medicine*. New York: Oxford University Press; 2012, Page 208.)

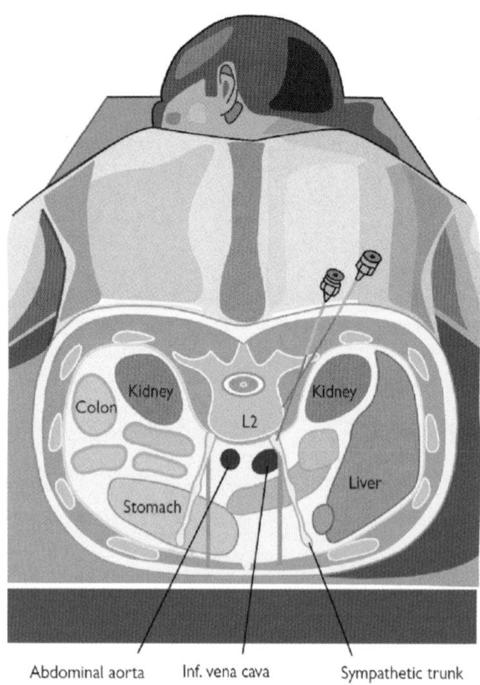

Figure 12.2 Right lumbar sympathetic block. (Reproduced with permission from Dinakar P, Michna E. Lumbar sympathetic nerve block. In: Gupta A, ed. *Interventional Pain Medicine*. New York: Oxford University Press; 2012, Page 221.)

Drugs, Dosages, Administration

Lidocaine 1% for skin and subcutaneous infiltration, radiopaque contrast dye (iohexol 180 mg/mL or equivalent). The injectate may be plain local anesthetic (consider 0.125–0.5% bupivacaine) or local anesthetic and steroid (consider dexamethasone). Local anesthetic should be dosed, giving consideration to the calculated toxic local anesthetic dose based on the patient's weight. Recommend a minimum of 5 mL and maximum of 10 mL of total injectate, excluding the volume of contrast dye. Based on the patient's body weight, also calculate an appropriate dose of adjuvant (if desired).

WARNING!! It is important to calculate the allowable total local anesthetic dose by weight and to stay below this maximum dose in order to decrease the risk for local anesthetic systemic toxicity (LAST). This calculation should include all local anesthetics, including that given by the surgeon, IV local anesthetic given by the anesthesiologist, and EMLA or subcutaneous lidocaine given before starting an IV. See Chapter 15 for information on Local Anesthetic Systemic Toxicity Treatment.

WARNING!! Inadvertent high spinal or epidural block may result in loss of consciousness and apnea; therefore, airway protection and ventilation equipment, resuscitation drugs and equipment, and intravenous sedation should be readily available.

WARNING!! Bilateral stellate ganglion blocks should NOT be performed; if the recurrent laryngeal nerve is blocked on both sides, this may lead to a loss of laryngeal reflexes and respiratory compromise.[10]

!! **Potential Complications:** Potential complications include pneumothorax, intravascular injection into the vertebral or carotid artery, blockade of the recurrent laryngeal nerve, neuraxial block, local anesthetic toxicity, seizures, esophageal perforation, and infection.

>> **Tip on Technique:** The most common approach is the anterior paratracheal approach at C6 using surface landmarks. Chassaignac's tubercle is readily palpable in most individuals.

Caution! Medial angulation of the needle may result in an intervertebral injection.

Caution! Diffusion of local anesthetic may block the ipsilateral recurrent laryngeal nerve, resulting in hoarseness and possible shortness of breath. The phrenic nerve is also commonly blocked and can lead to ipsilateral diaphragmatic paresis. Diffusion of local anesthetic posterior to the tubercle can result in a brachial plexus block as well.

>> **Tip on Technique:** Before starting the case, gather all of the necessary equipment. It may be useful to place equipment on a mobile flat surface, such as a Mayo stand, to use for equipment setup during the procedure.

Step-by-Step

1. **Position the patient and disinfect the insertion area.** The patient should lie supine facing the ceiling with a pillow under the upper back/lower neck to place the neck and head in a slight extension. Position the C-arm over the cervicothoracic junction without angulation. Disinfect the skin and apply a sterile drape over the insertion area. Use sterile equipment and sterile technique throughout the procedure.
2. **Identify the location for the stellate ganglion block and anesthetize the skin.** Chassaignac's tubercle is palpable in the groove at the level of C6. Identify Chassaignac's tubercle and infiltrate the adjacent skin and subcutaneous tissue with 1 to 2 mL of 1% lidocaine using the 25-gauge, 1.5-inch needle. Palpate the cricoid cartilage and then slide a finger laterally into the groove between the trachea and sternocleidomastoid muscle, retracting the muscle and adjacent carotid and jugular vessels laterally. Landmarks on the anteroposterior radiograph include the anterior tubercle and transverse process of C6 (Figure 12.3).

   !! **Potential Complications:** Local anesthetic injection into nearby vessels.

Caution! Although the block can be carried out at C6 or C7, it is important to recognize that the vertebral artery typically lies anterior to the transverse process at C7, and care must be taken to avoid puncturing the vertebral artery while performing a stellate ganglion block.

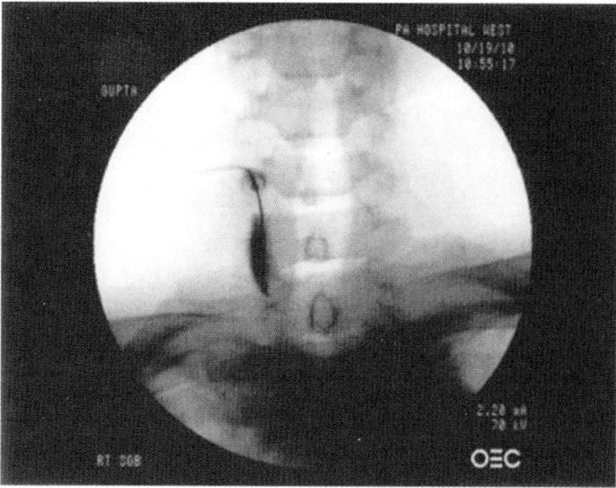

Figure 12.3 Anteroposterior radiograph of the cervical spine during stellate ganglion block. (Reproduced with permission from Diwan S, Baqai A. The stellate ganglion block. In: Gupta A, ed. *Interventional Pain Medicine*. New York: Oxford University Press; 2012, Page 215.)

3. **Advance the spinal needle to Chassaignac's tubercle.** Advance a 25-gauge, 3.5-inch needle through the skin and subcutaneous tissue until it is seated in a plane that is coaxial with the axis of the x-ray path. The needle is at the final position when contact is made with the surface of the vertebral body.

   >> **Tip on Technique:** The needle may not seat easily and can be held in a coaxial plane with a small clamp or hemostat

4. **Inject radiopaque contrast dye.** Rule out intravascular placement and confirm proper position with injection of radiopaque contrast dye.
5. **Inject local anesthetic with or without steroid.** Incrementally, inject up to 10 mL of local anesthetic with or without steroid.

   Pearl: Signs of a successful stellate ganglion block include Horner syndrome (miosis, ptosis), enophthalmos, anhidrosis, nasal congestion, venodilation in the hand and forearm, and an increase in the temperature of the blocked limb by at least 1° C.[10]

Postoperative Management Considerations

Patients should be monitored for at least 30 minutes after a stellate ganglion block because symptoms of inadvertent neuraxial injection may not appear for 15 to 20 minutes or longer.

Lumbar Sympathetic Block

Setup

Equipment

- C-arm for fluoroscopy
- 25-gauge 1.5-inch needle
- 22-gauge 5-inch spinal needle

Drugs, Dosages, Administration

Lidocaine 1% for skin and subcutaneous infiltration, radiopaque contrast dye (iohexol 180 mg/mL or equivalent). The injectate may be local anesthetic only (consider 0.125–0.5% bupivacaine) or local anesthetic and steroid (consider dexamethasone). Local anesthetic should be dosed giving consideration to the calculated toxic local anesthetic dose based on the patient's weight. It is recommended that 15 to 20 mL of injectate be used, excluding the volume of the contrast dye. Based on the patient's body weight, also calculate an appropriate dose of adjuvant (if desired).

WARNING!! It is important to calculate the allowable total local anesthetic dose by weight and to stay below this maximum dose in order to decrease the risk for local anesthetic systemic toxicity (LAST). This calculation should include all local anesthetics, including that given by the surgeon, IV local anesthetic given by the anesthesiologist, and EMLA or subcutaneous lidocaine given before starting an IV. See Chapter 15 for information on Local Anesthetic Systemic Toxicity Treatment.

!! **Potential Complications:** Potential complications include local anesthetic systemic toxicity, seizures, intravascular injection, neuraxial injection, infection, bleeding, intralymphatic injection, back pain, genitofemoral nerve injury, lumbar plexus injury, and neuritis.

>> **Tip on Technique:** The optimal location to place a single needle is over the anterolateral margin of the inferior portion of L2, the L2–3 interspace, or the superior margin of L3.

>> **Tip on Technique:** Before starting the case, gather all necessary equipment. It may be useful to set up needed equipment on a mobile flat surface, such as a Mayo stand.

Step-by-Step

1. **Position the patient and disinfect the insertion area.** Position the patient prone with his or her head turned to either side and a pillow placed under the lower abdomen and iliac crest to minimize lumbar lordosis. Position the C-arm is over the mid-lumbar region with a 20- to 30-degree oblique rotation. Disinfect the skin and apply a sterile drape over the insertion area.
2. **Identify and anesthetize the location for the lumbar sympathetic block.** Lumbar sympathetic blocks are best performed at the inferior border of L2, the L2–3 interspace, or the superior margin of L3. Infiltrate the adjacent skin and subcutaneous tissue with 1 to 2 mL of 1% lidocaine using a 25-gauge 1.5-inch needle.
3. **Advance the spinal needle toward the lumbar sympathetic chain.** Advance a 22-gauge 5-inch spinal needle coaxially toward the anterolateral surface of the L2 vertebral body (Figure 12.4).

   The direction of the needle is assessed and redirected by obtaining repeat images after every 1 to 1.5 cm of needle advancement.[10] Maintain the needle tip over the lateral border of the vertebral body. When the needle contacts bone, walk it off laterally and rotate the C-arm to obtain a lateral view. Proper needle position is verified in the anteroposterior view where the needle tip is medial to the lateral margin of the vertebral body.

4. **Inject radiopaque contrast dye.** Rule out intravascular placement and confirm proper position with injection of radiopaque contrast dye.
5. **Inject local anesthetic with or without steroid.** Incrementally, inject up to 20 mL of local anesthetic with or without steroid.

   Pearl: Signs of a successful lumbar sympathetic block include venodilation and an increase in the temperature of the blocked limb by at least 1° C.

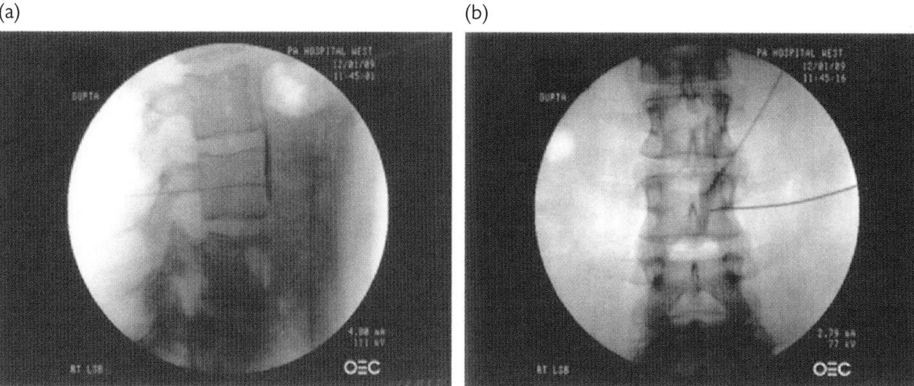

Figure 12.4 Right lumbar sympathetic block. a: Lateral view. b: Anteroposterior view. (Reproduced with permission from Dinakar P, Michna E. Lumbar sympathetic nerve block. In: Gupta A, ed. *Interventional Pain Medicine*. New York: Oxford University Press; 2012, Page 223.)

Postoperative Management Considerations

Monitor the patient per your local practice following this procedure.

Further Reading

Borucki A, Greco C. An update on complex regional pain syndromes in children and adolescents. *Curr Opin Pediatr*. 2015;27(4):448–452.

Merskey H, Bogduk N. *Classification of Chronic Pain*. 2nd ed. Seattle: IASP Press; 1994.

Weissman R, Uziel Y. Pediatric complex regional syndrome: a review. *Pediatr Rheumatol Online J*. 2016;14:29.

References

1. Wilder RT, Berde CB, Wolohan M et al. Reflex sympathetic dystrophy in children: clinical characteristics and follow-up of seventy patients. *J Bone Joint Surg Am*. 1992;74:910–919.
2. Benzon HT, Raja SN, Fishman SM, et al. Essentials of pain medicine. 3rd ed. Philadelphia: Elsevier/Saunders; 2011.
3. Logan DE, Conroy C, Sieberg CB, Simons LE. Changes in willingness to self-manage pain among children and adolescents and their parents enrolled in an intensive interdisciplinary pediatric pain treatment program. *Pain*. 2012;153:1863–1870.
4. Martinez-Silvestrini JA, Micheo WF. Complex regional pain syndrome in pediatric sports: a case series of three young athletes. *Bol Asoc Med P R*. 2006;98:31–37.
5. Martin DP, Bhalla T, Rehman S, Tobias JD. Successive multisite peripheral nerve catheters for treatment of complex regional pain syndrome type I. *Pediatrics*. 2013;131(1):e323–326.
6. Margic K, Pirc J. The treatment of complex regional pain syndrome (CRPS) involving upper extremity with continuous sensory analgesia. *Eur J Pain*. 2003;7(1):43–47.
7. Dadure C, Motais F, Ricard C, et al. Continuous peripheral nerve blocks at home for treatment of recurrent complex regional pain syndrome I in children. *Anesthesiology*. 2005;102(2):387–391.
8. Borucki A, Greco C. An update on complex regional pain syndromes in children and adolescents. *Curr Opin Pediatr*. 2015;27(4): 448–452.
9. Rathmell J. Stellate ganglion block. In: *Atlas of Image-Guided Intervention in Regional Anesthesia and Pain Medicine*. Philadelphia: Wolters Kluwer/Lippincott Williams & Wilkins Health; 2012:115–121.

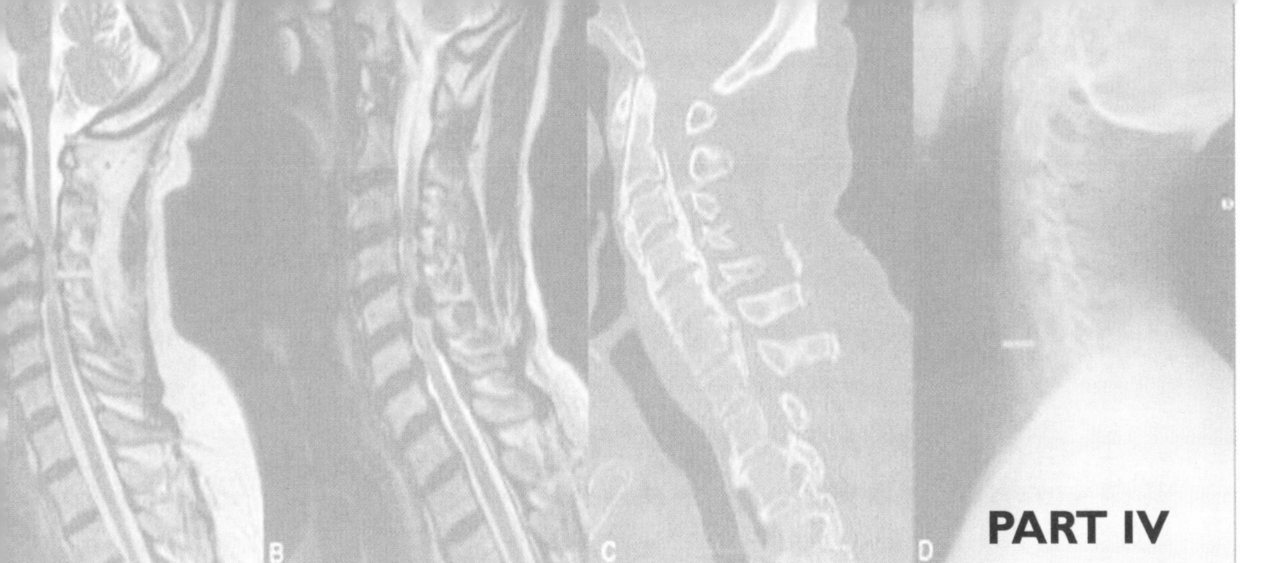

PART IV

PEDIATRIC EMERGENCIES

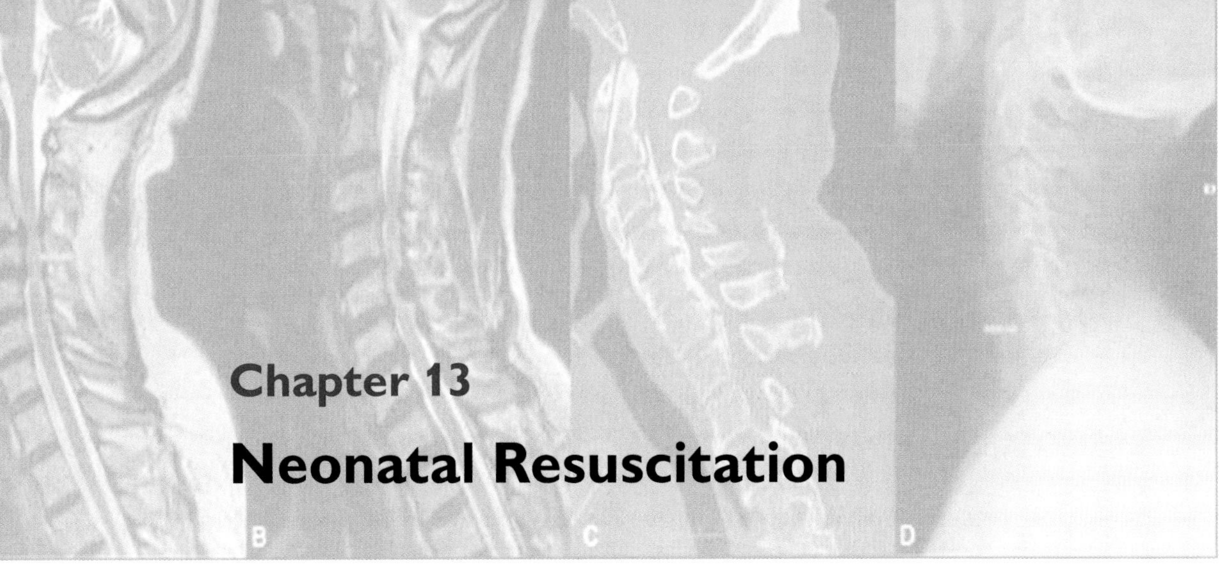

Chapter 13

Neonatal Resuscitation

Sarah Nizamuddin

Introduction

When a neonate is born, it is important to quickly recognize signs of infant distress. After birth, a newborn should be dried and warmed, evaluated for heart rate and breathing, and resuscitated as indicated. One out of 10 newborns will need help to take their first breath; one out of 100 newborns will need resuscitation medications and/or chest compressions.[1,2] Immediately after birth, the preductal SpO_2 can be as low as 60%, taking as long as 10 minutes to rise to a SpO_2 of 85 to 95% in the normal infant.[3] Meconium-stained amniotic fluid can mean that the fetus is in trouble—for these patients, the resuscitation team should be present, including someone with qualifications to intubate.

Clinical Applications

If ANY of the following are true in the newborn, begin evaluation: (1) <37 weeks gestation, (2) poor tone, or (3) not breathing or crying. The guidelines in this chapter are also applicable to infants with respiratory or cardiopulmonary collapse through first several weeks of life.

Setup

Personnel

At least one person should be present at all births whose sole responsibility is to take care of the infant and is capable of performing steps 1 and 2 (see later). In the case of increased risk factors for needing resuscitation (preterm, maternal infection, hypertension, oligohydramnios, non-reassuring fetal heart rate, meconium-stained amniotic fluid, emergency cesarean delivery),[4] other personnel with the ability to perform intubation, chest compressions, and umbilical vein catheterizations should be readily available.

Environment

Increase the room temperature and turn on a radiant warmer. If available and the need is anticipated, set up a thermal mattress and warmed humidified resuscitation gases.

Equipment

Immediately available:

- Bag mask or Neopuff
- Intravenous catheters/tubing/fluids
- Plastic wrap and a cap (for preterm infants)

Quickly available:

- Umbilical venous catheter kit

>> **Tip on Technique:** If there is a need for immediate intravenous access, the umbilical vein is often the most easily and quickly accessible location for clinicians with expertise in this technique.

!! **Potential Complications:** Incorrect placement of an umbilical venous catheter can lead to hepatic or pericardiac hematomas.

Step-by-Step

1. **The first minute: establish respirations and maintain normothermia.** Place the infant into the "sniffing" position to open the airway and tap the feet or rub the back to stimulate the infant to breathe.

Caution! If the infant is not breathing or crying, clamp and cut the umbilical cord right away so that resuscitation can be started immediately.[1]

Suctioning airway secretions is no longer recommended as a routine practice in infants who are born in either clear or meconium-stained amniotic fluid. However, suctioning secretions when copious or obstructing the airway or in depressed infants with meconium-stained amniotic fluid may be considered.[3]

Caution! Only suction the airway if needed—newborns have high vagal tone, and suctioning can cause bradycardia due to the vagal response.

Maintain normothermia (36.5°–37.5° C). Place the infant under a radiant warmer, dry the infant (if full-term), wrap the infant in clean plastic[5] (if preterm), and place a cap on the infant's head (if preterm) (Figure 13.1).

>> **Tip on Technique:** Immediately replace wet blankets with dry, warm blankets to keep the infant warm.

>> **Tip on Technique:** In a low resource environment, warming can also be achieved by initially placing the infant's torso in a clean food-grade plastic bag.[6] After the infant is stable and dry, skin-to-skin contact with the mother, with a blanket placed over both, is very useful for maintaining normothermia.

Pearl: Hypothermia in the newborn leads to increased mortality and is associated with developing respiratory problems, intraventricular hemorrhage, and possible sepsis.[3,7,8] Hypothermia can lead to failure to transition successfully from fetal to newborn circulation, causing persistent pulmonary hypertension of the newborn (PPHN), which, when untreated, is a terminal condition.

Caution! If the infant is not breathing, has labored breathing, is gasping, or has a heart rate under 100 bpm after a full minute of warming and drying, continue **quickly** to step 2.

2. **The second minute: continue resuscitation and, if needed, positive pressure ventilation** (go to '**Infant is UNSTABLE**' or '**Infant is Stable**' section as appropriate).

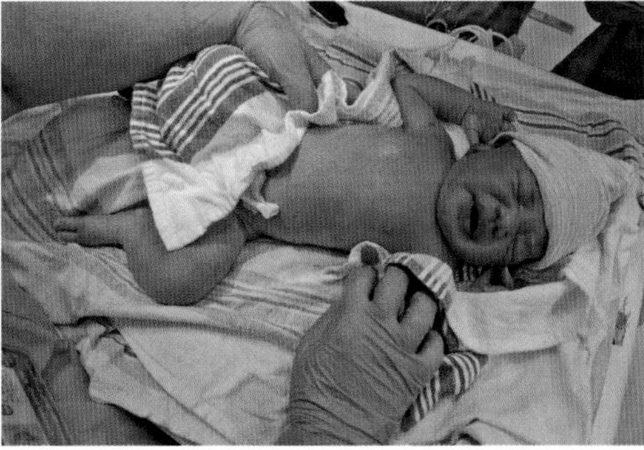

Figure 13.1 Drying and warming an infant at birth is important to maintain normothermia.

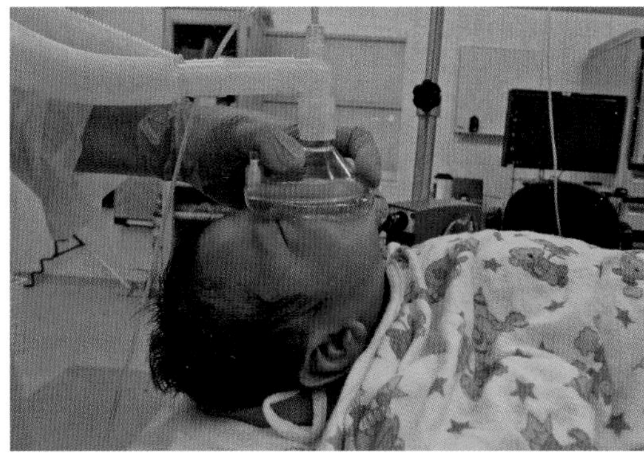

Figure 13.2 Placing the neonate in an appropriate sniffing position is necessary for proper ventilation.

Infant is UNSTABLE: If the heart rate remains below 100 bpm or breathing is labored or absent, place the infant in the "sniffing" position (Figure 13.2), immediately begin PPV with a bag mask device using an appropriately sized mask with or without an oral airway. Ventilate at 10 breaths/minute. Start with air and titrate supplemental oxygen as necessary. Have another provider continue warming, drying, and simulating. Ventilation is the most important component for resuscitating the newborn who is still compromised after warming, drying, stimulating, and clearing the airway.

Caution! If you are not seeing good chest rise with mask ventilation, consider repositioning, adding an oral airway, or intubating.

The most common reason for a low heart rate in a neonate is poor ventilation or hypoxia. However, if the heart rate remains below 60 bpm despite adequate PPV (by an endotracheal tube, if necessary), continue to Step 3.

Infant is stable: If the newborn remains stable with a heart rate above 100 bpm with nonlabored, regular breathing, continue keeping the infant warm and monitor for signs of distress (infant can stay with mother). The next steps in this chapter are not needed for a stable infant.

3. **The third minute: start chest compressions if the heart rate is below 60 bpm** (go to correct section below as per infant's heart rate).

Heart rate below 60 bpm: Increase oxygen to 100% and begin chest compressions on the lower third of the sternum at 100 compressions/minute. The depth of compressions should be about one-third of the chest's anteroposterior diameter. The preferred method is to compress with both thumbs and encircle the chest with both hands. (Figure 13.3). An alternate technique is to compress with two fingers with the other hand placed on the back for support.

WARNING!! Once started, it is important to continue the chest compressions at 100 per minute until the infant's heart rate rises above 100 bpm to assist the infant in achieving adequate cardiac output and circulation.

WARNING!! Watch for signs of compressor fatigue—change compressors frequently to ensure high quality CPR.

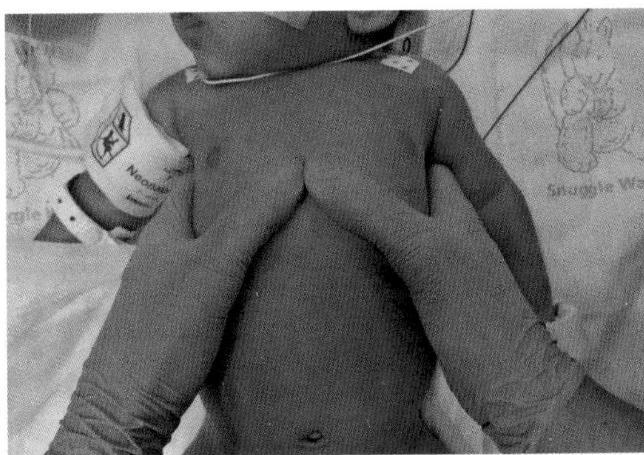

Figure 13.3 The two-hand compression technique is depicted, with both hands encircling the infant's chest to apply appropriate compressions.

>> **Tip on Technique:** Continue PPV during chest compressions—a 3:1 compression-to-ventilation ratio is recommended for neonatal resuscitation because the cause of arrest is most likely respiratory in origin. If a cardiac origin of cardiac arrest is likely, then a 15:2 ratio may be considered.[3]

>> **Tip on Technique:** An increase in the heart rate of a newborn is one of the best signs of a good response to resuscitation.[3,9] In addition to pulse oximetry, consider the use of a three-lead electrocardiogram for more accurate heart rate monitoring.[10]

Heart rate between 60 and 100 bpm: Continue PPV, monitoring, warming, drying, and stimulating.

Heart rate above 100 bpm, breathing well: Continue monitoring, warming, drying, and simulating. If the infant is not breathing well, continue PPV.

4. **Administer medications and/or fluids, as necessary.** If the heart rate remains below 60 bpm despite adequate ventilation and high-quality chest compressions, administer epinephrine every 3 to 5 minutes. The dose of epinephrine should be 0.01 to 0.03 mg/kg given intravenously. If IV access has not been established, consider 0.05 to 0.1 mg/kg through the endotracheal tube.[3]

>> **Tip on Technique:** Consider careful volume expansion with an isotonic crystalloid solution or blood if hypovolemia or blood loss is thought to be contributing to hemodynamic instability. A recommended starting dose is 10 mL/kg of fluid or packed red blood cells.

Postoperative Management Considerations

After the newborn infant is stabilized and ventilation and circulation established, arrange disposition, including neonatal intensive care, if needed, and communicate with the family. If the infant is older than 36 weeks' gestational age and has moderate to severe hypoxic ischemic encephalopathy, therapeutic hypothermia should be considered (based on current guidelines—see latest American Academy of Pediatrics guidelines for updates).[9]

Further Reading

Wyckoff MH, Aziz K, Escobedo MB, et al. Part 13: neonatal resuscitation: 2015 American Heart Association guidelines update for cardiopulmonary resuscitation and emergency cardiovascular care. *Circulation*. 2015;132:S543–560.

References

1. Lee AC, Cousens S, Wall SN, et al. Neonatal resuscitation and immediate newborn assessment and stimulation for the prevention of neonatal deaths: a systematic review, meta-analysis and Delphi estimation of mortality effect. *BMC Public Health.* 2011;11(Suppl. 3):S12.
2. Perlman JM, Risser R. Cardiopulmonary resuscitation in the delivery room: associated clinical events. *Arch Pediatr Adolesc Med.* 1995;149(1):20–25.
3. Wyckoff MH, Aziz K, Escobedo MB, et al. Part 13: neonatal resuscitation: 2015 American Heart Association guidelines update for cardiopulmonary resuscitation and emergency cardiovascular care. *Circulation.* 2015;132(18 Suppl. 2):S543–S560.
4. Aziz K, Chadwick M, Baker M, Andrews W. Ante- and intra-partum factors that predict increased need for neonatal resuscitation. *Resuscitation.* 2008;79(3):444–452.
5. Reilly MC, Vohra S, Rac VE, et al. Randomized trial of occlusive wrap for heat loss prevention in preterm infants. *J Pediatr.* 2015;166(2):262–268.
6. Berkelhamer SK, Kamath-Rayne BD, Niermeyer S. Neonatal resuscitation in low-resource settings. *Clin Perinatol.* 2016;43(3):573–591.
7. Laptook AR, Salhab W, Bhaskar B; Neonatal Research Network. Admission temperature of low birth weight infants: predictors and associated morbidities. *Pediatrics.* 2007;119(3):e643–649.
8. Van de Bor M, Van Bel F, Lineman R, Ruys JH. Perinatal factors and periventricular-intraventricular hemorrhage in preterm infants. *Am J Dis Child.* 1986;140(11):1125–1130.
9. Kattwinkel J, Perlman JM, Aziz K, et al. Part 15: neonatal resuscitation: 2010 American Heart Association guidelines for cardiopulmonary resuscitation and emergency cardiovascular care. *Circulation.* 2010;122(18 Suppl 3):S909–919.
10. Katheria A, Rich W, Finer N. Electrocardiogram provides a continuous heart rate faster than oximetry during neonatal resuscitation. *Pediatrics.* 2012;130(5):e1177–e1181.

Chapter 14

Infant and Pediatric Cardiopulmonary Resuscitation

Sarah Nizamuddin

Introduction

High-quality cardiopulmonary resuscitation (CPR) in children with cardiac arrest is vitally important to increase the chance of survival. The rate of return of spontaneous circulation from in-hospital cardiac arrests has improved between 2001 and 2013, from 39% to 77%.[1] In adults, cardiac arrest is most commonly due to primary cardiac causes. In contrast, the cause of pediatric cardiac arrest is often asphyxia resulting in hypoxia. Because of this difference, there is a greater level of importance given to ventilation during infant and pediatric CPR.[2,3] After recognition of the loss of pulse or blood pressure, quick initiation of CPR is necessary to provide blood flow to vital organs.

Clinical Applications

If ANY of the following are true, begin CPR: (1) loss of pulse or blood pressure or (2) unstable ventricular tachycardia or ventricular fibrillation.

Pearl: The 2010 American Heart Association guidelines changed the sequence of CPR from A-B-C to C-A-B in efforts to decrease the time to chest compressions (A = airway, B = breathing, C = compressions).

Pearl: According to the 2015 American Heart Association guidelines, performing CPR for an extended period of time is indicated because of newer evidence that surviving to discharge occurred in 12% of pediatric patients who received in-hospital CPR for greater than 35 minutes, with more than half of these children (60%) having a favorable outcome neurologically.[4] These guidelines are for witnessed, in-hospital arrests.

Setup

Equipment

Immediately available:

- Code cart with code drugs
- Defibrillator
- Mask, bag mask ventilator
- Endotracheal tube and laryngoscopes
- Backboard

WARNING!! Familiarize yourself with the defibrillator(s) in your institution before you need it, as significant differences exist among types and manufactures.

>> **Tip on Technique:** Assigning roles to team members in the room is critical in running an organized resuscitation.

>> **Tip on Technique:** Closed-loop communication may help decrease the chance of incorrect drug dosages or prolonged pauses in chest compressions. Closed-loop communication involves the following: when clinician A gives a direction to clinician B, clinician B repeats the direction back. Then, clinician A will confirm that clinician B repeated back the direction correctly. As an example: if clinician A says, "Clinician B, start chest

compressions," clinician B will repeat back, "Starting chest compressions." Then clinician A will repeat back "correct." Using the clinician's name or touching the clinician on the shoulder can also assist with having the communication heard in the loud, busy environment that occurs during a resuscitation.

Step-by-Step

1. **Position the patient.** When a patient requires CPR, it is best to place the patient supine if possible. However, prone or lateral CPR can be performed if necessary (Figure 14.1).

   >> Tip on Technique: Tailor patient position for CPR to the surgery being performed and according to whether there is an open incision at the time of arrest. Chest compressions can be performed with one hand on each side of the open incision if necessary. High-quality chest compressions are the priority.

2. **Determine whether the patient is breathing and has a pulse.** Quickly examine the patient for breathing and presence of a pulse (Figure 14.2). It is important to perform this initial step in no more than 10 seconds to minimize time to compressions. If additional people are present, ask someone to call for help while performing this initial step.

   >> Tip on Technique: A carotid or femoral pulse may be easiest to palpate.

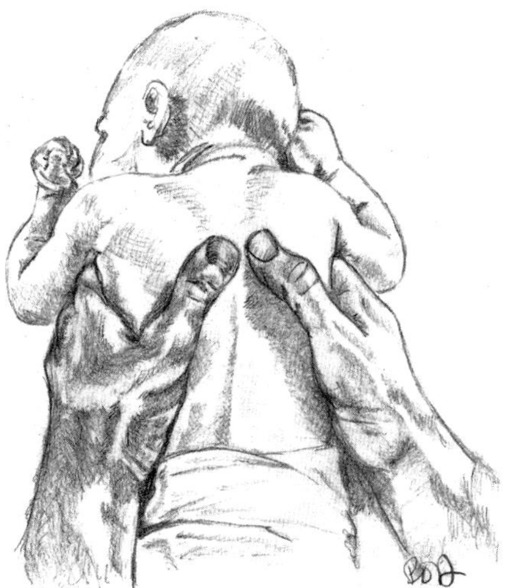

Figure 14.1 Prone cardiopulmonary resuscitation. (Original artwork by Brooke Trainer-Albright, MD.)

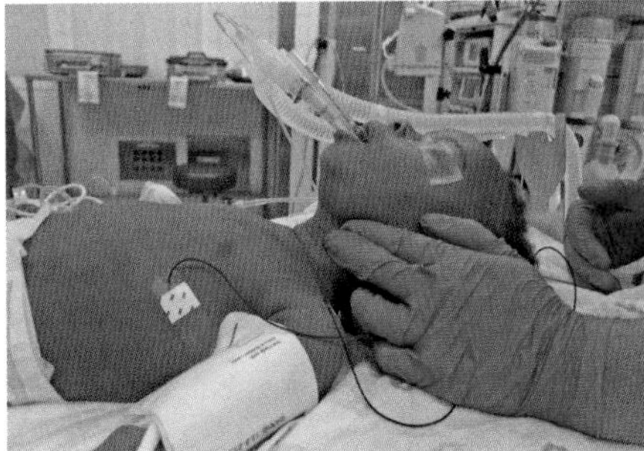

Figure 14.2 Check for a patient's pulse at the carotid (pictured), brachial, or femoral artery.

3. **Begin CPR.** If one rescuer is present, begin CPR at a ratio of 30 compressions to 2 breaths. If two or more rescuers are present, follow a 15:2 ratio of compressions to breaths for pediatric patients. Pulse and rhythm checks should be performed every 2 minutes.

WARNING!!	To decrease chance of compressor fatigue, change compressors every 2 minutes or more often if necessary while minimizing pauses in CPR.

>> **Tip on Technique:** For infants, hand placement is detailed in Chapter 13, Neonatal Resuscitation. For older pediatric patients, the compression location is two fingerbreadths above the inferior tip of the sternum (Figure 14.3). Compression rate should be between 100 and 120 per minute.[5] Compression depth should be at least one third of the anteroposterior diameter of the chest.

>> **Tip on Technique:** If the patient is not yet intubated, consider placement of an advanced airway, without interrupting compressions if possible. When in place, give 10 breaths/minute continuously.

4. **Attach defibrillator pads, shock if warranted.** As soon as possible, attach the defibrillator pads to the patient and evaluate the rhythm. If the patient is in a shockable rhythm (ventricular tachycardia or ventricular fibrillation), shock immediately, then resume compressions.

WARNING!!	After a shock is delivered, immediately resume compressions. Do NOT pause to evaluate for pulse/rhythm until the next rhythm check.
WARNING!!	Confirm that all rescuers are clear of the patient before administering shocks.

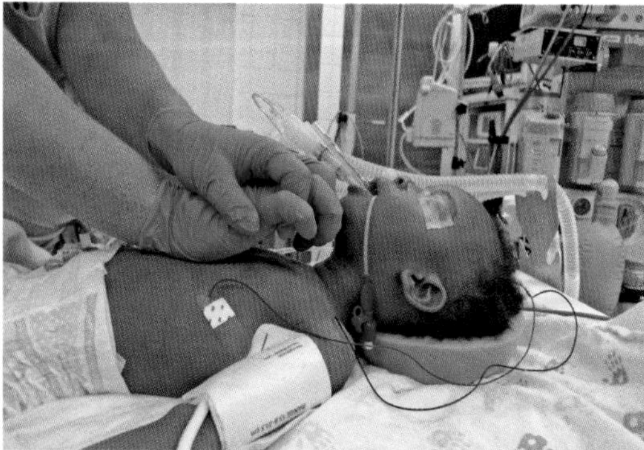

Figure 14.3 Correct hand placement for cardiopulmonary resuscitation in patients weighing more than approximately 10 kg.

>> **Tip on Technique:** Although paddles can also be used to deliver shocks, pads may be more convenient and assist with minimizing pauses in compressions.

>> **Tip on Technique:** An initial dose of 2 to 4 J/kg of monophasic or biphasic energy is recommended. For subsequent shocks, 4 J/kg may be reasonable. Higher energy levels up to 10 J/kg may be considered, using your clinical judgment.[6]

>> **Tip on Technique:** Ensure that the heart is between the two pads so that current can flow to the heart (Figure 14.4).

5. **Administer medications.** Intravenous (IV) epinephrine (0.01 mg/kg) should be administered every 3 to 5 minutes during CPR. For ventricular tachycardia and ventricular fibrillation refractory to defibrillation, IV amiodarone (5 mg/kg) may be administered.

>> **Tip on Technique:** Designating a person to keep track of medications administered and times of events can be very helpful during CPR.

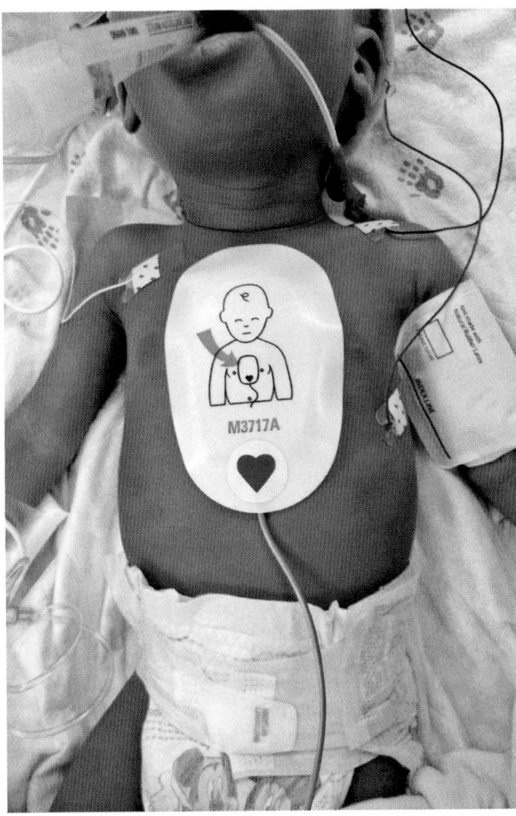

Figure 14.4 On smaller children, pads can be placed on the front and back of the patient to avoid overlap.

Table 14.1 Common Reversible Causes of Cardiac Arrest (H's and T's)

H's	T's
Hypovolemia	Tension pneumothorax
Hypoxia	Thrombosis, pulmonary
Hydrogen ion (acidosis)	Thrombosis, cardiac
Hyperkalemia/hypokalemia	Tamponade, cardiac
Hypoglycemia	Tamponade, pulmonary (breath stacking or excessive auto-PEEP)
Hypothermia	Toxins
Hypervagal	Trauma
malignant Hyperthermia	pulmonary hyperTension
	prolonged q-T

From Moitra VK, Elnav S, Thies KS, et al. Cardiac Arrest in the Operating Room: Resuscitation and Management for the Anesthesiologist: Part 1. *Anesth Analg*. 2018;126(3):876–888.

>> **Tip on Technique:** If the patient does not have IV access and obtaining access is difficult, consider placement of an intraosseous (IO) line (see Chapter 8, Pediatric Intraosseous Placement).

>> **Tip on Technique:** While the IV/IO route is preferred for epinephrine during CPR, epinephrine can also be administered through the endotracheal tube in intubated patients. In this case, the resuscitation dose is 0.1 mg/kg.

6. **Continue CPR; consider reversible causes.** Continue chest compressions while checking for a pulse and evaluating the rhythm every 2 minutes. Shock if necessary. Administer epinephrine every 3 to 5 minutes. Consider reversible causes of arrest while performing CPR. Common reversible causes are shown in Table 14.1. Consider initiation of extracorporeal membrane oxygenation (ECMO) if appropriate.

Postoperative Management Considerations

When the patient has achieved return of spontaneous circulation (ROSC), ensure that the appropriate intensive care unit bed and care are secured. Meet with patient's family to discuss events and plans for further care. Debrief with the resuscitation team.

>> **Tip on Technique:** Consider initiation of therapeutic hypothermia (see American Heart Association guideline).

Further Reading

Atkins DL, Berger S, Duff JP, et al. Part 11: pediatric basic life support and cardiopulmonary resuscitation quality: 2015 American Heart Association guidelines update for cardiopulmonary resuscitation and emergency cardiovascular care. *Circulation*. 2015;132:S519–S525.

de Caen AR, Berg MD, Chameides L, et al. Part 12: pediatric advanced life support: 2015 American Heart Association guidelines update for cardiopulmonary resuscitation and emergency cardiovascular care. *Circulation*. 2015;132:S526–S542.

References

1. Girotra S, Spertus JA, Li Y, et al. Survival trends in pediatric in-hospital cardiac arrests: an analysis from Get With the Guidelines-Resuscitation. *Circ Cardiovasc Qual Outcomes.* 2013;6(1):42–49.
2. Goto Y, Maeda T, Goto Y. Impact of dispatcher-assisted bystander cardiopulmonary resuscitation on neurological outcomes in children with out-of-hospital cardiac arrests: a prospective, nationwide, population-based cohort study. *J Am Heart Assoc.* 2014;3(3):e000499.
3. Kitamura T, Iwami T, Kawamura T, et al. Conventional and chest-compression-only cardiopulmonary resuscitation by bystanders for children who have out-of-hospital cardiac arrests: a prospective, nationwide, population-based cohort study. *Lancet.* 2010;375(9723):1347–1354.
4. Matos RI, Watson RS, Nadkarni VM, et al. Duration of cardiopulmonary resuscitation and illness category impact survival and neurologic outcomes for in-hospital pediatric cardiac arrests. *Circulation.* 2013;127(4):442–451.
5. Atkins DL, Berger S, Duff JP, et al. Part 11: pediatric basic life support and cardiopulmonary resuscitation quality: 2015 American Heart Association Guidelines update for cardiopulmonary resuscitation and emergency cardiovascular care. *Circulation.* 2015;132(18 Suppl 2):S519–S525.
6. de Caen AR, Berg MD, Chameides L, et al. Part 12: pediatric advanced life support: 2015 American Heart Association guidelines update for cardiopulmonary resuscitation and emergency cardiovascular care. *Circulation.* 2015;132(18 Suppl 2):S526–S542.
7. Moitra VK, Einav S, Thies KC, et al. Cardiac arrest in the operating room: resuscitation and management for the anesthesiologist part 1. *Anesth Analg.* 2018;127(3):e49–e50.

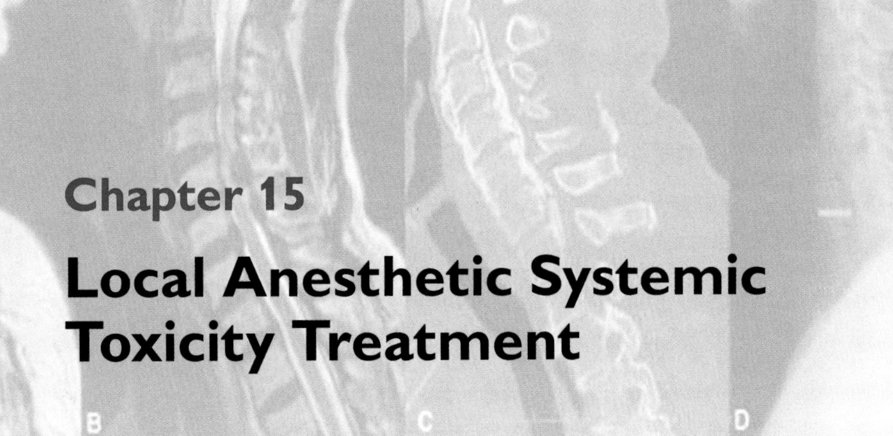

Chapter 15

Local Anesthetic Systemic Toxicity Treatment

Anna Clebone

Introduction

Local anesthetic systemic toxicity is a systemic adverse reaction to the administration of any local anesthetic. Children are at particular risk for local anesthetic systemic toxicity given their smaller body weight. Additionally, because local anesthetics are highly protein bound, infants, who have lower levels of plasma proteins, may be at even greater risk. Under general anesthesia, some of the early central nervous system signs of local anesthetic systemic toxicity, such as altered consciousness and seizures, may be masked, and the first indicator of local anesthetic systemic toxicity may be hemodynamic instability or cardiac arrest. Nevertheless, in a multicenter database of more than 100,000 consecutive pediatric regional anesthetics, local anesthetic systemic toxicity did not occur more often in pediatric patients undergoing regional anesthesia under general anesthesia compared with patients undergoing regional anesthesia awake or under sedation, and was overall very rare (2.2/10,000 and 15.2/10,000, respectively).[1,2] In cases of cardiac arrest from local anesthetic systemic toxicity, prolonged chest compressions or extracardiac membrane oxygenation (ECMO) may be required because toxicity may last for several hours or more. In addition to resuscitation, early administration of intralipid is the most important step.

Clinical Applications

Local anesthetic systemic toxicity can occur any time that a local anesthetic is given. It is recommended that a cognitive aid containing the treatment steps for local anesthetic systemic toxicity be immediately available when local anesthetic is given. The Society for Pediatric Anesthesia[3] and the American Society of Regional Anesthesia and Pain Medicine have published such aids.[4] Figure 15.1 shows another option containing similar information, a cognitive aid designed to support both a step-by-step response, when the aid is accessed at the beginning of the event, and "sampling," for those cases in which the clinician only accesses the cognitive aid for a discrete piece of information, such as a drug dose.[5] In this human factors–informed design, clinicians can easily go directly to the block containing the specific information that they are looking for, instead of having to spend time during a critical event reading through information that is not needed in that moment. Clinicians can go directly to the purple block for "Treatment" ideas, the gold block for "Differential" diagnosis suggestions, or the blue block when only "Drug/Dosage" information is needed. Additionally, "Crisis Management" information is identified in the red block, which makes it easy to identify crisis actions when needed. Note that when step-by-step guidance is desired, however, it is still supported through the aid by clinicians accomplishing the bulleted items in each block in order, starting with the green block.

Critical Physiology

Any local anesthetic may cause local anesthetic systemic toxicity; however, bupivacaine is particularly cardiotoxic. Local anesthetic systemic toxicity can occur with any route of local anesthetic absorption, including intravenous (IV), tissue, topical, or mucous membrane. Cardiac toxicity occurs as a result of the fact that local anesthetics block calcium, sodium, and potassium channels. These blockages lead to decreased contraction of the heart, decreased tone of the vasculature, and disturbances in conduction. Intralipid may work by binding the local anesthetic molecule, then moving it away from vulnerable sites (e.g., heart and brain); as a "lipid sink"; or through effects on sodium channels.[6] Lipidrescue.org provides further information on this physiology, as well a registry for reporting local anesthetic systemic toxicity events and the use of intralipid.

7 Local Anesthetic Systemic Toxicity PEDS

7

Local Anesthetic Systemic Toxicity PEDS

VERIFY DX–STABILIZE PATIENT

- Verify Local Anesthetic Systemic Toxicity (LAST):
  - CNS symptoms (may not occur): tinnitus, metallic taste, seizures
  - CV collapse: rhythm disturbance, altered consciousness
- Give 100% O_2, evaluate ventilation, stop N_2O and volatiles
- Stop local anesthetic
  - What was given? Drug, dose, site? Does this = a crisis or not?
  - If crisis, **request intralipid** (available in CCD block cart, DCAM block room, CLI carts, pharmacy)
- Ensure adequate IV access, monitoring of continuous ECG, BP, and SaO_2
- **AVOID** propofol, vasopressin, calcium channel blockers

TREATMENT	
Address ALL That Apply:	**Action**
Need for seizure suppression	▪ Midazolam 0.05–0.1 mg/kg IV
Hypotension	▪ Epinephrine 1 MICROgram/kg IV/IO, as needed, may need infusion 0.02–0.2 MICROgrams/kg/min
Acidosis, hyperkalemia	▪ Draw serial ABGs, consider a-line ▪ Hyperkalemia tx, see **CARD 5**

DIFFERENTIAL (Partial)

- Fat, thrombotic, cement embolus: See AIR EMBOLUS, **CARD 1**
- Anaphylaxis: see **CARD 2**

DRUG/DOSAGE SUMMARY

- **Intralipid 20%** 1.5 mL/kg IV over 1 min, repeat until stable (see orange box below)
- **Epinephrine** 1 MICROgram/kg IV/IO
- **Midazolam** 0.05–0.1 mg/kg IV

INTRALIPID DOSING

- Bolus **Intralipid 20% 1.5 mL/kg IV** over 1 minute. Repeat every 3–5 minutes, until hemodynamically stable
  - Start infusion **0.25 mL/kg/min**, increase as needed to 0.5 mL/kg/min
- **Continue infusion for at least 10 min** after hemodynamic stability is restored.
- Max dose of intralipid 20% is 10 mL/kg over first 30 min. If not responding, reconsider if other diagnosis or inadequate resuscitation

CRISIS MANAGEMENT (If Severe)

- Notify surgeon, call for help and code cart
- Check pulse. If cardiac instability occurs:
  - Start chest compressions (lipid must circulate)
  - Give epinephrine 1–10 MICROgrams/kg IV/IO
  - If cardiac arrest, see **CARD 4**
  - Consider ECMO (pager #7722)

Figure 15.1 Cognitive aid for pediatric local anesthetic systemic toxicity to support "sampling". (Adapted with permission from content authored by the Society for Pediatric Anesthesia Checklist Subcommittee and Quality and Safety Committee.)

Setup

Equipment

- Intralipid should be readily available any time that local anesthetic is being used. An initial dose of intralipid should be kept on every block cart.
- Standard American Society of Anesthesiologists (ASA) monitors should be placed on the patient at all times if more than minimal amounts of local anesthetic (e.g., minimal amounts for anesthetizing the skin before an IV placement) are being administered.
- Standard resuscitation equipment should be available at any anesthetizing location.

>> **Tip on Technique:** A checklist should be used before the administration of any regional or neuraxial anesthetic. This checklist should include a discussion of previous recent regional anesthetics given as well as the immediate availability of the local anesthetic systemic toxicity (LAST) treatment kit and intralipid (Figure 15.2).[7]

Drugs, Dosages, Administration

Intralipid is used to counteract the effects of local anesthetic systemic toxicity. Benzodiazepines, such as midazolam, may be needed to treat seizures, if they occur. Small doses of epinephrine (e.g., 1 MICROgram/kg) may be needed to treat hypotension.

Pediatric Regional Anesthesia Time-Out Checklist

PREOPERATIVELY

Patient:
- Site marked
- Consider allergies (including sterile prep)
- Consider anticoagulation
- Consider bleeding tendency

Equipment:
- Available and set up
- **LAST*** treatment kit available

IMMEDIATELY BEFORE PROCEDURE+

- Patient Name...________
  MRN...________
  Birthdate...________
  Weight...________
- Surgery type...________
- Block type(s)...________
- Laterality...________
- Dose and timing of other local anesthetics..........________
  (By surgeon, by anesthesia, in ED, on floor, topical, or IV)
- Maximum allowable local anesthetic for block......________

NOTE: **LAST** can occur with appropriate doses.
Carefully titrate for individualized patient conditions.

For treatment of suspected LAST – Flip card

*Local Anesthetic Systemic Toxicity
+Perform for each procedure if new position, different team, or time delay

Figure 15.2 Pediatric Regional Anesthesia Time Out Checklist. ED = emergency department; IV = intravenous; LAST = local anesthetic systemic toxicity; MRN = medical record number. (Reproduced with permission from Clebone A, Burian B, Polaner D. A time-out checklist for pediatric regional anesthetics. *Reg Anesth Pain Med*. 2017;42[1]:105–108. Available at: https://journals.lww.com/rapm/Abstract/2017/01000/A_Time_Out_Checklist_for_Pediatric_Regional.15.aspx.)

To decrease the likelihood of having local anesthetic systemic toxicity occur in the first place, carefully calculate the maximum allowable local anesthetic dose. Take into account the fact that the patient may have received other local anesthetics on the floor or may receive more in the operating room for the induction of anesthesia (when applicable) or from the surgical team. Be cognizant that extra local anesthesia may be given by the surgeon, if needed, during the surgery.

Step-by-Step

1. **Recognize local anesthetic systemic toxicity.** In an awake patient, the clinician may see central nervous system signs first, which may include the patient noticing a metallic taste in his mouth, numbness around the mouth, nervousness, changes in mental status, twitching of the muscles, changes in vision, or even seizures. Later central nervous system signs include depression of respirations, sleepiness, and loss of consciousness.

   The first cardiovascular sign is variable. Tachycardia and hypertension may occur first owing to a sympathetic surge. Sometimes, however, local anesthetic systemic toxicity may initially manifest as hemodynamic depression as evidenced by bradycardia and hypotension. If toxicity continues, ventricular tachycardia, ventricular fibrillation, and asystole may occur.[3]
2. **Stop local anesthetic, request intralipid, and perform initial stabilization.** Stop injecting local anesthetic (during block or by surgeon), and stop any local anesthetic infusions. Wipe off EMLA cream if present. Immediately request the intralipid kit (**and administer intralipid as soon as available**). Next, if the patient is not already intubated, secure the airway and administer 100% oxygen. Confirm that the electrocardiogram (ECG) and SaO_2 are being monitored continuously, along with blood pressure every minute. Confirm or establish adequate IV access (not infiltrated).[3]
3. **AS SOON AS POSSIBLE, administer intralipid.**

   Intralipid dosing:
   - Administer bolus intralipid 20% 1.5 mL/kg over 1 minute.
   - Start infusion 0.25 mL/kg/min.

   - Repeat bolus every 3 to 5 minutes up to 4.5 mL/kg total dose until circulation is restored.
   - Double the rate to 0.5 mL/kg/min if blood pressure remains low.
   - Continue infusion for 10 minutes after hemodynamic stability is restored.
   - MAX total intralipid 20% dose: 10 mL/kg over first 30 minutes.
4. **Treat seizures and hypotension, if present.** Seizures should be treated with a benzodiazepine (for example, the Society for Pediatric Anesthesia recommends midazolam 0.05 to 0.1 mg/kg IV).[3] When a benzodiazepine is administered, be prepared to treat resultant hypoventilation. Treat hypotension with small doses of epinephrine, 1 mcg/kg. **Avoid** higher doses of epinephrine, vasopressin, calcium channel blockers, beta-blockers and propofol.[3]

   Pearl: Local anesthetic systemic toxicity is a pro-arrhythmogenic state; for this reason, higher dose boluses of epinephrine are not recommended by the American Society of Regional Anesthesia.[8]
5. **Treat cardiac instability.** If cardiac instability occurs: Start cardiopulmonary resuscitation (CPR)/pediatric advanced life support (PALS). Continue chest compressions (lipid must circulate). You may need to perform prolonged compressions. Consider alerting nearest cardiopulmonary bypass/ECMO center and intensive care unit if no return of spontaneous circulation (ROSC) after 6 minutes.

6. **Monitor and correct electrolyte abnormalities.** Monitor and correct acidosis, hypercarbia, and hyperkalemia.
7. **Consider other diagnoses.** In any crisis, consider the differential diagnosis. In particular, if hemodynamic stability is not restored after administering 10 mL/kg of intralipid over the first 30 minutes, then consider the possibility that the instability may be due to another diagnosis (review the Hs and Ts).

Postoperative Management Considerations

Monitor the patient in the intensive care unit.

Further Reading

Neal JM, Bernards CM, Butterworth JF, et al. ASRA practice advisory on local anesthetic systemic toxicity. *Reg Anesth Pain Med.* 2010;35(2):152–161.

References

1. Taenzer AH, Walker BJ, Bosenberg AT, et al. Asleep versus awake: does it matter?: Pediatric regional block complications by patient state: a report from the Pediatric Regional Anesthesia Network. *Reg Anesth Pain Med.* 2014;39(4):279–283.
2. Walker BJ, Long JB, Sathyamoorthy M, et al. Complications in pediatric regional anesthesia: an analysis of more than 100,000 blocks from the Pediatric Regional Anesthesia Network. *Anesthesiology.* 2018;129(4):721–732.
3. Gonzalez LP, Braz JR, Modolo MP, et al. Pediatric perioperative cardiac arrest and mortality: a study from a tertiary teaching hospital. *Pediatr Crit Care Med.* 2014;15(9):878–884.
4. McGreevy MW. *A Practical Guide to Interpretation of Large Collections of Incident Narratives Using the Quorum Method.* NASA Technical Memorandum, NASA TM1997/112190. Moffett Field, CA: NASA Ames Research Center; 1997.
5. Burian BK, Clebone A, Dismukes RK, Ruskin KJ. More than a tick box: medical checklist development, design, and use. *Anesth Analg.* 2018;126(1):223–232.
6. White JL. Emergency manuals and flight 1549. *Anesth Analg.* 2014;118(6):1388.
7. Clebone A, Burian BK, Polaner DM. A time-out checklist for pediatric regional anesthetics. *Reg Anesth Pain Med.* 2017;42(1):105–108.
8. Neal JM, Bernards CM, Butterworth JF, et al. ASRA practice advisory on local anesthetic systemic toxicity. *Reg Anesth Pain Med.* 2010;35(2):152–161.

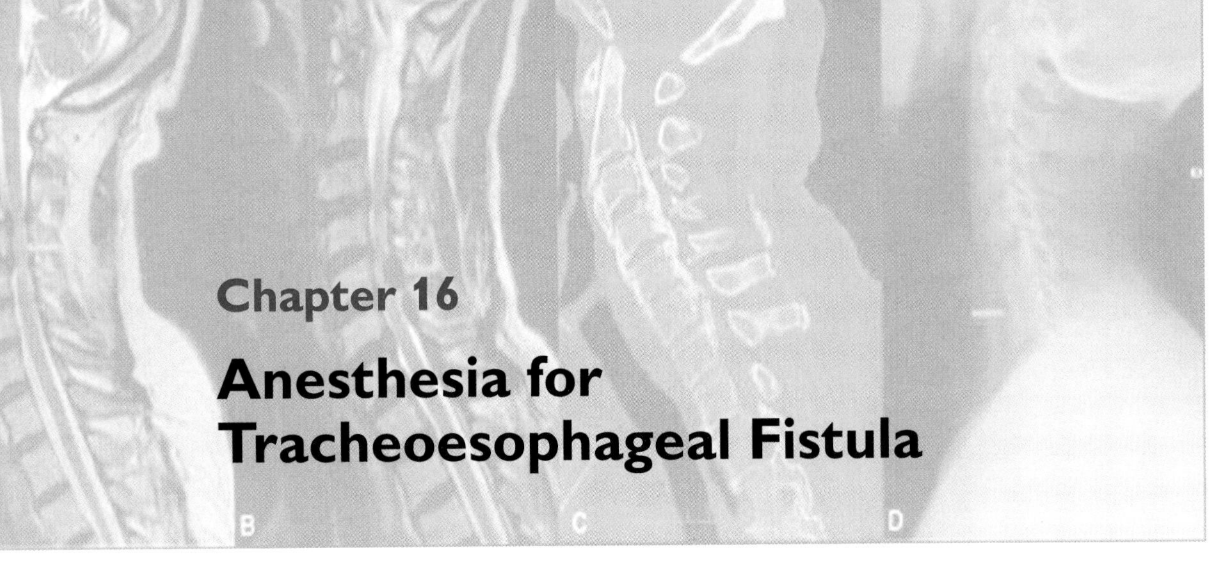

Chapter 16

Anesthesia for Tracheoesophageal Fistula

Ajay D'Mello and Vidya T. Raman

Introduction

A tracheoesophageal fistula (TEF) is a communication that is congenital or acquired between the trachea and esophagus. The reported incidence of TEF or esophageal atresia (EA) is roughly one to two per 5,000 live births.[1] The first successful surgery for TEF was in 1939. Presently, owing to progress made in surgical techniques, neonatal intensive care, and neonatal anesthesia, the majority of neonates with TEF/EA who do not have severe associated congenital anomalies are expected to have satisfactory outcomes.[2]

Critical Anatomy

The most common types of TEF as described by Gross are illustrated (Figure 16.1).[3] Coexisting congenital abnormalities occur in 30 to 50% of patients with TEF/EA. Congenital anomalies are more common in patients with isolated esophageal *atresia* (65%) compared with isolated tracheoesophageal *fistula* (10%).[4,5]

Additional anomalies associated with TEF often occur in the spectrum known as **VACTERL**:

Vertebral anomalies
Anal atresia
Cardiac defects (ventricular septal defect, atrial septal defect, tetralogy of Fallot, right-sided arch, patent ductus arteriosus)
Tracheo**E**sophageal fistula
Renal anomalies
Limb abnormalities

Step-by-Step

1. **Perform an initial evaluation.** Infants with TEF/EA present with a classic triad of symptoms that include choking and cyanosis during feeding, recurrent lower respiratory tract infection, and abdominal distension.[6] The diagnosis, if not established prenatally, is suspected with failure to pass an oral suction tube more than 10 cm.[7] A chest radiograph with a nasogastric tube coiled in the esophagus and an air bubble in the stomach confirms the presence of a TEF (except in cases of isolated esophageal atresia, in which the air bubble in the stomach will not be seen). Perform a physical exam, including neurologic, heart, and lung exams. Also perform a preoperative echocardiogram to exclude cardiac anomalies and to exclude an abnormal right-sided aortic arch, which would change the surgical approach.

   Lab samples should be obtained to determine baseline values for the following: complete blood count, electrolyte levels, venous blood gas concentrations, blood urea nitrogen and serum creatinine, blood glucose level, serum calcium level, arterial blood gas concentrations as necessary, and type and screen.

> **WARNING!!** Owing to the prevalence of congenital heart disease, a preoperative electrocardiogram and echocardiogram are mandatory in all patients with TEF/EA.

>> **Tip on Technique:** Neonates with a TEF are at risk for other airway anomalies, including tracheomalacia, bronchomalacia, and tracheal stenosis. The position of the fistula and potential for more than one fistula also affect surgical management. Many surgeons now proceed with bronchoscopy to help define airway anatomy before surgical repair (Figure 16.2).[8,9]

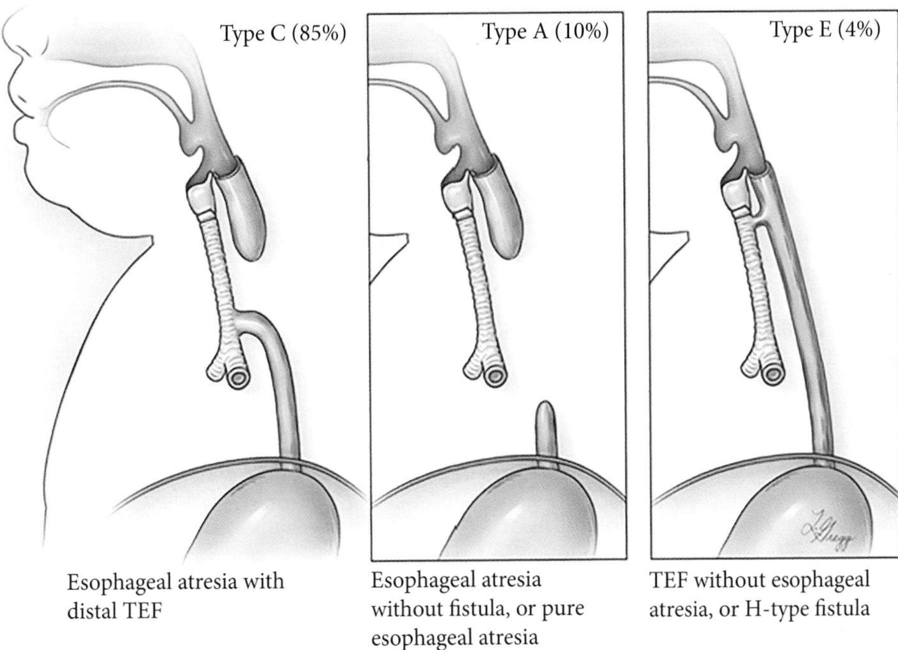

Figure 16.1 Anatomic variants of tracheoesophageal fistula (Tracheoesophageal Fistula (TEF) variants reproduced with permission by Lydia Gregg.).

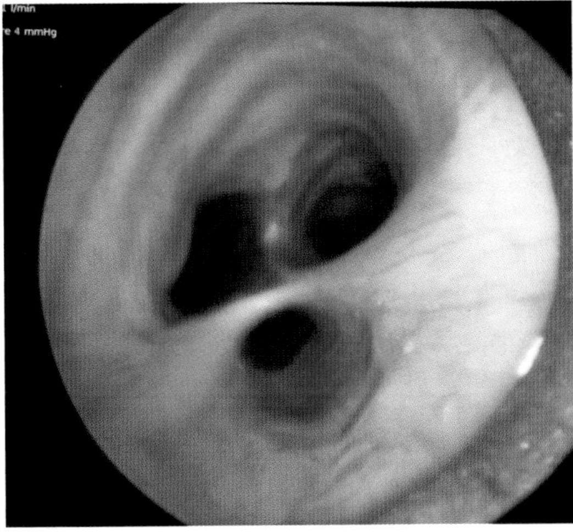

Figure 16.2 Bronchoscopic view of a large tracheoesophageal fistula near the carina.

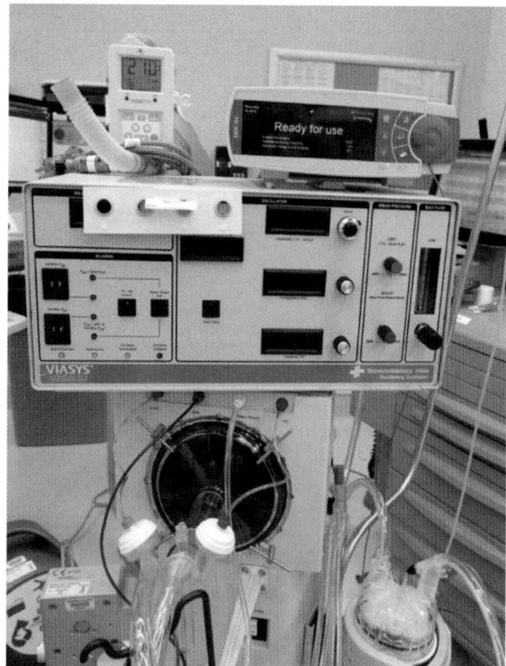

Figure 16.3 Oscillatory ventilator.

Caution! A thorough evaluation of pulmonary status is necessary to determine if one-lung ventilation will be tolerated during surgery. One-lung ventilation has the advantage of creating a still operative field for thoracotomy or thoracoscopic repairs. However, unacceptable desaturations may occur (despite a high FiO_2 and continuous positive airway pressure to the dependent lung), requiring termination of one-lung ventilation. Successful ventilation may require a specialized ventilator, such as an oscillatory ventilator (Figure 16.3), during the procedure.

Caution! Neonates with a sacral dimple would benefit from lumbar ultrasound to assess for tethered cord. This is particularly important if a caudal catheter is planned for postoperative pain management because a tethered cord and other spinal abnormalities are contraindications for caudal anesthesia.

Caution! Electrolytes should be checked often because they may become deranged as a result of large volumes of suctioned secretions and IV fluid replacement.

2. **Conduct initial management.** After the diagnosis of TEF has been established and while other coexisting anomalies are being investigated, implement the following interventions to protect the lungs from aspiration pneumonia:
   - Designate the infant as NPO (nothing per os),

- Place the infant in an upright position with his or her head elevated to at least 30 degrees to minimize reflux through the fistula; this position should be maintained, if possible, until the airway is secured.
- Suction the upper pouch, intermittently, and
- Administer appropriate antibiotics to treat aspiration pneumonia or sepsis.[10]

Repair of TEF/EA is not a surgical emergency. However, neonates with severe respiratory distress must be intubated preoperatively. It should be noted that intubation does not protect the child from aspiration of gastric contents through the fistula.[11]

3. **Position the patient.** Position the patient supine and head-up for induction to decrease the risk for aspiration. If a nasogastric tube is in situ, it should be placed on gentle suction. After induction and intubation for the surgical procedure, in most cases the patient will be placed in the left lateral decubitus position so that a right thoracotomy can be performed (Figure 16.4).
4. **Manage the patient's temperature.** Meticulous attention to temperature is essential to prevent the neonate from developing hypothermia and to minimize temperature shifts. All neonates easily become hypothermic owing to their high surface area to body mass ratio, thin skin, low body fat, and inability to shiver.[5] The neonate should be transported to the operating room in a warmed incubator. Use all modalities of temperature maintenance available: increase the operating room temperature (prewarm the room to >75° F) and use a forced-air warmer (typically underbody), fluid warmer, infrared warming lights, heated and humidified circuit, and warmed surgical irrigation.

WARNING!!	Aggressive temperature management is a must! Closely monitor the patient to avoid hypothermia or hyperthermia.
WARNING!!	When using infrared warming lights, ensure that they remain the required distance from the patient according to the manufacturer to avoid burns.

>> **Tip on Technique:** Avoid an oral/esophageal temperature probe because it may interfere with the surgery and/or cause displacement of the endotracheal tube. Ideally, monitor rectal or bladder temperature.

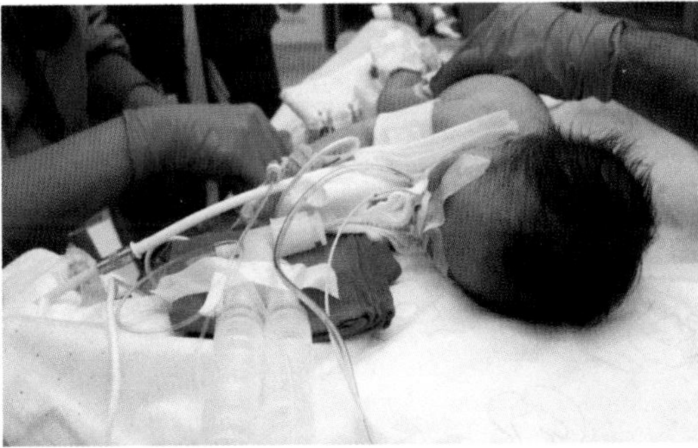

Figure 16.4 Patient positioned for right thoracoscopic repair.

!! **Potential Complications:** Care with positioning is very important during neonatal procedures. An infant's relatively thin skin is easily damaged. Be careful about cords, lines, and tubing lying over the infant's limbs. Circulation to an infant's limbs is easily compromised by external pressure.

!! **Potential Complications:** Pay attention to where the infant is located beneath the surgical drapes. It is easy for surgeons and assistants to accidently apply pressure on the infant's face, chest, and limbs. It is also common for surgical instruments to be unknowingly placed on the infant's face or limbs.

5. **Apply monitors.** Standard noninvasive monitors should include an ECG, pulse oximeter, blood pressure, end-tidal CO_2, and temperature. Invasive arterial line monitoring (umbilical or radial) for blood gas and hemodynamic monitoring is often indicated, especially in patients with comorbid congenital heart or pulmonary disease. A precordial stethoscope positioned in the left axilla during a right thoracotomy allows for monitoring of breath sounds and adequacy of ventilation of the dependent lung. Additionally, the placement of two pulse oximeters, one preductal (right hand) and one postductal (foot), will provide useful data in the event of shunting and pulmonary hypertension.
6. **Establish intravenous (IV) access.** A preinduction peripheral IV is recommended. Additional IV access should be placed after induction of anesthesia. Arterial line placement (umbilical or radial) for blood gas and hemodynamic monitoring should be placed before incision if not already placed in the neonatal intensive care unit (NICU).

>> **Tip on Technique:** If a right-sided thoracotomy is being performed, avoid placing lines in the right arm if possible because this arm will most likely be elevated with limited access during surgery.

7. **Determine anesthetic type and method of induction.** General endotracheal anesthesia is used for surgical repair of a TEF. For induction, many anesthesiologists use a deep inhalational technique with the infant kept breathing spontaneously with or without gentle assistance of each breath to minimize atelectasis (Figure 16.5).

The anesthetic goal is to secure the airway with the lowest possible inspiratory pressures needed to inflate the lungs while avoiding atelectasis and distension of the abdomen. Positive pressure mask ventilation is best avoided to minimize gastric distension from shunting of

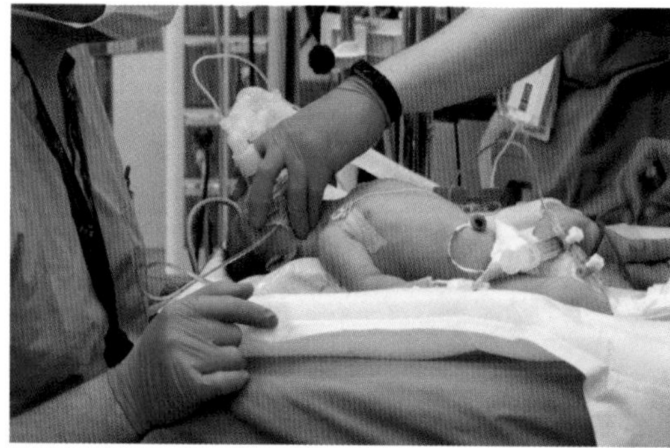

Figure 16.5 Induction of anesthesia with spontaneous ventilation and minimal positive pressure ventilation.

inspired gases through the fistula and into the stomach.[12] If the stomach accidentally becomes severely inflated, compromising ventilation, an emergency gastrostomy or gastric needle decompression can be performed by the surgeon (or if a gastrostomy tube is already in place, the gastrostomy tube can be vented).

Caution! The placement of a gastrostomy may result in ineffective ventilation owing to a low-pressure leak because the resistance to ventilating through the fistula will now be decreased. The leak could be significant if the patient's lungs are noncompliant because of pneumonia or respiratory distress syndrome.[7]

>> **Tip on Technique:** If the neonate has or requires a gastrostomy tube, the distal end can be placed under a water seal or connected to an extra capnography monitor. The presence of bubbles in the water or expiratory gases on the capnograph indicates ventilation through the fistula or that the endotracheal tube is proximal to the fistula, necessitating repositioning of the endotracheal tube.

8. **Perform a bronchoscopy (by surgeon) and determine the approach to intubation.** After induction and before intubation, some surgeons will perform a bronchoscopy to determine the number, location, and size of the fistulas and to look for bronchial anomalies and tracheomalacia (Figure 16.6). A carefully titrated IV anesthetic infusion is needed during the bronchoscopy to keep the infant breathing spontaneously yet deeply enough to tolerate the stimulus. Oxygenation can often be achieved through a nasal cannula or through a port in the bronchoscope. In cases for which a bronchoscopy after the induction of anesthesia is not needed, possible techniques for induction and intubation include an awake intubation with small doses of narcotics or a rapid sequence intubation to minimize mask ventilation. Clinical judgment must be used when deciding on an induction and intubation technique, particularly because the intubation technique chosen will depend on the location and size of the fistula (choose one of the following, as appropriate).

   If the fistula above the carina: If the fistula is high enough in the trachea, and the surgeon does not prefer one-lung ventilation, only a regular intubation with a cuffed endotracheal tube is required. In other words, with a high-enough fistula that is above the carina,

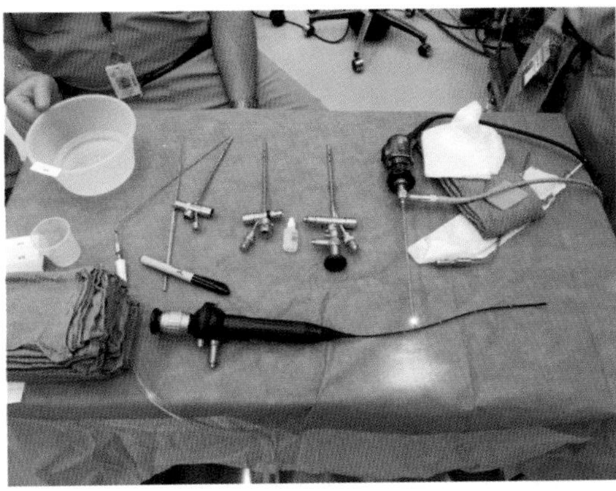

Figure 16.6 Bronchoscopy setup.

the tip of the endotracheal tube will lie distally to the fistula itself, and the fistula will not be ventilated. An endotracheal tube without a Murphy eye is often desired so that the fistula will not be inadvertently ventilated through the Murphy eye.

>> **Tip on Technique:** One technique for endotracheal tube positioning, to ensure that the endotracheal tube is as occlusive as possible, is to mainstem the endotracheal tube, then gradually pull it back while listening to the lung that is not being ventilated (typically the left side). Stop pulling back as soon as bilateral lung sounds are achieved. Then rotate the endotracheal tube so that the beveled (shorter) side is facing forward to maximize the endotracheal tube surface area that is occluding the fistula. Lung ultrasound, looking for pleural sliding, can also be used to determine whether each lung is being ventilated during endotracheal tube positioning. (see Chapter 2, 'Lung Ultrasound' in Ultrasound Guided Procedures and Radiologic Imaging for Pediatric Anesthesiologists, eds. Clebone, Burian, and Finkle, Oxford University Press 2021)

If the fistula is close to or at the carina or if the surgeon prefers one-lung ventilation: A purposeful mainstem intubation may be desirable to isolate the operative lung. An infant-sized fiberoptic bronchoscope can be useful for placing the endotracheal tube into the mainstem bronchus, although a small-enough fiberoptic bronchoscope may not be available. (See Chapter 3, Fiberoptic, Video Laryngoscope, and Nasal Airway Procedures, Table 3.1 for fiberoptic bronchoscope and corresponding ETT sizes) Typically, a right thoracotomy is performed (if a right-sided aortic arch is not present), and therefore, a left mainstem intubation is required; this can be technically difficult to achieve.

If the surgeon wishes to occlude the fistula: Another option is, in conjunction with the surgeon, to use a Fogarty catheter to occlude the fistula (this can be used as the primary means of fistula occlusion, or later in the surgery as a rescue) (Figure 16.7).[7] A Fogarty catheter may be particularly useful to improve ventilation in unstable patients with large fistulas.[12–16] Use of a Fogarty catheter may be of benefit in both minimally invasive and open surgical approaches. An advantage of using a Fogarty catheter is the ability to control the fistula early during surgery.[17] The Fogarty catheter can be directed by the surgeon to occlude the fistula during rigid bronchoscopy or can be guided with a fiberoptic bronchoscope either alongside or within an endotracheal tube (Figures 16.8 and 16.9).

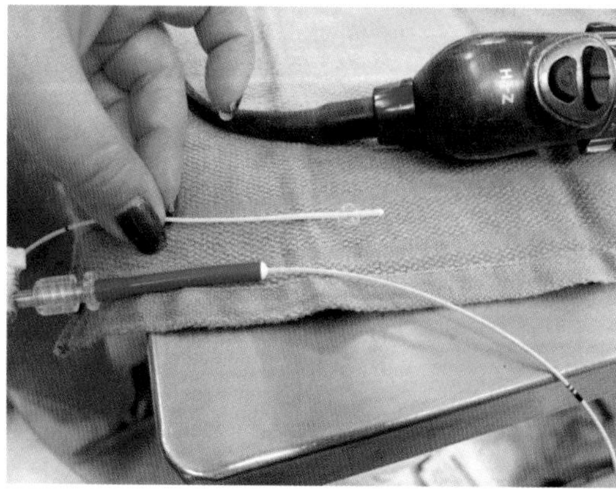

Figure 16.7 Fogarty catheter.

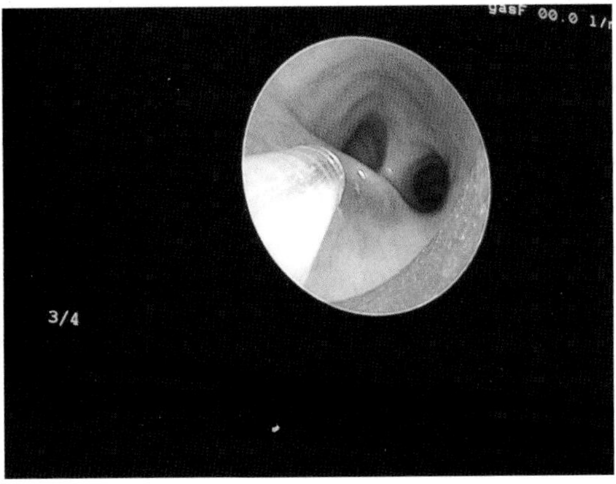

Figure 16.8 Fogarty catheter approaching a pericarinal tracheoesophageal fistula.

WARNING!!	It is important to continually assess ventilation. If a Fogarty catheter is used, during positioning or surgical manipulation, the Fogarty catheter may dislodge, precipitating complete airway obstruction if not promptly recognized and treated.[18]

If the previous options are not practical: Oscillatory ventilation is another option for ventilation during surgery for an infant with a TEF. An oscillatory ventilator delivers very rapid, very low tidal volume breaths with a theoretically lower risk for insufflating the esophagus and stomach through the fistula. A ventilator capable of this mode (often available from the NICU) should be used by personnel familiar with this equipment (may be a respiratory therapist or NICU physician).

>> **Tip on Technique:** Confirmation of endotracheal tube position following patient positioning is recommended to ensure that there is no displacement.

9. **Maintain anesthesia and monitor for possible surgical complications.** Good communication between the surgeon and anesthesiologist is crucial because significant ventilatory and hemodynamic compromise can occur during the repair.

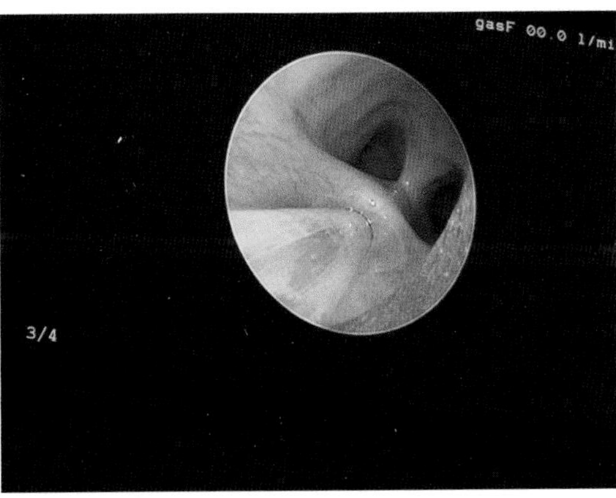

Figure 16.9 Fistula occluded with a Fogarty catheter.

Complications affecting surgical exposure, ventilation, and hemodynamics include but are not limited to:

- Displacement of the endotracheal tube either distally into the mainstem bronchus or proximally above the fistula
- Atelectasis due to lung retraction leading to desaturations requiring intermittent re-expansion of the lung
- Obstruction of the endotracheal tube with blood requiring frequent suctioning
- Hypercarbia despite best efforts to maintain normocarbia compounded by surgical insufflation of CO_2 during thoracoscopy
- Airway obstruction from surgical retraction
- Hemodynamic compromise due to surgical compression of the mediastinum.

Additionally, the surgical procedure itself will often involve ligation of the TEF (or multiple TEFs), followed by reanastomosis of the esophagus, if possible, or insertion of a feeding tube into the stomach, if anastomosis is not possible because of the anatomic length of the esophagus or the patient's size.

WARNING!!	Inadequate ventilation may occur due to migration of the endotracheal tube into the fistula or preferential ventilation through the fistula resulting in massive gastric distension.[13]

10. **Determine ongoing surgical blood loss and blood and fluid requirements.** Ensure that blood is available from the blood bank. The blood bank should take the usual neonatal precautions to reduce white blood cell and potassium load from the units that are given. Estimated blood loss can vary greatly and depends on the surgical plan.

WARNING!!	What may seem to be a small amount of absolute blood loss can be hemodynamically significant in an infant. Because of the small total blood volume of these patients, significant blood loss may not be recognized. Total blood volume is estimated to be 85 mL/kg for a full-term neonate. An infant has an estimated blood volume of 80 mL/kg. Preterm infants have an estimated blood volume of 95 mL/kg. Blood from surgical losses may pool under the drapes, increasing the difficulty of detection.

Maintenance fluids should consist of glucose solutions after the child has been made NPO because neonates are prone to hypoglycemia. Administering a maintenance rate using an infusion pump helps avoid hypoglycemia during the surgical procedure. Blood glucose monitoring should be performed at regular intervals during the anesthetic. Isotonic solutions (crystalloid and/or colloid) should be used to replace insensible losses or small volumes of blood loss. A maintenance rate using an infusion pump helps to avoid hypoglycemia during the surgical procedure. Insensible losses should be estimated at 3 to 4 mL/kg/hr and replaced with isotonic solution.

Postoperative Management Considerations

Generally, after repair of a TEF/EA, infants will remain intubated in the immediate postoperative period and managed in the NICU. An intubated neonate can also be more aggressively treated for postoperative pain. For infants who will remain intubated: if the tip of the endotracheal tube is in the mainstem bronchus, it should be pulled back to above the carina, and the lung should be reinflated under direct vision from the surgical thoracoscope if possible. The endotracheal tube should be gently suctioned.

WARNING!!	Aggressive suctioning of the endotracheal tube after the repair could lead to disruption of surgical sutures.

In infants with underlying lung disease from aspiration or prematurity, prolonged postoperative intubation may be necessary. Communicate with the surgeon, who may wish to have the endotracheal tube positioned 1 cm or more from the repaired fistula site.

!! **Potential Complications**: Extubation can be complicated by tracheomalacia and bronchomalacia. Pneumonia and atelectasis can also complicate the postoperative period.

Further Reading

Broemling N, Campbell F. Anesthetic management of congenital tracheoesophageal fistula. *Pediatr Anesth*. 2011;21:1092–1099.

Davis PJ, Cladis FP, Motoyama EK, eds. *Smith's Anesthesia for Infants and Children*. 8th ed. Philadelphia: Elsevier Mosby; 2011:574–579.

References

1. Depaepe A, Dolk H, Lechat MF. The epidemiology of tracheooesophageal fistula and oesophageal atresia in Europe. EUROCAT Working Group. *Arch Dis Child*. 1993;68:743–748.
2. Choi PJ, Jun HJ, Lee YH, et al. Surgical treatment of the congenital esophageal atresia. *Korean J Thorac Cardiovasc Surg*. 1999;32:567–572.
3. Gross R. *The Surgery of Infancy and Childhood*. Philadelphia: WB Saunders; 1957.
4. Spitz L. Oesophageal atresia. *Orphanet J Rare Dis*. 2007;2:24.
5. Krosnar S, Baxter A. Thoracoscopic repair of esophageal atresia with tracheoesophageal fistula: anesthetic and intensive care management of a series of eight neonates. *Pediatr Anesth*. 2005;15:541–546.
6. Crabbe DC. Isolated tracheo-oesophageal fistula. *Paediatr Respir Rev*. 2003;4:74–78.
7. Broemling N, Campbell F. Anesthetic management of congenital tracheoesophageal fistula. *Pediatr Anesth*. 2011;21:1092–1099.
8. Kosloske AM, Jewell PF, Cartwright KC. Crucial bronchoscopic findings in esophageal atresia and tracheoesophageal fistula. *J Pediatr Surg*. 1988;23:466–470.
9. Shoshany G, Vatzian A, Ilivitzki A, et al. Near-missed upper tracheoesophageal fistula in esophageal atresia. *Eur J Pediatr*. 2009;168:1281–1284.
10. Davis PJ, Cladis FP, Motoyama EK, eds. *Smith's Anesthesia for Infants and Children*. 8th ed. Philadelphia: Elsevier Mosby; 2011.
11. Hammer GB. Pediatric thoracic anesthesia. *Anesth Analg*. 2001;92:1449–1464.
12. Andropoulos DB, Rowe RW, Betts JM. Anaesthetic and surgical airway management during tracheoesophageal fistula repair. *Pediatr Anaesth*. 1998;8:313–319.
13. Ratan SK, Rattan KN, Ratan J, et al. Temporary transgastric fistula occlusion as salvage procedure in neonates with esophageal atresia with wide distal fistula and moderate to severe pneumonia. *Pediatr Surg Int*. 2005;21:527–531.
14. Chang JW, Choo OS, Shin YS, et al. Temporary closure of congenital tracheoesophageal fistula with Fogarty catheter. *Laryngoscope*. 2013;123:3219–3222.

15. Richenbacher WE, Ballantine TV. Esophageal atresia, distal tracheoesophageal fistula, and an air shunt that compromised mechanical ventilation. *J Pediatr Surg*. 1990;25:1216–1218.
16. Filston HC, Rankin JS, Grimm JK. Esophageal atresia: prognostic factors and contribution of preoperative telescopic endoscopy. *Ann Surg*. 1984;199:532–537.
17. Pepper VK, Boomer LA, Thung AK, et al. Routine bronchoscopy and Fogarty catheter occlusion of tracheoesophageal fistulas. *J Laparoendosc Adv Surg Tech A*. 2017;27(1):97–100.
18. Goudsouzian NG, Ryan JF. Bronchoscopy and occlusion of tracheoesophageal fistula. *Anesth Analg*. 1996;82:1308.
19. Buchino JJ, Keenan WJ, Pietsch JB, et al. Malpositioning of the endotracheal tube in infants with tracheoesophageal fistula. *J Pediatr*. 1986;109:524–525.

Chapter 17

Anesthesia for Neonatal Myelomeningocele

Anna Clebone

Introduction

Myelomeningocele, also known as spina bifida aperta (often shortened to the nonspecific name "spina bifida"), is a congenital disorder of the spine. One out of 10,000 infants born alive in the United States will have a myelomeningocele.[1] In infants with a myelomeningocele, the neural tube has not closed, and the vertebral arches have not fused during development, leading to spinal cord and meningeal herniation through the skin. Because of the high potential for injury and infection of the exposed spinal cord, which could lead to lifetime disability, these lesions are typically repaired in the first 24 to 48 hours after birth (Figures 17.1 and 17.2. In those infants with associated hydrocephalus, a ventriculoperitoneal shunt may be placed during the same surgery as the myelomeningocele repair.

Critical Anatomy

A myelomeningocele occurs before day 28 of human fetal development and is an abnormality in which the posterior neural tube closes incompletely. The outcome is a vertebral column deformity, through which the meningeal-lined sac herniates. After the bony defect is created, the hypothesized mechanism of meningeal herniation is that the pulsations of cerebrospinal fluid act progressively to balloon out the spinal cord.[1] If the sac is filled with spinal nerves or the spinal cord, it is known as a myelomeningocele; if the sac is empty, it is called a meningocele (Figure 17.3). Myelomeningoceles occur most often at the lumbar level, although higher lesions do exist and are associated with more severe disability. All infants with a myelomeningocele will have a Chiari II malformation, which is a constellation of hindbrain anomalies that includes brainstem and cerebellar vermian herniation through the foramen magnum. Only one third of children with a myelomeningocele, however, will be symptomatic from a Chiari II malformation.[2] Associated hydrocephalus occurs in 80% of infants with a myelomeningocele, although this cause of hydrocephalus is not entirely understood. Myelomeningocele may be diagnosed prenatally, and fetal magnetic resonance imaging can be useful in the prediction of the severity of the syndrome in an individual child.

Step-by-Step

1. **Conduct a preoperative evaluation and prepare for the procedure.** Perform a physical exam, including neurologic, heart, and lung exams. Infants with associated hydrocephalus may have a bulging fontanelle, and neurologic deficits may exist, including sensory and motor deficits and foot malformations.[1] Evaluate for associated congenital abnormalities.

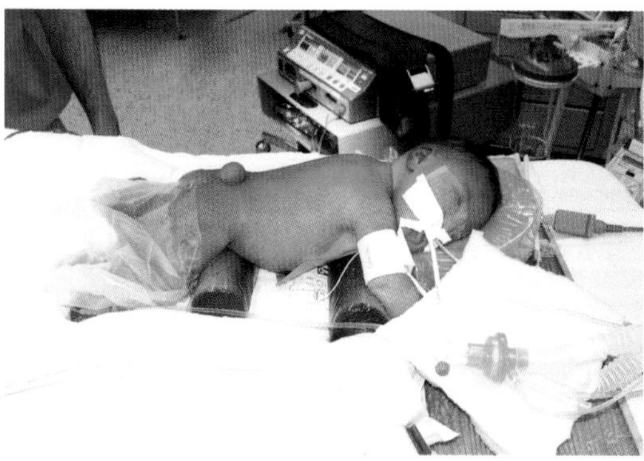

Figure 17.1 Infant with a closed myelomeningocele. (Courtesy of Ron Litman.)

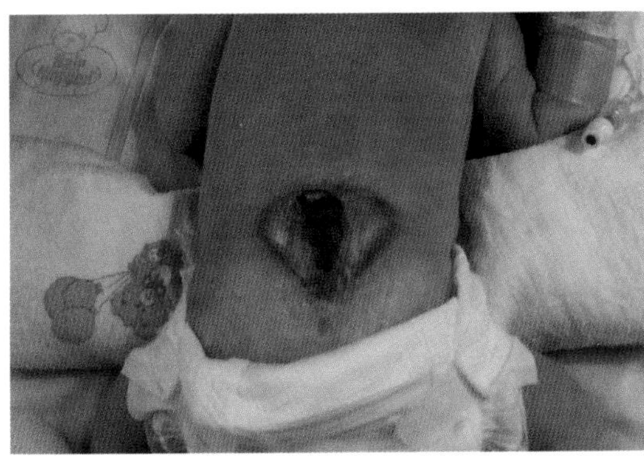

Figure 17.2 Infant with an open myelomeningocele. (Courtesy of Ron Litman.)

An echocardiogram, abdominal ultrasound, and renal ultrasound should be performed in infants with a myelomeningocele, owing to the association with cardiac, renal, and intestinal abnormalities. One third of patients with a myelomeningocele will also have congenital heart disease, with the most frequently found associated disorders being ventricular septal defect and the secundum type of atrial septal defect.[2] Myelomeningocele can be also associated with scoliosis, restrictive lung disease from scoliosis, tethered cord, syringomyelia, and renal abnormalities.

Infants with a severe Chiari II malformation that is symptomatic may be intubated preoperatively in the neonatal intensive care unit. A severe Chiari II malformation will cause associated symptoms from compression of the brainstem, including bradycardia and disordered breathing, or even apnea (from disruption of the medullary respiratory center).[1] Other symptoms that may occur in patients with a symptomatic Chiari II malformation include cranial nerve IX dysfunction causing dysphagia and a decreased gag reflex, cranial nerve X dysfunction causing stridor on inspiration, a feeble cry, hypotonia, nystagmus, or opisthotonos.[2]

WARNING!! Clinicians must avoid using latex because many children with a myelomeningocele will require multiple genitourinary procedures, with a high lifetime risk for allergy.

>> **Tip on Technique:** Fluid resuscitation should occur preoperatively as well, especially given that insensible fluid loss may occur preoperatively from the exposed myelomeningocele. Labs drawn preoperatively should include a hemoglobin and type and screen, and glucose should be monitored in any patient younger than 3 months.

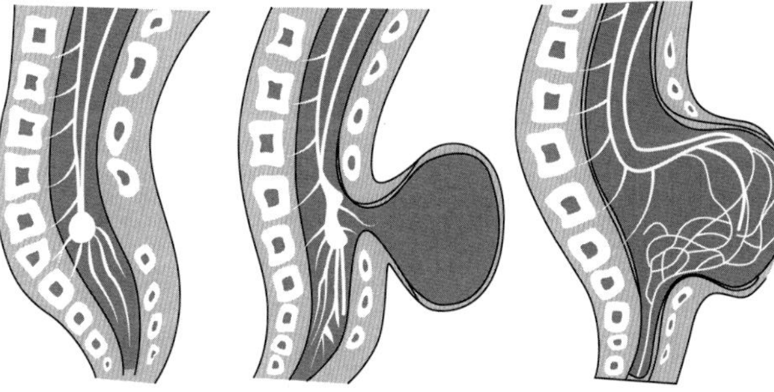

Figure 17.3 Sagittal section through the lumbosacral spine of newborns with the three common forms of spinal dysraphism. (From Samandouras G. Congenital abnormalities. In: Samandouras G, ed. *The Neurosurgeon's Handbook*. Oxford: Oxford University Press; 2010, Page 713.)

2. **Position the patient for induction and intubation.** The infant will typically have saline-soaked sterile gauze placed over the myelomeningocele at birth, and the gauze should be kept moist until surgery. The myelomeningocele must be protected from injury, which may be particularly challenging during induction and intubation. Additionally, the neck must be handled carefully during intubation and positioning in any child, but especially in infants with a myelomeningocele, owing to the potential for spinal cord and brainstem compromise. Keep in mind that one third of patients will have neurologic symptoms resulting from the Chiari II malformation.[2] If the infant is supine for intubation, myelomeningocele protection can be accomplished by the use of rolled-up towels with a hole in the center or a soft pillow with a hole in the center, with the myelomeningocele sitting in the hole without any pressure on the myelomeningocele itself. Alternatively, the infant can be induced and intubated in the right lateral decubitus position, again to avoid any pressure on the myelomeningocele itself.
3. **Manage the patient's temperature.** All neonates easily become hypothermic because of their high surface area to body mass ratio, thin skin, low body fat, and inability to shiver. Use all modalities of temperature maintenance available: increased operating room temperature, forced-air warmer (typically underbody), fluid warmer, infrared warming lights, and heated and humidified circuit.

WARNING!!	Aggressive temperature management is a must! Closely monitor the patient to avoid hypothermia or hyperthermia.
WARNING!!	When using infrared warming lights, ensure that the lights remain the required distance from the patient according to the manufacturer's directions to avoid burns.

4. **Apply monitors.** Standard American Society of Anesthesiologists (ASA) monitors and a core temperature probe (esophageal or rectal) are required for this procedure. After induction, place a second intravenous (IV) line. Use an arterial line for procedures involving a large flap or in patients with significant preoperative cardiac or pulmonary compromise.
5. **Determine anesthetic type, induce patient, and ensure access.** Use general endotracheal anesthesia for surgical repair of a myelomeningocele. The infant's neck must be handled carefully during intubation and positioning because one third of patients will have symptoms resulting from the Chiari II malformation and from associated brainstem and cervical spine compression, and additional compromise can occur from neck flexion.[2] If a significant degree of hydrocephalus exists, the infant's head may be large, making intubation more challenging. These infants may also have a shorter than usual trachea (which may be seen on chest radiograph); caution should be taken with intubation and positioning to ensure that the endotracheal tube position is not mainstem or supraglottic.

   After induction, place a second IV line. In cases in which the myelomeningocele is large and hemodynamic compromise or significant blood loss is anticipated, also place an arterial line for the beat-to-beat blood pressure monitoring and/or frequent blood draws for arterial blood gas monitoring.

   Pearl: Arterial access is important for larger surgeries so that arterial blood gases can be easily drawn to monitor blood loss and adequacy of ventilation.

6. **Position the patient for the surgical procedure.** After induction, intubation, and line placement, carefully place the patient prone for the surgical procedure and avoid injury. Place

foam or gel rolls (or rolled-up towels) underneath the infant's hips and chest. If these rolls are incorrectly placed or migrate to a position under the abdomen, intra-abdominal pressures may increase, which could result in engorged epidural veins and increased bleeding from the surgery as well as compromised ventilation.[2]

Caution! Care with positioning is very important during neonatal procedures. An infant's relatively thin skin is easily damaged. Be careful about cords, lines, and tubing lying over the infant's limbs. Circulation to an infant's limbs is easily compromised by external pressure.

Caution! Pay attention to where the infant is located beneath the surgical drapes. It is very easy for surgeons and assistants to accidently put pressure on the infants face, chest, and limbs. It is also common for surgical instruments to be unknowingly placed on the infant's face or limbs.

7. **Maintain anesthesia and monitor for possible surgical complications**. Use tandard agents for the maintenance of anesthesia. Often, neuromonitoring is performed during the procedure. The specific anesthetic required to facilitate neuromonitoring varies based on the institution, but often, muscle relaxant must be avoided. This is particularly challenging because any movement of the child during the surgery could lead to spinal cord injury. Anesthetic depth must be carefully managed, however, because more IV-adminsitered or inhaled anesthetic than is needed will cause a lower blood pressure, which may lead to cerebral ischemia.[3]
8. **Monitor blood loss and requirements for blood and fluid replacement.** Estimated blood loss can vary greatly and depends on the size of the myelomeningocele and the surgical plan. If a myocutaneous flap is required, blood loss may increase—communicate with the surgeon about the possible and ongoing blood loss preoperatively and throughout the case.

WARNING!! What may seem to be a small amount of absolute blood loss can be hemodynamically significant in an infant. Because of the small size of total blood volume in these patients, significant blood loss may not be recognized. Total blood volume is estimated to be 85 mL/kg for a full-term neonate. An infant has an estimated blood volume of 80 mL/kg. Preterm infants have an estimated blood volume of 95 to 100 mL/kg. Blood from surgical losses may pool under the drapes, increasing the difficulty of detection.

>> **Tip on Technique:** Maintenance fluids should consist of glucose containing solutions because neonates are prone to hypoglycemia. Blood glucose monitoring should be performed at regular intervals during the anesthetic. Isotonic solutions (crystalloid and/or colloid) should be used to replace insensible losses or small volumes of blood loss. Insensible losses will likely be 3 to 4 mL/kg/hr.

Postoperative Management Considerations

Clinicians can often extubate patients after a myelomeningocele repair. An exception is if the repair was large or if associated cardiac or respiratory conditions exist. Continue cardiopulmonary monitoring for at least 24 hours after the last anesthesia or opioids. If a ventriculoperitoneal shunt was not placed intraoperatively, the patient should be evaluated frequently postoperatively for the possibility of the development of hydrocephalus.[4]

Acknowledgments

The author would like to thank Dr. David Frim and Dr. Corey Scher for their generous assistance with this chapter.

Further Reading

Samandouras G. Congenital abnormalities. In: Samandouras G, ed. *The Neurosurgeon's Handbook*. Oxford: Oxford University Press; 2010.

References

1. Samandouras G, ed. *The Neurosurgeon's Handbook*. Oxford: Oxford University Press; 2010.
2. Boat A, Sadhasivam S. Myelomeningocele repair. In: Goldschneider K, Davidson A, Wittkugel E, et al., eds. *Clinical Pediatric Anesthesia: A Case-Based Handbook*. New York: Oxford University Press; 2012.
3. Clebone A, Scher C. Does a low mean blood pressure in the neonate under anesthesia lead to cognitive deficits? In: Scher C, Clebone A, Miller S, et al., eds. *You're Wrong, I'm Right*. New York: Springer; 2016, Pages 109–110.
4. Hamid RK, Newfield P. Pediatric neuroanesthesia. Hydrocephalus. *Anesthesiol Clin North Am* 2001;19(2):207–218.

Chapter 18

Anesthesia for Gastroschisis or Omphalocele Repair

Caitlin Aveyard

Introduction

Gastroschisis and omphalocele are congenital defects in the abdominal wall. These two conditions have different embryologic origins, but anesthetic management is similar for both. Gastroschisis is a full-thickness abdominal wall defect resulting in extrusion of abdominal viscera into the amniotic space without amniotic membrane coverage. The defect is usually to the right of the umbilicus.[1,2] Omphalocele is a defect in the abdominal wall in the umbilical area in which the extruded abdominal contents (intestine, liver, spleen, bladder) are covered in a thin sac (Figure 18.1).[2] Infants with an omphalocele often have associated syndromes or chromosomal abnormalities. With either gastroschisis or omphalocele, the extruded abdominal contents must be covered and kept moist before surgical correction.

There are several options for closure of gastroschisis or omphalocele lesions: (1) primary surgical closure, (2) closure in stages with the use of a silo, or (3) the "sutureless" closure technique. Primary closure may be performed as early as during the first few hours of birth if the defect is small enough to be reduced without putting the infant at risk for abdominal compartment syndrome. Alternatively, a silo can be placed over the abdominal wall defect in an awake infant. The abdominal contents can then be gradually reduced into the abdomen, and then the defect is surgically corrected at a later time after the viscera "fit" into the abdomen. With sutureless closure techniques, the abdominal contents are reduced or covered with a silo if the intestines cannot be fully reduced into the abdomen. The umbilical cord is kept moist to avoid desiccation. When the abdominal contents are fully reduced, the umbilical cord is stretched across the abdominal wall defect and taped in place. After approximately 2 weeks, the defect covered by the umbilical cord contracts, leaving an umbilicus.[1] The sutureless closure technique has become increasingly used because with this technique, general anesthesia can often be completely avoided (Figure 18.2). Avoiding general anesthesia is advantageous in infants because of

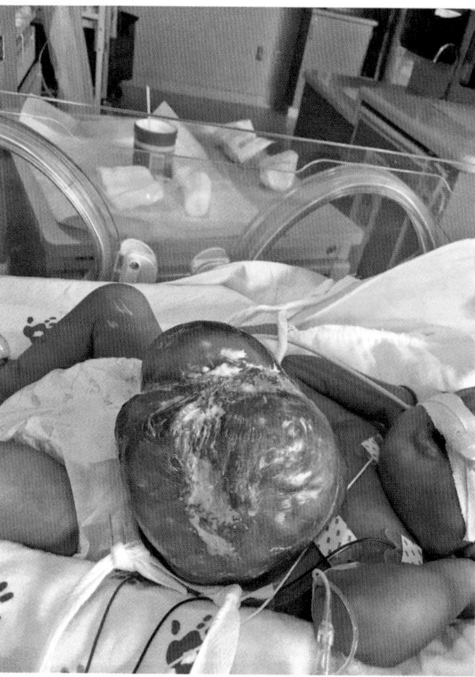

Figure 18.1 An unrepaired giant omphalocele.

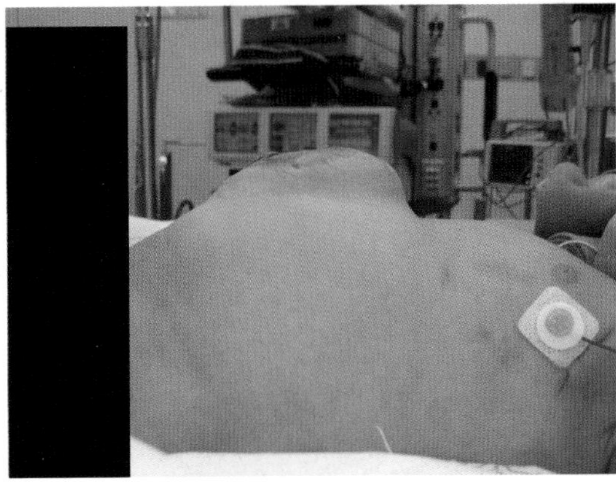

Figure 18.2 A sutureless omphalocele closure.

the high risk in this population as well as the concern for neurotoxicity.[3] Many of the steps for anesthetic management of gastroschisis or omphalocele repair are also relevant for other large abdominal surgeries in infants.

Critical Anatomy

The abdominal wall defect in gastroschisis is to the right of the umbilicus, while it is in the umbilical region in patients with an omphalocele. Infants with an omphalocele have a greater risk for associated syndromes or chromosomal abnormalities than infants with gastroschisis.

Step-by-Step

1. **Prepare for the procedure.** Obtain the following labs: hemoglobin, basic metabolic panel, liver enzymes (if liver involvement is present, which occurs in some cases of omphalocele), and a blood type and screen. Evaluate the patient for other congenital abnormalities. Infants with omphalocele often have additional non-gastrointestinal abnormalities. Congenital cardiac anomalies can occur in up to 30% of infants with an omphalocele. These anomalies may include an atrial septal defect, ventricular septal defect, tetralogy of Fallot, dextrocardia, or patent ductus arteriosus. Additionally, infants with an omphalocele may also have abnormal chest wall and abdominal wall mechanics as well as pulmonary hypoplasia.[4]

> **WARNING!!** Infants with one abnormality may have others. Check for the presence of cardiac anomalies and perform a full preoperative exam, including auscultation, palpation for upper and lower extremity pulses, four limb oxygen saturations and blood pressures, and an echocardiogram, when indicated.

>> **Tip on Technique:** The infant should be adequately resuscitated with fluid and electrolytes whenever possible before anesthesia.

> **WARNING!!** Aggressive temperature management is a must! Closely monitor the patient to avoid hypothermia or hyperthermia.

WARNING!!	When using infrared warming lights, ensure that they remain the required distance from the patient, according to the manufacturer, to avoid burns.

2. **Position the patient and set up equipment to manage the patient's temperature.** Position the patient supine. All neonates easily become hypothermic because of their high surface area to body mass ratio, thin skin, low body fat, and inability to shiver.[5] Infants undergoing abdominal surgery in particular also lose heat through their exposed abdominal contents. Use all modalities of temperature maintenance available: increased operating room temperature, forced-air warmer (typically underbody), fluid warmer, infrared warming lights, and heated and humidified circuit.

   !! **Potential Complications:** Care with positioning is very important during neonatal procedures. An infant's relatively thin skin is easily damaged. Be careful about cords, lines, and tubing lying over the infant's limbs. Circulation to an infant's limbs is easily compromised by external pressure.

Caution!	Pay attention to where the infant is located beneath the surgical drapes. It is very easy for surgeons and assistants to accidently put pressure on the infant's face, chest, and limbs. It is also common for surgical instruments to be unknowingly placed on the infant's face or limbs.

3. **Set up monitors.** Standard American Society of Anesthesiologists (ASA) monitors, with the possible addition of an arterial line, and a core temperature probe (esophageal or rectal) should be used. Abdominal pressure, as well as peak airway pressure, may increase significantly with the closure of a large abdominal wall defect.[6] Consider placing an arterial line to aid in the evaluation of perfusion if primary closure of a large defect is planned. A second pulse oximeter (so that the patient has one on an upper extremity and one on a lower extremity) can be useful. If abdominal pressures significantly increase with abdominal closure, decreased perfusion to the lower extremities may occur.[6] Loss of a lower extremity pulse oximeter waveform could identify this decreased perfusion.
4. **Determine the anesthetic type, evaluate and ensure adequate access, and induce the patient.** Typically, general endotracheal anesthesia is used for surgical repair of a gastroschisis or omphalocele. Because of the likelihood for increased gastric contents, a rapid sequence induction/intubation or awake intubation should be considered. The nasogastric/orogastric tube should be suctioned before induction. Or, if not in situ, a nasogastric or orogastric tube should be placed and suctioned after intubation. After induction, a second intravenous (IV) line should be placed. In cases in which the defect is large and hemodynamic compromise or significant blood loss is anticipated, an arterial line should also placed for the purpose of beat-to-beat blood pressure monitoring and/or frequent blood draws for arterial blood gas monitoring. If the patient has umbilical venous or arterial access, these lines will likely need to be removed before the surgical procedure and will thus not be available for use after the surgery has commenced.

Caution!	If a significant increase in intra-abdominal pressure occurs with abdominal wall closure, perfusion to the intra-abdominal contents and lower limbs may decrease. The increased intra-abdominal pressure may also limit venous

drainage from the lower extremities. Obtaining at least one upper extremity peripheral IV line is advisable. Arterial access is important for larger surgeries to monitor the arterial blood gas for PO_2 as part of ventilation monitoring during and after the closure of the abdominal wall because ventilation may become more difficult with the increase in abdominal pressure.

Caution! Consider the possibility that a child with an omphalocele may also have Beckwith-Wiedemann syndrome, which is also associated with airway anomalies and the potential for difficult intubation.[7]

6. **Maintain anesthesia and monitor for possible surgical complications.** Standard agents should be used for the maintenance of anesthesia. Nitrous oxide should be minimized or avoided because of its diffusion into the bowel cavity, which may cause bowel edema and increase surgical difficulty. While the gut is being reduced back into the abdomen, as well as during closure of the abdominal fascia, the intra-abdominal pressure will increase. Depending on how much this pressure increases, there may be a compromise of ventilation, intra-abdominal organ perfusion, venous return, and lower extremity perfusion. The anesthesiologist must carefully watch for increased airway pressures and loss of lower extremity pulse oximetry and communicate with the surgeon; if pressures are excessively increased with attempted closure leading to compromise, the abdomen must be left open.

   >> Tip on Technique: With the expected intravascular volume shifts during the repair of abdominal wall defects, hemodynamic lability frequently occurs. A dopamine infusion may be useful to temporize the patient while fluid and/or blood resuscitation is occurring.[5]

7. **Communicate with the surgical team regarding patient blood loss and carefully monitor blood and fluid replacement requirements.** Estimated blood loss can vary greatly and depends on the size of the abdominal wall defect and the surgical plan. Communicate with the surgeon about the possible and ongoing blood loss preoperatively and throughout the case.

WARNING!! What may seem to be a small amount of absolute blood loss can be hemodynamically significant in an infant. Because of the small size of total blood volume of these patients, significant blood loss may not be recognized. Total blood volume is estimated to be 85 mL/kg for a full-term neonate. An infant has an estimated blood volume of 80 mL/kg. Preterm infants have an estimated blood volume of 95 mL/kg.

Significant fluid resuscitation is required during gastroschisis or omphalocele repair due to large insensible fluid losses from exposed bowel. Maintenance fluids should consist of glucose solutions because neonates are prone to hypoglycemia. Blood glucose monitoring should be performed at regular intervals during the anesthetic. Isotonic solutions (crystalloid and/or colloid) should be used to replace insensible losses or small volume blood loss. Administration of 10 mL/kg/hr (or more) of an isotonic solution may be necessary intraoperatively.[5]

!! Potential Complications: It is critical to maintain normovolemia. Hypovolemia and metabolic acidosis can easily occur if the patient is under-resuscitated. Conversely, over-resuscitating with intravascular fluids or blood can lead to increased difficulty closing the abdominal defect, prolonged postoperative ventilation, prolonged neonatal intensive care unit stays, or even congestive heart failure.[2]

Note: Do not forget to replace gastric fluid losses.

Postoperative Management Considerations

Patients are often left intubated after omphalocele or gastroschisis procedures. After abdominal wall closure, peak airway pressures are expected to increase with decreased thoracic compliance. Also, keep in mind that an intubated neonate can be treated more aggressively for postoperative pain than one who is not intubated.

References

1. Skarsgard E. Management of gastroschisis. *Curr Opin Pediatr.* 2016;28:363–369.
2. Islam S. Clinical care outcomes in abdominal wall defects. *Curr Opin Pediatr.* 2008;20:305–310.
3. Ko R, Pinyavat T, Stylianos S, et al. Optimal timing of surgical procedures in pediatric patients. *J Neurosurg Anesthesiol.* 2016;28:395–399.
4. Krishnamurphy G, Ratner V, Bacha E, Aspelund G. Comorbid conditions in neonates with congenital heart disease. *Pediatr Crit Care Med.* 2016;17:S367–S376.
5. Maxwell L. Anesthetic management for newborns undergoing emergency surgery. *ASA Refresher Courses.* 2007;35:107–126.
6. Yaster M, Buck J, Dudgeon D, et al. Hemodynamic effects of primary closure of omphalocele/gastroschisis in human newborns. *Anesthesiology.* 1998;69:84–88.
7. Morton N, Fairgrieve R, Moores A, Wallace E. Anesthesia for the full-term and ex-premature infant. In: Gregory G, Andropoulos D, eds. *Gregory's Pediatric Anesthesia*. 5th ed. Oxford: Blackwell Publishing Ltd; 2012:503–506.

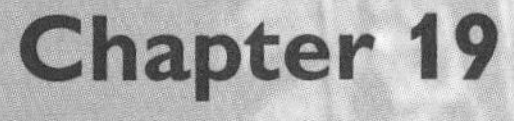

Chapter 19

Anesthesia for Congenital Diaphragmatic Hernia Repair in Infants

Chirag Shah, Anna Clebone, and Caitlin Aveyard

Introduction

A congenital diaphragmatic hernia (CDH) is a congenital condition in which a developmental defect in the diaphragm allows abdominal contents to migrate into the thoracic cavity. This leads to lung underdevelopment and hypoplasia in utero. It occurs in about 1 in 2,000 newborns.

Critical Anatomy

A defect in the diaphragm usually occurs on the left side, most commonly in the posterolateral region, and is known as a Bochdalek hernia. A defect in the anterior region is known as a Morgagni hernia. On a chest radiograph of an infant with a left congenital diaphragmatic hernia, you will typically see a smaller left lung, shift of the heart and mediastinum rightward (leading to a compressed right lung), and bowel contents in the left side of the thorax (Figures 19.1 and 19.2). Obtaining a prenatal diagnosis is not always possible because visualization of a congenital diaphragmatic hernia may be difficult on fetal ultrasound; 11% are not diagnosed until after birth.[2]

Note: Lung hypoplasia and the abnormal development of pulmonary vasculature resulting in pulmonary hypertension contribute to the morbidity and mortality associated with a congenital diaphragmatic hernia.

>> **Tip on Technique:** Prenatal ultrasound can be used to diagnose a congenital diaphragmatic hernia. The diagnosis is made when abdominal contents are not in their usual location and may be noted in the thorax. Fetal surgery for congenital diaphragmatic hernia is performed in some centers.

>> **Tip on Technique:** Extracorporeal membrane oxygenation (ECMO) is an option for congenital diaphragmatic hernia patients who cannot be optimized on medical therapy. Criteria for starting ECMO may include the inability to maintain preductal and postductal oxygen saturations, hypotension refractory to fluids and vasopressors, and acidosis despite optimal ventilator management (Figure 19.3).[3]

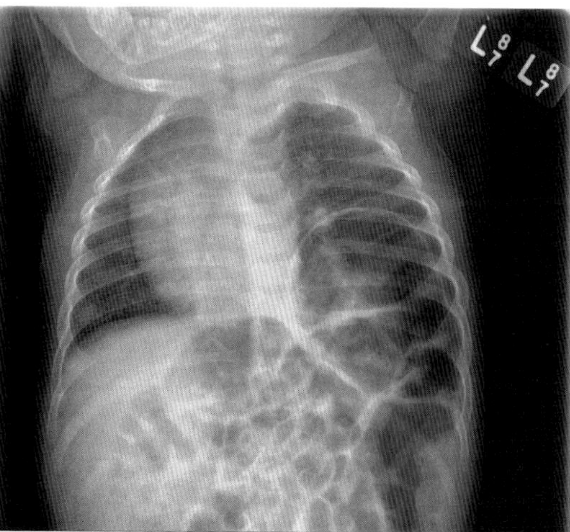

Figure 19.1 Radiograph of an infant with a left-sided congenital diaphragmatic hernia.

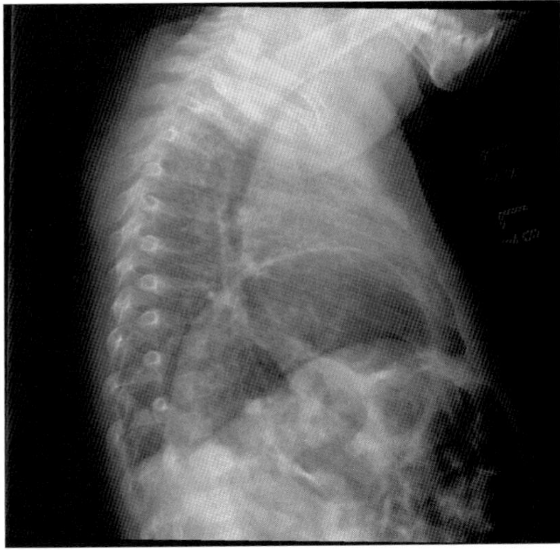

Figure 19.2 Lateral view: radiograph of an infant with a left-sided congenital diaphragmatic hernia.

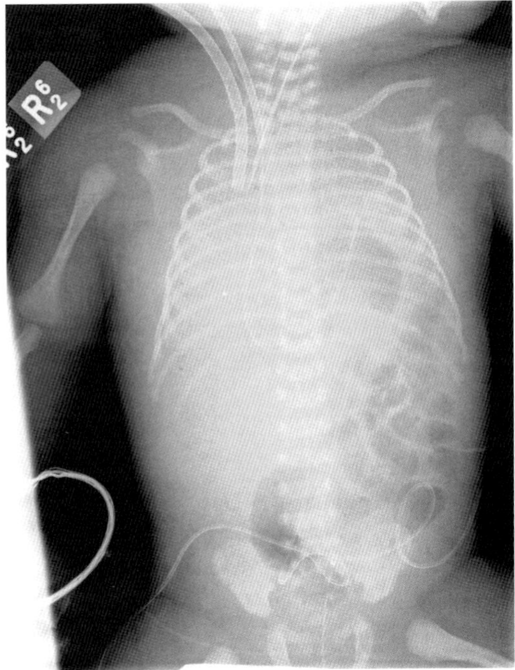

Figure 19.3 Note expected opacification of the chest after ECMO initiation (as well as bowel gas in the chest).

Step-by-Step

1. **Conduct a preoperative evaluation and prepare for the procedure.** Preoperatively, evaluate the extent of disease and the extent to which the pulmonary and gastrointestinal systems are compromised. Evaluate the patient for associated congenital abnormalities, which may involve the cardiovascular, renal, gastrointestinal, and central nervous systems. At birth, infants with a congenital diaphragmatic hernia will have

decreased or absent lung sounds over the thorax on the side of the hernia, tachypnea due to lung compromise, and a scaphoid abdomen due to the abdominal contents being displaced into the thorax.

Pearl: Liver herniation into the chest and a significant degree of lung hypoplasia are poor prognostic indicators (Figure 19.4).[4]

WARNING!! Infants with one abnormality may have others. Check for the presence of cardiac anomalies and perform a full preoperative exam, including performing auscultation, palpating upper and lower extremity pulses, obtaining oxygen saturations and blood pressures in all four limbs, and acquiring an echocardiogram when indicated.

WARNING!! Syndromes associated with a congenital diaphragmatic hernia include trisomy 18, trisomy 13, Cornelia de Lange syndrome, Pallister-Killian and Marfan syndromes, spina bifida, hydrocephaly, anencephaly, congenital heart disease, and multiple malformation syndromes.[2]

Obtain the following labs: complete blood count including hemoglobin, hematocrit, and platelets; basic metabolic panel; lactate; liver enzymes (if the liver has herniated into the

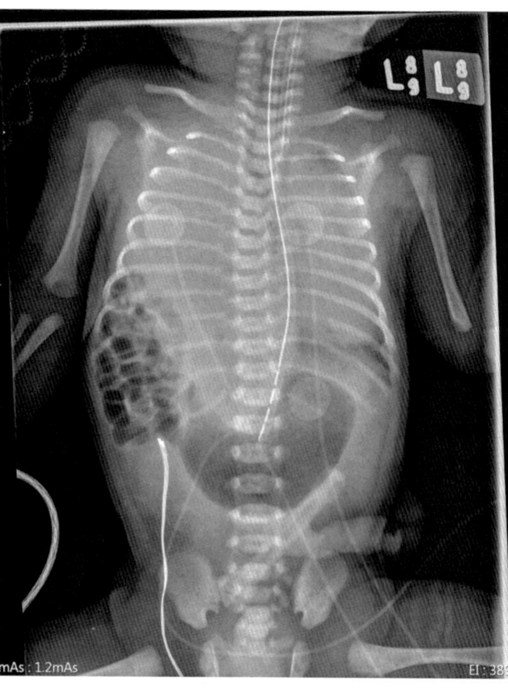

Figure 19.4 Right-sided hernia containing the liver.

chest); and hematologic type and screen. Surgery is usually performed after the neonate has been medically stabilized, including resuscitation with fluids and electrolytes.

2. **Position the patient and manage the patient's temperature.** The patient should be positioned supine for the induction of anesthesia. All neonates easily become hypothermic because of their high surface area to body mass ratio, thin skin, low body fat, and inability to shiver.[5] Use all modalities of temperature maintenance available: increased operating room temperature, forced-air warmer (typically underbody), fluid warmer, infrared warming lights, and a heated and humidified breathing circuit.

WARNING!! Aggressive temperature management is a must! Closely monitor the patient to avoid hypothermia or hyperthermia.

WARNING!! When using infrared warming lights, ensure that they remain the required distance from the patient, according to the manufacturer, to avoid burns.

!! Potential Complications: Care with positioning is very important during neonatal procedures. An infant's relatively thin skin is easily damaged. Be careful about cords, lines, and tubing lying over the infant's limbs. Circulation to an infant's limbs is easily compromised by external pressure.

>> Tip on Technique: Pay attention to where the infant is located beneath the surgical drapes. It is very easy for surgeons and assistants to accidently put pressure on the infant's face, chest, and limbs. It is also common for surgical instruments to be unknowingly placed on the infant's face or limbs, which can lead to injury.

3. **Apply monitors.** Standard American Society of Anesthesiologists (ASA) monitors and a core temperature probe (esophageal or rectal) should be used. Monitor the patient's preductal and postductal oxygen saturations.

>> Tip on Technique: The focus of monitoring should be on end-organ perfusion, including heart rate, urine output, and lactate levels.

4. **Determine anesthetic type, induce the patient and secure the airway, and ensure vascular access.** Most neonates with a congenital diaphragmatic hernia will present to the operating room already intubated. In neonates who are not already intubated, many practitioners avoid bag mask ventilation after the induction of anesthesia, if possible, for two reasons: (1) high positive pressures may damage the fragile, hypoplastic lung, or even cause a pneumothorax; and (2) any distension of the stomach caused by mask ventilation will limit expansion of the already hypoplastic lung.[6] If mask ventilation is necessary, peak pressures should not exceed 20 mmHg. During transport to and from the operating room, use a T-piece ventilation device (Figure 19.5) that delivers a controlled and limited target peak inspiratory pressure with each breath, such as the Neopuff.

   After intubation, place an orogastric or nasogastric tube to suction to help with decompression of the stomach. After induction, place a second intravenous line. A central line should be considered for patients with larger defects when the need for vasopressors is anticipated. In cases in which the defect is large and hemodynamic compromise or significant blood loss is anticipated, an arterial line should also be placed for the purpose of beat-to-beat blood pressure

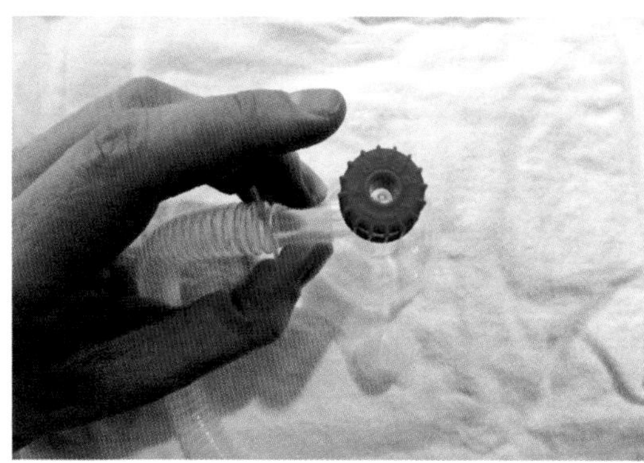

Figure 19.5 T-piece ventilation device.

monitoring and/or frequent blood draws for arterial blood gas monitoring. Furthermore, an arterial line will aid in the evaluation of oxygenation and perfusion and may be especially useful for patients with larger hernias who will have a greater degree of lung hypoplasia. If the patient has umbilical venous or arterial access, these lines will likely need to be removed before the surgical procedure and thus will not be available for use after the surgery has commenced.

WARNING!! If the patient is hypoxemic, this may be a result of a right to left shunt (through a patent foramen ovale) because of pulmonary hypertension.[1] In hypoxemic patients, an echocardiogram is indicated before surgery to look for the possibility of a right-to-left shunt. Increased systemic blood pressures can help to reduce the shunt.

>> **Tip on Technique:** Owing to the presence of a fragile, hypoplastic lung, patients with a congenital diaphragmatic hernia are at high risk for lung injury or even pneumothorax if high peak ventilation pressures are used. To prevent high peak pressures, these infants are often ventilated with lower than normal tidal volumes, and permissive hypercapnia is often tolerated.

5. **Maintain anesthesia and monitor for possible surgical complications.** Use standard agents for the maintenance of anesthesia. Nitrous oxide should be avoided because of its diffusion into the bowel, which may cause bowel expansion and increase the difficulty of both ventilation and removal of the bowel from the thoracic cavity. Use of a muscle relaxant will likely aid in optimizing surgical conditions.

>> **Tip on Technique:** If the patient is hypotensive, a crystalloid or albumin bolus (10–20 mL/kg) may spare the need to start vasopressors.

6. **Estimate anticipated blood loss and determine likely blood and fluid requirements.** Estimated blood loss can vary greatly and depends on the size of the hernia and the surgical plan. Communicate with the surgeon about the possible and ongoing blood loss preoperatively and throughout the case.

WARNING!!	What may seem to be a small amount of absolute blood loss can be hemodynamically significant in an infant. Because of the small size of total blood volume of these patients, significant blood loss may not be recognized. Total blood volume is estimated to be 85 mL/kg for a full-term neonate. An infant has an estimated blood volume of 80 mL/kg. Preterm infants have an estimated blood volume of 95 mL/kg.
WARNING!!	It is critical to maintain normovolemia. Hypovolemia and metabolic acidosis can easily occur if the patient is under-resuscitated. Conversely, over-resuscitating with intravascular fluids or blood can lead to increased difficulty closing the abdominal defect, prolonged postoperative ventilation, prolonged neonatal intensive care unit stays, or even congestive heart failure.[2]

>> **Tip on Technique**: Maintenance fluids should consist of glucose-containing solutions because neonates are prone to hypoglycemia. Blood glucose monitoring should be performed at regular intervals during the anesthetic. Isotonic solutions (crystalloid and/or colloid) should be used to replace insensible losses or small volumes of blood loss.

Postoperative Management Considerations

Patients are often left intubated after a congenital diaphragmatic hernia repair with the same ventilator parameters as in the operating room. Remember that the patient's lungs are still hypoplastic, fragile, and prone to pneumothorax even after the diaphragmatic hernia is repaired. If a transport ventilator is not available, peak ventilation pressures should be carefully titrated with each breath using a T-piece device that delivers limited and controlled peak inspiratory pressures, or using a pressure gauge on the manual bag device. An advantage to having the patient remain intubated after surgery is that doing so allows the neonate to be more aggressively treated for postoperative pain.

Further Reading

Gallot D, Marceau G, Coste K, et al. Congenital diaphragmatic hernia: a retinoid-signaling pathway disruption during lung development? *Birth Defects Res A Clin Mol Teratol.* 2005;73(8):523–531.

Hilgendorff A, Apitz C, Bonnet D, Hansmann G. Pulmonary hypertension associated with acute or chronic lung diseases in the preterm and term neonate and infant. The European Paediatric Pulmonary Vascular Disease Network, endorsed by IS HLT and DGPK. *Heart.* 2016;102(Suppl. 2):ii49–56.

Kadir D, Lilja HE. Risk factors for postoperative mortality in congenital diaphragmatic hernia: a single-centre observational study. *Pediatr Surg Int.* 2017;33(3):317–323.

Maxwell L. Anesthetic management for newborns undergoing emergency surgery. *ASA Refresher Courses.* 2007;35:107–126.

Morini F, Capolupo I, van Weteringen W, Reiss I. Ventilation modalities in infants with congenital diaphragmatic hernia. *Semin Pediatr Surg.* 2017;26(3):159–165.

Reiss T, Schaible L, van den Hout. Standardized postnatal management of infants with congenital diaphragmatic hernia in Europe: the CDH EURO Consortium Consensus. *Neonatology*. 2010;98:354–364.

Snoek KG, Capolupo I, Morini F, et al. Score for Neonatal Acute Physiology-II predicts outcome in congenital diaphragmatic hernia patients. *Pediatr Crit Care Med*. 2016;17(6):540–546.

Snoek KG, Reiss IK, Greenough A, et al. Standardized postnatal management of infants with congenital diaphragmatic hernia in Europe: the CDH EURO Consortium Consensus—2015 update. *Neonatology*. 2016;110(1):66–74.

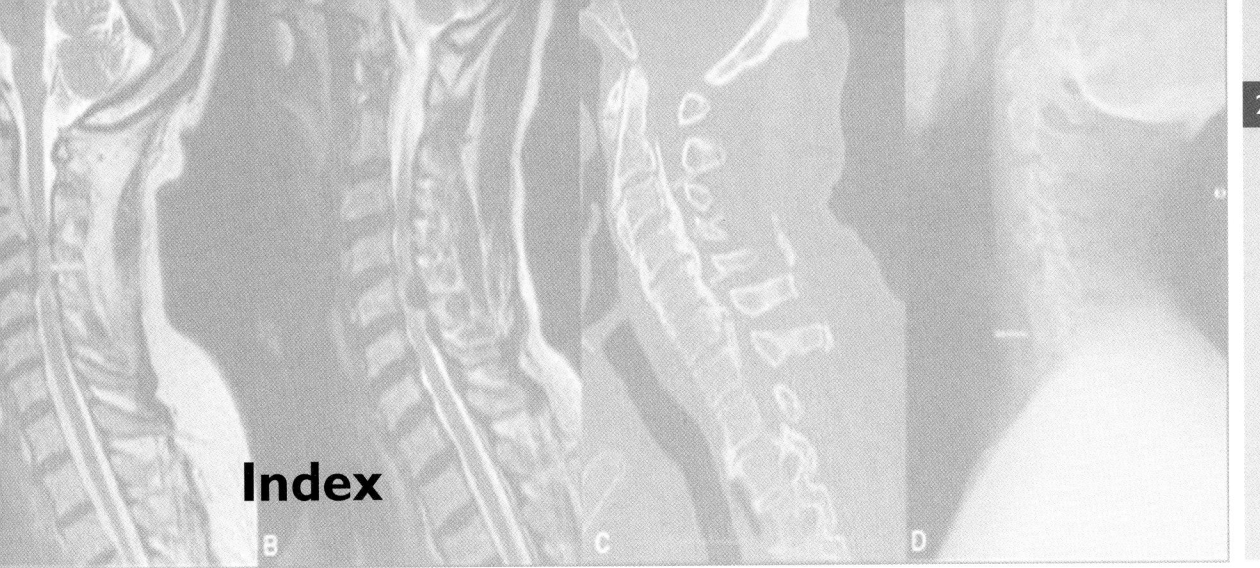

Index

For the benefit of digital users, indexed terms that span two pages (e.g., 52–53) may, on occasion, appear on only one of those pages.
References to tables and figures is denoted by an italic *t* or *f* following the page number.